Optimizing Care
for Young Children with Special Health Care Needs

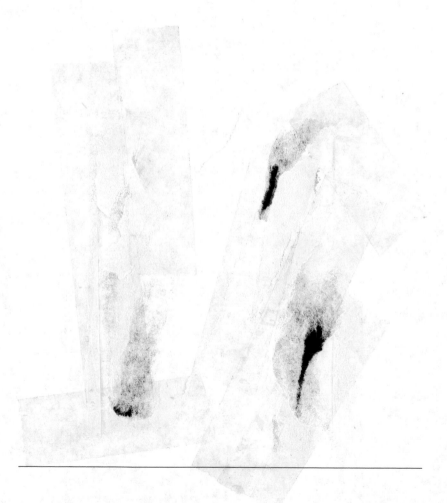

Optimizing Care
for Young Children
with Special Health
Care Needs

Knowledge and Strategies
for Navigating the System

edited by

Elisa J. Sobo, Ph.D.
San Diego State University

and

Paul S. Kurtin, M.D.
Rady Children's Hospital

San Diego, California

with invited contributors

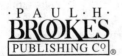

·P A U L·H·
BROOKES
PUBLISHING C°®

Baltimore • London • Sydney

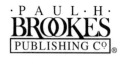

Paul H. Brookes Publishing Co.
Post Office Box 10624
Baltimore, Maryland 21285-0624

www.brookespublishing.com

"Paul H. Brookes Publishing Co." is a registered trademark of
Paul H. Brookes Publishing Co., Inc.

Typeset by Maryland Composition, Inc., Glen Burnie, Maryland.
Manufactured in the United States of America by
Versa Press, Inc., East Peoria, Illinois.

Excerpts from personal communications are used by permission of the
authors of the communications.

Library of Congress Cataloging-in-Publication Data

Optimizing care for young children with special health care needs:
  knowledge and strategies for navigating the system / edited by Elisa
  J. Sobo and Paul S. Kurtin.
    p.   cm.
  Includes bibliographical references and index.
  ISBN-13: 978-1-55766-854-7 (alk. paper)
  1. Children with disabilities—Rehabilitation.   2. Infants with disabilities—
Rehabilitation.   3. Children with disabilities—Medical care.   4. Infants
with disabilities—Medical care.   I. Sobo, Elisa Janine, 1963–   .
II. Kurtin, Paul S., 1951–   .
  [DNLM: 1. Child Health Services.   2. Disabled Children.   3. Child,
Exceptional.   4. Child, Preschool.   5. Infant, Newborn.   6. Infant.
WA 320 062 2007]
RJ138.068 2007
362.4083'2—dc22   2006034300

British Library Cataloguing in Publication data are available from the British
Library.

CONTENTS

About the Editors

Elisa J. Sobo, Ph.D., Associate Professor, Department of Anthropology, San Diego State University, 5500 Campanile Drive, San Diego California 92182-6040

Dr. Sobo specializes in medical anthropology. In addition to children with special health care needs, her areas of interest include biomedical and other medical cultures, organizational issues in health care and health research, patient–provider communication, health disparities and cultural competence, health-related stigma and identity, risk perception, reproductive and sexual health, childhood and child health, nutrition and foodways, qualitative methods (including ethnographic and rapid assessment methods), and Jamaican culture. Dr. Sobo has authored, coauthored, or coedited nine books, and her articles have appeared in a wide variety of peer-reviewed journals including *Journal of Health Services Research, Medical Anthropology Quarterly,* and *Social Science and Medicine.* She is working on *Culture and Meaning in Health Services Research (HSR): An Applied Anthropological Approach,* a methodology textbook that is concurrently an ethnographic study of the health services research arena. Dr. Sobo serves on the board of the Society for Medical Anthropology, is a Fellow of the Society for Applied Anthropology, and has served on the medical committee of the Royal Anthropological Institute. She is an affiliated faculty member of San Diego State University's Graduate School of Public Health and an associate clinical professor of pediatrics and of family and preventive medicine at the University of California, San Diego School of Medicine.

Paul S. Kurtin, M.D., Chief Quality and Safety Officer, Rady Children's Hospital San Diego, and Research Professor, Graduate School of Public Health, San Diego State University, San Diego, California 92182-4443

Dr. Kurtin, a board-certified adult and pediatric nephrologist, is also director of the Maternal Child Health Initiative at San Diego

State University's Graduate School of Public Health. His research interests have focused on quality of care and outcomes assessment and management. He is the founding medical director of the Child Health Accountability Initiative. This collaborative of children's hospitals works together to improve the care of hospitalized children and children with special health care needs. In his present position at Rady Children's Hospital, Dr. Kurtin focuses on designing, implementing, evaluating, and continuously improving health services throughout a large pediatric integrated delivery system. He has spoken widely on these topics, including presentations at the Institute of Medicine and numerous national and international meetings.

About the Contributors

Sheila Bloom, M.S., Research Coordinator, Center for Child and Adolescent Health Policy, MassGeneral Hospital *for* Children, Boston, Massachusetts 02114

For 20 years, Ms. Bloom's research has focused on health policy and related issues involving children with special health care needs. A main research activity has involved surveying families of children with special health needs regarding their care and coordinating multi-site, national studies. She is a coauthor of numerous book chapters and journal articles as well as the book *Home and Community Care for Chronically Ill Children* (Oxford University Press, 1993). Ms. Bloom is also an editorial associate of *Ambulatory Pediatrics,* the journal of the Ambulatory Pediatric Association.

W. Carl Cooley, M.D., Medical Director, Crotched Mountain Foundation, One Verney Drive, Greenfield, New Hampshire 03047

Dr. Cooley codirects the Center for Medical Home Improvement at Crotched Mountain Foundation in Greenfield, New Hampshire, where he also is the medical director. He also is Associate Professor of Pediatrics at the Dartmouth Medical School. Dr. Cooley, the recipient of the 2006 American Academy of Pediatrics's first annual Cal Sia Medical Home Leadership and Advocacy award, the 2005 Maternal and Child Health Bureau's Director's Award, and New Hampshire's 2001 Pediatrician of the Year award, has interests in Down syndrome, autism, and family resilience and adaptation to having a child with special needs. He has developed a widely adopted quality improvement method for primary care practices interested in implementing the medical home model as well as a quality improvement instrument called the Medical Home Index to measure the *medical homeness* of individual practices. He is coauthor of *Preventive Care for Children with Genetic Disorders: Providing a Medical Home* (Cambridge University Press, 2006).

Denise Dougherty, Ph.D., Senior Advisor, Child Health and Quality Improvement, U.S. Department of Health and Human Services, Agency for Healthcare Research and Quality (AHRQ), 540 Gaither Road, Rockville, Maryland 20850

Dr. Dougherty has published on outcomes, quality measurement, and quality improvement in children's health. She is a consistent voice in the field on the need for evidence-based practice and the translation of research findings into policy and practice to improve children's health. Prior to working at AHRQ, Dr. Dougherty led the Program on Education and Human Resources at a congressional agency and wrote reports for Congress on a variety of public policy topics, including adolescent health, children's mental health, AIDS/HIV, blood policy and technology, and Indian health. Before getting her Ph.D. in social psychology from Boston University, Dr. Dougherty was a municipal finance analyst on Wall Street.

Kristin Gist, M.S., Director, Developmental Services, Rady Children's Hospital San Diego, San Diego, California 92123

In 1974, Ms. Gist founded the Developmental Evaluation Clinic specifically for premature infants in the Neonatal Intensive Care Unit at Rady Children's Hospital. The program grew to support all children at risk and to include assessment and intervention programs for children in foster care and those with autistic spectrum disorders. Ms. Gist provided developmental and psychological evaluations for more than 15,000 children before moving into leadership of a large division that combines developmental and rehabilitation services. Her special interests include universal developmental and behavioral screening, early intervention for children at risk, and support for parents of children with disabilities and other special needs.

Charles J. Homer, M.D., M.P.H., President and CEO, National Initiative for Children's Healthcare Quality (NICHQ), 20 University Road, 7th Floor, Cambridge, Massachusetts 02138

In addition to leading the National Initiative for Children's Healthcare Quality, an action-oriented organization exclusively dedicated to improving the quality of health care for children, Dr. Homer is Associate Professor, Department of Society, Human Development and Health,

Harvard School of Public Health, and Associate Clinical Professor of Pediatrics, Harvard Medical School. He was a member of the third U.S. Preventive Services Task Force from 2000 to 2002, served as chair of the American Academy of Pediatrics Steering Committee on Quality Improvement and Management from 2001 to 2004, and is a member of the Ambulatory Steering Committee of the National Quality Forum. Prior to his position at NICHQ, Dr. Homer was director of the Clinical Effectiveness Program at Children's Hospital Boston, and served as program director of the first federally supported fellowship training programs in pediatric health services research.

Karen Kuhlthau, Ph.D., Associate Director, Center for Child and Adolescent Health Policy, and Assistant Professor of Pediatrics, Harvard Medical School, 50 Staniford Street, Suite 901, Boston, Massachusetts 92114

Dr. Kuhlthau has published more than 25 articles in pediatric and public health journals. She conducts research on pediatric health policy, health services use by children with special health care needs, and the quality of life of the children and their parents. Her current research is on the influence of child health status on parent well-being and on the long-term quality of life of survivors of childhood brain tumors. Dr. Kuhlthau is an associate editor of *Ambulatory Pediatrics.*

Gail Landsman, Ph.D., Associate Professor, Department of Anthropology, State University of New York at Albany, 1400 Washington Avenue, Albany, New York 12222

Dr. Landsman's research on U.S. mothers of children diagnosed with or at risk for disability has appeared as articles in peer-reviewed journals, including *Social Science and Medicine, Journal of Medical Humanities,* and *Signs,* and as chapters in a number of edited volumes. Dr. Landsman has collaborated with the New York State Department of Health Early Intervention Program, serving as a parent member on its Motor Disorders Clinical Guidelines Panel and as a core advisory group member on an Individuals with Disabilities Education Act grant to enhance Part C outcome indicators as well as on its Parent Involvement Committee. She is a member of the Family Workgroup of the Early Childhood Outcomes Center and has served on the steering committee of the Council on Anthropology and Reproduction. Dr. Landsman is the mother of three children, one of whom has cerebral palsy.

Laurel K. Leslie, M.D., Associate Research Scientist and Behavioral/
Developmental Pediatrician, Child and Adolescent Services Research
Center, 3020 Children's Way, MC 5033, San Diego, California 92123

Dr. Leslie's areas of interest include the interface between primary care
and subspecialty care; effective methods of identifying and treating the
developmental and behavioral problems of children in community settings; children in foster care; racial/ethnic disparities in the use of developmental, educational, and mental health services; and the impact of
Medicaid managed care on access to care. She currently is on several
national task forces addressing the developmental and mental health
needs of children and improvements in residency education to address
these needs.

Monica Marthell, B.S., Point of Care Tech, TriCore Reference Labora-
tories, Albuquerque, New Mexico 87108

Ms. Marthell graduated from the New Mexico Highlands University in
Las Vegas, New Mexico, where she was a biology major. She plans to
attend medical school and specialize in pediatrics and to pursue an M.S.
in public health. Ms. Marthell intends to work in disparities reduction,
especially in diabetes care. While working on this book, she was a fellow
in the Harvard Medical School's Health Policy Summer Program.

Thomas K. McInerny, M.D., Associate Chair for Clinical Affairs and
Professor of Pediatrics at the University of Rochester School of
Medicine/Golisano Children's Hospital at Strong, 601 Elmwood Ave-
nue, Box 777, Rochester, New York 14642

At the University of Rochester School of Medicine, Dr. McInerny works
closely with the primary care pediatricians in the Rochester region. He
has more than 30 years of experience as a primary care pediatrician,
was chief medical officer for a large individual practice association in
Rochester for 3 years, and is a certified physician executive with the
American College of Physician Executives. Dr. McInerny has published
more than 30 peer-reviewed articles on a variety of subjects, including
caring for children with chronic illness, mental health problems in
children, and quality improvement in pediatric practice. He is also the
editor-in-chief of the fifth edition of Hoekelman's *Primary Pediatric Care*
(Mosby, 2001).

Hodon Mohamed, Columbus, Ohio

Ms. Mohamed is a graduate of Denison University in Ohio. She is currently enrolled in the Ohio University College of Osteopathic Medicine. While working on this book, she participated in the 2005 Summer Research Trainee Program, which was sponsored by the Multicultural Affairs Office of the Massachusetts General Hospital, where she worked at the Center for Child and Adolescent Health Policy.

John M. Neff, M.D., Director, Center for Children with Special Needs, Children's Hospital and Regional Medical Center, and Professor of Pediatrics, University of Washington School of Medicine, Metropolitan Park West M/S: MPW5-2, 1100 Olive Way, Suite 500, Seattle, Washington 98101

Dr. Neff is a graduate of Pomona College and Harvard Medical School. He trained in pediatrics at Johns Hopkins Hospital and in virology and infectious diseases at Children's Hospital Boston and was medical director of Children's Hospital and Regional Medical Center in Seattle from 1981 to 1998. Dr. Neff has broad interests in child health and advocacy, especially with regard to smallpox and smallpox vaccination and the question of how to best serve children with special health care needs in our current environment. He has served on many state and national committees as well as with the Epidemic Intelligence Service of the Public Health Service. Notably, he chaired a statewide advisory committee on children with special needs during the Washington State health care reform initiatives from 1994 to 2000, the Committee on Hospital Care of the American Academy of Pediatrics from 1999 to 2003, and the Smallpox Vaccine Safety Work Group of the Advisory Committee on Immunization Practice of the Centers for Disease Control and Prevention and of the Armed Forces Epidemiological Board of the Department of Defense from 2003 to 2004.

Robert M. Sheets, M.D., Pediatric Rheumatologist, Children's Specialists of San Diego, Division of Rheumatology, and Assistant Clinical Instructor in Pediatrics, University of California, San Diego School of Medicine, 3020 Children's Way, MC #5113, San Diego, California 92123

Dr. Sheets earned his medical degree from Baylor College of Medicine in Houston, Texas. Prior to developing his 15-year career in pediatric rheumatology, Dr. Sheets practiced general pediatrics. He was affiliated with two large HMOs and was in charge of the pediatric portion of family practice programs in Merced and Salinas, California. Before joining Children's Specialists of San Diego in June 2000, Dr. Sheets was medical director of Loma Linda University Children's Hospital Team Center Clinics.

Lisa A. Simpson, M.B., B.Ch., MPH., FAAP, National Director, Child Health Policy, National Initiative for Children's Healthcare Quality, 20 University Road, 7th Floor, Cambridge, Massachusetts 02138

Dr. Simpson is All Children's Hospital Guild Endowed Chair in Child Health Policy at the University of South Florida, where she launched the Florida Initiative for Children's Healthcare Quality and conducts research focused on health care quality and disparities, health information technology, and regional and national improvement in the quality of care for children and adolescents. A board-certified pediatrician with training in public health, health services research, and health policy, Dr. Simpson was formerly the deputy director at the Agency for Healthcare Research and Quality (AHRQ) at the U.S. Department of Health and Human Services (DHHS). During her 7 years as AHRQ deputy director, she spearheaded numerous initiatives to increase the quality and quantity of child health services research sponsored by the agency. Dr. Simpson publishes and speaks frequently on the quality and outcomes of care for children. She has received numerous awards including the Excellence in Public Service Award from the American Academy of Pediatrics, the Senior Executive Service Meritorious Presidential Rank Award, and the DHHS Secretary's Distinguished Service Award.

Ruth E.K. Stein, M.D., Professor, Department of Pediatrics, Albert Einstein College of Medicine and the Children's Hospital at Montefiore, 111 East 210 Street, Bronx, New York 10467

Dr. Stein works in research and advocacy for children, especially those with chronic health conditions. Her research has been supported by the Maternal and Child Health Bureau; the National Institute of Mental Health; the Assistant Secretary for Planning and Evaluation, Health Resources and Services Administration; and numerous foundations.

She has written more than 150 publications and serves on several editorial boards as well as on the research committees of the Ambulatory Pediatric Association and the Society for Developmental and Behavioral Pediatrics. Dr. Stein is a past president of the Ambulatory Pediatric Association and a member of the Research Consortium on Children with Chronic Conditions. She recently served on the boards of Children, Youth and Families of the National Academy of Science and the Institute of Medicine and cochaired its Committee on the Evaluation of Child Health.

Marcia Van Riper, RN, Ph.D., Associate Professor, University of North Carolina at Chapel Hill School of Nursing and the Carolina Center for Genome Sciences, Carrington Hall CB #7460, Chapel Hill, North Carolina 27599

Dr. Van Riper has conducted numerous studies concerning families of children with Down syndrome, one study concerning families with twins, and one study concerning families with preterm infants. She recently completed a K01 study (Mentored Research Scientist Career Development Award) examining how families define and manage the ethical issues that emerge during four types of genetic testing: maternal serum screening for Down syndrome, carrier testing for cystic fibrosis, BRCA1&2 testing for families at high risk for breast cancer, and mutation analysis for Huntington disease. Dr. Van Riper collaborated on a study about feeding issues in children with Down syndrome and received funding for two pilot studies on how minority families make sense of and use the results of genetic testing.

Nora Wells, M.S.Ed., Director of Programs, Family Voices, 1135 Tremont Street, Suite 420, Boston, Massachusetts 02120

Ms. Wells directs programs for Family Voices, a national organization of families and friends of children with special health care needs. Ms. Wells is a frequent public speaker and has contributed chapters to *Children with Disabilities, Fifth Edition* (Paul H. Brookes Publishing Co., 2002) and *Health Care Choices for Today's Consumer, Guide to Quality and Cost* (Living Planet, 1994) and has published articles in peer-reviewed journals. In her work at Family Voices, Ms. Wells has managed a variety of projects and activities related to how families experience health care systems. She currently codirects the Family Voices National Center on

Family Professional Partnerships and is leading the Family Voices partnership with the Oregon Health & Science University in the design and
implementation of a data resource center to provide consumer access
to survey data on children and youth. Ms. Wells is the mother of three
young adult sons, the oldest of whom has cerebral palsy.

FOREWORD

Optimizing Care for Young Children with Special Health Care Needs: Knowledge and Strategies for Navigating the System builds upon a rich history in this country's efforts to ensure that all children, including children with special health care needs (CSHCN), and their families can and do receive the services and supports necessary for children to live, play, and grow to become productive citizens in their own homes and communities. The book's multiperspective, noncategorical approach provides unique insights into many of the perplexing issues facing families of CSHCN and their service providers in today's health care system, while its strong emphasis on family–professional partnerships provides a testament to the power of collaboration.

BACKGROUND AND COMMUNITY SYSTEMS BUILDING BLOCKS

Through its federal agencies, the United States has taken the initial steps to ensure implementation in every state of family-centered, culturally competent, comprehensive, and community-based service systems. The development of these systems has a long history, from the original Social Security Act (SSA) legislation in 1935, which called for Maternal and Child Health (MCH) Title V Programs to "locate, diagnose and treat crippled children," to our current recognition that the health of children must be addressed in the context of the family and the community environment in which the children live.

We learned many lessons during the journey. We have moved from disease-specific to population-based approaches, using a generic definition of children with special health care needs inclusive of children needing services beyond those required by typically developing children. We also have moved from the medical model to a comprehensive care model of interprofessional team care, from a deficit- to a strength-based perspective, from a doctor–patient relationship to a family–professional collaboration model, and from separate silos to integrated models of service delivery. We have demonstrated over and over that family-centered, community-based care is the model of practice for achieving the child and family outcomes we desire. This book will help to drive the much-needed diffusion and implementation of these ideals along the health care continuum.

The ideals themselves emerged through the efforts of many people in both the public and private sector over the past several decades. During the 1980s, the U.S. Surgeon General's Office and the Maternal and Child Health Bureau (MCHB) developed a national agenda to establish comprehensive, coordinated, culturally competent, community-based systems of care. These efforts were based on the principles of family-centered care and family–professional partnerships. By the early 1990s, with grant funding from MCHB, Family Voices, a national grass roots organization for families of CSHCN, was established and would have significant influence on national and state polices related to children with special health care needs and their families.

Early on, MCHB and the American Academy of Pediatrics (AAP) joined forces to launch a national initiative to promote a medical home for every child, and in 1994 the original medical home project, initiated in Hawaii, became the foundation for a National Center on the Medical Home in the AAP Department of Community Pediatrics, where it continues to play a major role.

MCHB and AAP, as well as several other major private and public organizations, increasingly acknowledged the role of caring communities in the lives of CSHCN and their families. For example, AAP set up community development efforts such as Community Access to Child Health (CATCH). Family Voices, Access to Care Through the Medical Home, and Community Systems Initiatives have become the core building blocks in current efforts in systems building.

Establishing the Mandate

In 1989, the Omnibus Budget Reconciliation Act (OBRA) amended Title V of the SSA to extend its authority and responsibility to provide and promote family-centered, community-based, coordinated care for CSHCN and to facilitate the development of "community based systems of services for such children and their families" (Omnibus Budget Reconciliation Act of 1989). In addition, *Healthy People 2000* and *Healthy People 2010*, which represent the health goals for the nation, similarly required that we "increase the proportion of States and territories that have service systems for CSHCN" (U.S. Department of Health and Human Services, 1991, 2000). Finally, in March 2002, *Delivering on the Promise* (U.S. Department of Health and Human Services, 2002) was published to report on the progress of federal agencies toward achieving the New Freedom Initiative. This initiative, the result of a presidential executive order, was based on the Supreme Court decision in *Olmstead v. L.C.* (1999) calling for options for community living for all persons with disabilities. *Delivering on the Promise* charged MCHB with the development and implementation of community-based systems for children and youth with special health care needs and their families. Thus, through legislative and judicial requirements and our national health goals, we have clear responsibilities and authorities to complete the implementation of community-based systems. The reality that families and providers face on a daily basis must be brought closer to the ideal described in these goals and requirements.

Defining the Population

An important challenge was the need for a new definition of the populations requiring such service systems. Through MCHB's partnership with families, AAP, and other major policy groups, a comprehensive definition of CSHCN was developed and published in the July 1998 issue of *Pediatrics*. Children with special health care needs are defined as "those who have or are at increased risk for a chronic physical, developmental, behavioral, or emotional condition and who also require health and related services of a type or amount beyond that required by children generally" (McPherson et al., 1998). This definition is purposely broad and inclusive of those children who need not only medical services but also related services (e.g., early intervention, special education, behavioral health, family support). The definition recognizes that a community system of services requires community development across sectors to integrate the multiple fragmented services needed by these children. The hope is that families can use the services easily and that communities can provide the services in a comprehensive, integrated way.

Defining the Service System

Perhaps the greatest challenge was to identify the care components for the community-based system of services. These were needed to measure national progress in putting in place the services and supports needed for successful outcomes. From many discussions came six simple concepts:

1. Families of CSHCN must partner in decision making at all levels and will be satisfied with the services they receive.

2. CSHCN must receive coordinated, ongoing, comprehensive care within a medical home.

3. Families of children with special health care needs must have ade-
    quate private and/or public insurance to pay for the services they
    need.

4. All children must be screened early and continuously for special
    health care needs.

5. Community-based service systems must be organized so that fami-
    lies can use them easily.

6. Youth with special health care needs must receive the services nec-
    essary to make transitions to all aspects of adult life, including adult
    health care, work, and independence.

When operationalized, these care components provide for accountability, as required by the Government Performance and Results Act
(GPRA) of 1993.

MEASURING THE PROGRESS

Indicators based on the definition of CSHCN just described have now
been developed, and in January 2004, data were released from the
first National Survey of CSHCN, funded by MCHB and conducted in
collaboration with the National Center for Health Statistics (U.S. Department of Health and Human Services, 2003). We now have state
and national prevalence estimates for CSHCN as well as baseline measurements on the six community-based system of services care component outcome indicators as follows:

*   Family participation and satisfaction: 57%

*   Access to a medical home: 51%

*   Access to affordable insurance: 60%

*   Early and continuous screening: 52%

*   Easy access to community-based services   74%

*   Services necessary to transition to adulthood   6%

We can describe the results as the glass being half full: Outcomes for
five of the six indicators are at 50% or beyond. We can also acknowledge that we have much more to do, particularly for the core outcome
on transition to adulthood. The survey has been revised to strengthen
some questions based on gaps identified and is now in the field for the
second time. In 2007, new data will be available to track progress and
hopefully to measure success.

REACHING THE GOAL

The creation of community-based systems of services provides a solution to many of the issues this country continues to face. Ensuring that all of our children, including those with special health care needs, receive the comprehensive array of services in their own communities 1) reduces the current fragmentation and inefficiencies; 2) leaves no child behind; and 3) achieves for the United States a children's system of services based on the principles of equity, universality, and sustainability.

Is it possible to achieve success by 2010? Of course it is. Partial implementation exists in all states, and coalitions are working to weave together programs that address the six critical core outcomes. If we are to succeed, children and youth must have access to high-quality primary health care through a medical home, with appropriate referrals to specialty and community resources; screening and surveillance for early identification must be strengthened in all states; communities must be supported to provide total inclusion opportunities; and youth must be assisted in the transition to productive adulthood. Achieving success will take partnerships among families, professionals, health, education, social services, and many other public, business, and voluntary organizations committed to this common agenda. This volume, which brings together a diversity of important information and perspectives in a comprehensive and accessible format to facilitate communication and dialogue, encourages such partnerships.

Merle G. McPherson, M.D., FACPM, FAAP
Director, Services for Children with Special Health Care Needs
U.S. Department of Health and Human Services
Health Resources and Services Administration
Rockville, Maryland

REFERENCES

Government Performance and Results Act (GPRA) of 1993, PL 103-62, 31 U.S.C. §§ 1115 *et seq.*

McPherson, M., Arango, P., Fox, H., Lauver, C., McManus, M., Newacheck, P.W., et al. (1998). A new definition of children with special health care needs. *Pediatrics, 102,* 137–140.

Olmstead v. L.C., 527 U.S. 581 (1999).

Omnibus Budget Reconciliation Act (OBRA) of 1981, PL 97-35, 95 Stat. 357.

Social Security Act of 1935, PL 74-271, 42 U.S.C. §§ 301 *et seq.*

U.S. Department of Health and Human Services. (1991). *Healthy People 2000: National health promotion and disease prevention objectives* (DHHS Publication No. [PHS] 91-50212). Washington, DC: Author.

U.S. Department of Health and Human Services. (2000, January). *Healthy People 2010* (Conference Edition in Two Volumes). Washington, DC: Author.

U.S. Department of Health and Human Services. (2002). *Delivering on the promise: Self-evaluation to promote community living for people with disabilities* (Report to the President on Executive Order 13217). Washington, DC: Author. Retrieved from http://www.hhs.gov/new freedom/final/hhs.html

U.S. Department of Health and Human Services, Health Resources and Services Administration, Maternal and Child Health Bureau. (2003). The National Survey of Children's Health. Rockville, MD: Author.

van Dyck, P.C., McPherson, M., Strickland, B., Nesseler, K., Blumberg, S.J., Cynamon, M.I., & Newacheck, P.W. (2002). The National Survey of Children with Special Health Care Needs. *Ambulatory Pediatrics, 2,* 29–37.

PREFACE

Optimizing Care for Young Children with Special Health Care Needs: Knowledge and Strategies for Navigating the System focuses on children ages birth to 5 living with chronic or disabling conditions. Appropriate care and services during these early years is crucial to promoting the most favorable outcomes for these exceptional children, referred to in this book as *children with special health care needs* (CSHCN).

WHY THIS BOOK?

It is our belief that a broader discussion of what appropriate care consists of—a discussion including the range of disciplinary and stakeholder perspectives and emphasizing engagement with the various opinions and experiences represented—is essential to improving that care. We have worked together toward this end for 7 years now, combining the anthropological and biomedical perspectives on a variety of projects assessing and improving care for CSHCN. In the course of this work, we heard many stories from parents, guardians, and providers who felt confused and stymied by the complexities of the health care and social services systems. We also heard from clinicians frustrated at their own inability to provide the best quality care or to make the system work for the families they served. The stories these people told validated the findings of our research and evaluation projects. Moreover, these stories resonated with our personal experiences of the aggravating process of securing high-quality care for young children with special health care needs.

The United States has one of the most scientifically and technologically advanced medical systems in the world. Our initial work asked why, then, is getting good care for children with disabilities or who are chronically ill such a challenge? What is it about our health care system that forces people to struggle to obtain the care to which they are entitled? We learned that once people understand the system, even with its multiple challenges, they can manipulate it to get care and services for their children. Unfortunately, the learning process could be painfully slow and the system could take years to master. So we began to wonder: What can be done to accelerate parental and health care professional learning? What can those new to the system learn from those who have dealt with it in the past?

We created this book in our quest to achieve high-quality care for CSHCN to encourage dialogue among all the stakeholders in the system. We invited leading child health experts in clinical care and public policy as well as parents of children with chronic conditions to each prepare a chapter on a specific aspect of providing care for the children. This book represents the culmination of these efforts. Although some of the contributors are nationally prominent scholars and applied child-health service researchers, others are parents, primary care physicians, and specialists directly involved in caring for CSHCN—front-line experts whose important, practical knowledge gained over years of caregiving is generally missing from the current literature.

Through this approach, we strove to create a comprehensive framework for understanding families' experiences and the most effective approaches providers can use to improve care and services for children and their families. The collection provides a critical summation of issues that cut across boundaries between specific chronic or disabling childhood conditions, overriding particular diagnostic labels. Chapters highlight the universal or noncategorical issues that CSHCN and their families must face. Such knowledge can be used to accelerate the adaptation process that all families must go through when a child is born with special needs and to enhance care coordination and family–provider communication. We hope, too, that the book can identify emerging trends and call attention to areas that remain problematic, thereby providing a platform for the next decade's efforts to advance research, policy, and service and care provision for children with special health care needs.

The book is divided into four sections. Section I provides overall context. It reviews the various definitions of CSHCN, showing that childhood disability and illness categories are clearly both sociocultural and medical constructions, and it provides overviews and explorations of the demographics and differential epidemiology of CSHCN, of the economics involved (e.g., financial costs to families, practitioners, systems of care), and of relevant policy and program issues (e.g., Title V of the Individuals with Disabilities Education Improvement Act of 2004, PL 108-446).

Section II, The Parent Experience, shifts the focus from the macro to the micro level, while acknowledging that the two are intimately intertwined. It opens with a chapter on household and familial issues such as parental and sibling stresses and goes on to discuss the ways that various cultural factors (e.g., biomedicine's curative stance, the disability rights movement) affect household and family responses to CSHCN. A chapter focusing on the parental perspective discusses the various roles (e.g., advocate, care coordinator) parents play in ensuring that their child receives needed and quality care, the nature of the parent–provider relationship and how it can be improved, common barriers that parents encounter, and how parents can become better advocates for their children and more effectively navigate the health care system (e.g., by sharing with and learning from other parents).

In Section III, The Provider Experience, primary care physicians (PCPs) and specialists discuss the systems within which they have worked, ways that each has tried to improve the system, and strategies to further strengthen systems of care for CSHCN. The section also discusses the roles and expectations of clinicians when it comes to care coordination, advocacy, the medical home, family-centered care, and other critical issues. Specialists often play a more significant role than PCPs in the care of CSHCN but generally are not prepared to offer more routine and standardized pediatric care (e.g., immunizations, well-child checks) in addition to their specialized services. The chapters in this section discuss the realities of given system constraints in caring for CSHCN (e.g., managed care, limited time, inadequate reimbursement, difficult referral processes), as well as concerns about specialist-to-specialist, specialist-to-PCP, and provider–parent relationships and communication.

In the book's final section, Present Strategies, Future Directions, modifiable factors are identified and practical improvement processes outlined. Emerging trends are reviewed and areas that remain problematic highlighted. The research implications of what parents, PCPs, and specialists report or request are examined. A discussion of links between the book's conclusions and the program-planning and policy-making processes make the book useful not only for those who provide direct care for CSHCN but also for those interested in implementing research-driven system changes to ensure that CSHCN and their families receive the support they need and deserve.

Together, the chapters address a number of the many questions that must be answered to optimize care for children with special health care needs; for example:

- Can learning curves for families and professionals be accelerated? At which points in these curves might interventions be most effective?

- How can the voice of the family best be heard and respected? How can the family be involved in care decisions even when those decisions must take into account complex medical information?

- How can all aspects of care—including care offered by a developmental specialist such as a speech or occupational therapist—be most effectively, efficiently, and consistently coordinated?

- How can families and providers most effectively work together to advocate for CSHCN?

This book is intended as a critical summation of issues and is not meant as a textbook on specific conditions that CSHCN and their families encounter. However, basic information regarding particular conditions is provided as needed in the context of discussions. The facts provided are presented to serve the broader aim of the book, which is to summarize the state of thinking on the subject today, describe the agenda for the future, and prepare readers to meet the goals of that agenda.

The book addresses neither terminal conditions nor issues specific to children over the age of 5. As such, it addresses only in passing mental health issues (most of which occur in children older than 5 years of age), sexuality, employment and independent living, and transition from pediatric to adult care. Its discussion of school issues is limited to those entailed in initial educational placement. The authors feel that by staying focused on only young children and infants, the book can give in-depth treatment to the issues most pertinent to that age range.

There is as yet only minimal and fragmented literature for health care professionals regarding CSHCN. Despite increasing recognition of the value of a noncategorical approach focusing on issues that affect all special child health conditions, much of the relevant literature is scattered and split up by the large diversity of conditions considered rather than coordinated through cross-condition similarities. Existing works typically focus on the particulars of recommended medical care, selected interventions, or required services for a specific condition or special health need (e.g., recommended schedule of tests or assessment for children with diabetes, how to address challenging behaviors in children with autism, reconstructive surgery for children with craniofacial malformations). Although such works provide important and vital information, they do so using a narrowly focused lens. They fail to show the broader perspective on how to optimize the care of CSHCN—one that takes into account the experiences and learning curves of both families and health care providers and that asks how families and providers can work together more effectively to care for children with special health care needs.

Furthermore, the experiences of parents and guardians of children with disabilities have received little attention except in the narrow terms of parental coping and adjustment—for example, in the relationship between caring for such children and the parents' own physical and mental health status or divorce rates. The literature has not adequately addressed parents' unpaid roles as managers and coordinators of care for children with disabilities (whether or not the family explicitly chooses to play such a role), nor has it explored the expertise the parents gain regarding their own child's condition. The literature by and for care providers rarely situates parents as educators of providers, and it has failed to explore their passage from novices to masters in navigating the health care system—except in the most anecdotal fashion.

To address these gaps and other system issues that conspire against coordinated, high-quality care for CSHCN, this book examines such children comprehensively and noncategorically, with a focus on the early years of the child's life and the ways in which parents learn to navigate the complex, confusing, and often uncoordinated health care system that their children depend upon. The book provides a much-needed blueprint for the development of applied research and policy designed to improve health outcomes for CSHCN.

It will be clear by now that rather than seeking to convey a single perspective in isolation, such as that of the parent or PCP, we incorporated and examined the perspectives and experiences both of parents of CSHCN and of the various physicians and specialists who care for the children. The book's key contribution will (we hope) thereby be a deeper understanding of the various needs, concerns, challenges, constraints, expectations, and goals of all involved. Our intended readers include pediatricians and family practice physicians who provide primary care for CSHCN; specialists (including therapists) and hospital house staff who treat the children; those involved in the children's case management; and allied health, nursing, and medical students who will serve the children later. The book should prepare its readers to better serve and advocate for CSHCN as well as to educate and counsel families regarding the journey that caring for a child with special needs entails. Its secondary audience, researchers and policy makers, are advised regarding strategic areas for action, which we hope will give this book a research and policy impact.

We could not have completed this project without the help of many organizations and individuals, including Michael Seid, whose discussions with us in the early stages of book planning were instrumental in shaping the form of the collection; and Kimberly Dennis, Erica Prussing, and Elizabeth Walker, who were critical members of the Down syndrome project from which this book stemmed. We also thank all of the chapter authors as well as those experts who, while they could not provide chapters, did provide guidance, advice, and support. We thank the families and children who have participated, whether directly or indirectly, in our improvement work. We thank Ruth and Sol Gerber for their generous support of research activities that formed a main impetus for this book and Jon Kurtin for helping to make that support possible. We thank the Alliance Health Care Foundation (Grant #99-10) and the California Endowment (Grant #20023662) for supporting parts of the book preparation process. And we thank our readers for persevering with the task of health care improvement, exerting pressure through research, advocacy, caregiving, and policy work so that children with special needs receive the high-quality health care that they, like all children, deserve.

PROLOGUE

Twenty-three years ago, Hank was in the first year of his orthopedic surgery residency studying muscle disease and biomechanics and Jill was three months pregnant. Out for a walk in a suburban Denver mall, we came across a live telethon raising money for United Cerebral Palsy. We paused to watch the activities long enough to reflect on disabling conditions like cerebral palsy and muscular dystrophy. We talked about what kind of lives children (and adults) with these diagnoses and their families led. Four months later one of our twins died *in utero* and we were the parents of a premature son born with cerebral palsy.

What transpired between our son Sean's birth and our writing this prologue could fill a book. Our lives changed in extraordinary ways, as do the lives of all individuals who become parents. (In addition to Sean, we have another son, Reid, born without disabilities.) Jill became busier as a caregiver for her first child than she ever expected to be; she also became an active advocate for children with disabilities and their families. Hank became board certified in pediatric orthopedic surgery, traveling throughout the United States and abroad lecturing about his specialty: cerebral palsy.

As new parents of a son with disabilities, we were scared, hurt, and unprepared for the challenges of raising a child with significant disabilities. At the same time, we were filled with hope and love. We also had many, many questions about how we were to proceed with the care of our son.

From the beginning, our most immediate need was to ensure Sean's good health. As a 3-pound preemie with heart and intestinal complications, he needed a team of NICU doctors to get him safely through four surgeries. And although it was a great joy when he finally came home after 3 months, it also was a great adjustment.

Through the years of caring for our son and through numerous surgeries and hospitalizations, we learned that what was most lacking was not medical expertise but coordination of care. Without the aid of what is now termed a *medical home,* and without the services of a developmental pediatrician (an arena that is only now gaining acceptance within pediatrics), we were left with the difficult task of managing, and in some cases directing, the care that Sean received from a multitude of specialists who did not communicate with one another. Hank inevitably assumed the medical care coordinator role, placing himself in the uncomfortable and ill-advised position of being both our son's father and his managing doctor. Having said that, however, Hank was better prepared than most to assume such a role because of his experience, however limited initially, within the health care system.

Our second most pressing need in those early years was information. In the days before the Internet, information was much harder to obtain. That parents of children with disabilities are a diverse group is a given. That each parent experiences the shock, grief, and acceptance of anomalous birth in different ways is also clear. Some parents shy away from information at first, needing more time to process or accept the situation. However, most of the parents we met on our journey with Sean were hungry for information. Our information needs were broad. We required answers to basic questions such as "What is cerebral palsy?" "What causes it?" "What should we expect as our child develops?" But we also needed specialized information on specific therapies, surgeries, medication, and equipment.

We were faced on a daily basis with choices about different therapies and surgeries with only limited knowledge of how or even if they worked. But when faced with these choices, parents often ask themselves questions such as, "If I don't authorize this surgery (or this treatment, or this brace, or this medicine), will my child miss an opportunity to have a better life?" "How will we afford it?" "How will it affect our family?" The information we were able to gather helped us to think our options through and to become better advocates for Sean. We could more fully and effectively participate in decision making that affected him not only medically but also educationally and socially. We could better connect with community resources not provided by or accessed through clinical medicine (e.g., school resources, respite care).

Our dominant and ultimately our most centering need was to create a healthy family life. Within a short period of time we had amassed enough experience with the medical emergencies and day-to-day crises entailed in Sean's cerebral palsy to know that normal, or typical, was not necessarily our goal for him.

Having a second child taught us to step back and consider: We were a family of four, not one. Sean may have had special needs, but the rest of us had needs as well. Focusing all the attention on one family member caused resentment and problems for everyone. Yes, Sean did need special assistance and, yes, he often required more time and attention. This was one reality. But another reality was that in addition to critical medical and therapeutic care, Sean needed as much of a typical home environment as could be provided. To achieve this required a lot of vigilance, mostly on Jill's part, as she assumed the primary care-giving role. Deciding how many therapy sessions and doctors' appoint-ments a week were manageable without disrupting everyone's life at home was a constant balancing act but one that got easier with time and experience. Sometimes taking a family trip to the beach to allow Sean (as well as the rest of us) to experience the variety of textures, sounds, and experiences that the warm sand and cool water had to offer was more therapeutic than having two cranky babies and a stressed mother endure another hour-long therapy session in which Sean was forced into uncomfortable positions on a mat in a hot room.

Learning to pay attention to what Sean could teach us about his own needs proved to be invaluable, especially as he grew older. Care-fully watching and listening to Sean even when he was a young child revealed much, often guiding us to make better choices on how to spend time and energy. To this day, one of our family's fondest memo-ries is of a game we spontaneously created from what started out to be routine time spent on the floor in the evenings with Sean sitting in therapeutic positions reaching for a Nerf ball, shifting weight, throwing the ball, and so forth. With the eager insistence of an energetic little brother who also wanted some attention and fun, our family sponta-neously combined our creativity and resourcefulness to invent what evolved into a high-spirited game we all loved to play. We moved the activity to the hallway where the walls kept Sean's wild throws in-bounds and where the doorways served as natural goals. Our nightly family game of halley-ball often found us eventually in a pile on the floor giggling and wrestling, with Sean screeching the loudest of all. Our halley-ball games and similar innovative family activities proved to be the therapy we all most needed to infuse ourselves with the energy, resilience, and team spirit we would require over the long haul.

Twenty-two years after Sean's birth, we have found our family's journey to be unpredictable, bittersweet, and profoundly challeng-ing—but always full of opportunities for laughter, gratitude, and joy. However, our family and the families of children with disabilities that Hank has worked with were, and are, confronted with challenges and hurdles that few of us are prepared by our culture to handle. Fear and sometimes a crushing sense of loss can contribute to the stress that unprepared families must face on a sometimes daily basis. How can our health care system and local communities better reach out to help these families? How can families be empowered to help themselves? How can we best serve, learn from, and celebrate our exceptional children? These are the central issues of this book, and the resolutions are often complex and context-specific. An essential part of our family's journey has been to help refine the quality and range of responses that families, experts, and society in general have to share with other families of children with special health care needs. The chapters in this volume contribute significantly to this end.

—Jill and Hank Chambers

Jill Chambers has been an active advocate for children and adults with special needs and has spoken regionally, nationally, and internationally regarding her experiences as the mother of a son with a disability. She has served on several boards of directors and committees including Kids Included Together (San Diego), United Cerebral Palsy of San Diego, and the Lawrence Family Jewish Community Center, all of which named her Volunteer of the Year.

Hank Chambers, M.D., is director of the Cerebral Palsy Center and the Motion Analysis Laboratory at Children's Hospital and Health Center in San Diego. Dr. Chambers is also associate clinical professor of Orthopedic Surgery at the University of California San Diego's School of Medicine and serves on the board of directors of United Cerebral Palsy. He was recently elected president of the American Academy for Cerebral Palsy and Developmental Medicine.

Optimizing Care
for Young Children
with Special Health
Care Needs

I

SETTING THE STAGE FOR CHANGE

An estimated 15% to 20% of U.S. children have a significant on-going health care need related to a chronic condition. Most of these children require long-term services from a variety of health care professionals and organizations and use substantially more pediatric health services than their healthy peers (Newacheck et al., 1998); indeed, their care accounts for the majority of pediatric health care costs (Ireys, Anderson, Shaffer, & Neff, 1997).

The overall costs of health care for children are low, however, and for this and other reasons, not much attention has been paid to the health care needs of children in general let alone children with special health care needs (CSHCN; Forrest, Simpson, & Clancy, 1997).[1] The relative dearth of child-focused health services research as well as the broader scholarly bias favoring the adult perspective even in studies that ostensibly deal with children (Castaneda, 2002; Mayall, 2002) has led to a situation in which adult standards are all too often applied within the field of children's health.

The service standard usually applied to adults provides only for treatment of specific, discrete conditions. It does not provide for services to enhance developmental potential, which, theoretically, already has been achieved in adults (see Castaneda, 2002). The service standard does not include treatments or interventions in the present to offset the high probability of future impairment. And there is no explicit role for the family in the adult-focused service approach.

Perhaps more important, the focus of adult medicine on disease and cure, as opposed to prevention and development in pediatrics, and the differential epidemiology associated with childhood conditions, in which numerous conditions exist but each affects only a few children, has stifled interest in CSHCN. In the context of the U.S. medical community's penchant for specialization (Good, 1998), differential epidemiology also has meant that the typical approach to care for CSHCN

---

[1]The term *children with special health care needs* and the acronym *CSHCN* are used interchangeably throughout the book.

has been *categorical* in nature; that is, it has been driven by a child's specific special health diagnosis—his or her category of disease—and not by the child's overall health needs or the needs of the family.

Even relatively common specific health conditions (e.g., Down syndrome, cerebral palsy) are unusual enough that an individual primary care physician may follow only one or two affected children at a time (Cooley, 1999). As such, primary care physicians may feel that they lack the necessary expertise or experience with a given condition to treat and monitor it properly. In more complex cases, collaboration by the primary care physician with other health care providers is probable, given that no single provider can arrange or deliver all the needed services (Perrin, 2002). This is due in part to the fragmented nature of today's health care system, and in part to the time and fiscal constraints imposed by managed care that make it unlikely that a general pediatrician or family physician can keep current with the condition-specific literature and meet all of the patients' specialized needs. U.S. Secretary of Health and Human Services Tommy G. Thompson has noted, "Even providers with appropriate training find our current service system offers few incentives to ensure appropriate health care for children and adults with special needs" (p. iii; U.S. Public Health Service, 2002).

We should therefore reconsider estimates regarding the size and composition of the CSHCN population. As pediatrician Ruth Stein explains in Chapter 1, and as subsequent chapters demonstrate, the actual number of CSHCN depends on one's definition. Definitions have implications for program access because they determine who can receive what care, where, when, from whom, and for how long—and who will pay for that care (Beers, Kemeny, Sherritt, & Palfrey, 2003). Some classification schemes focus on impairments, others on etiologies. Further, the breakdown in terms of specific conditions depends on how comorbidities are classified. In recent years, major efforts have been made to increase consistency in how *children with special health care needs* is defined for government, program, and research purposes. In any case, asthma, seizure disorder, cerebral palsy, mental retardation, and attention-deficit/hyperactivity disorder (ADHD) are among the most common conditions; other, less common conditions include congenital heart disease, spina bifida, sickle cell disease, arthritis, hemophilia, and AIDS (Perrin, Kuhlthau, Gortmaker, Beal, & Ferris, 2002).

In Chapter 1, Ruth Stein focuses on defining the CSHCN population, and in Chapter 2, health service researchers Karen Kuhlthau, Sheila Bloom, Monica Marthell, and Hodon Mohamed discuss the organization, administration, and evolution of key policies affecting health care service delivery for children with special health care needs. Numerous federally supported programs exist to meet specific needs of CSHCN and their families, but these programs, the policies behind them, and the services they support are variable and complex.

In Chapter 3, pediatrician John Neff ties the CSHCN demographic profile and policy issues to the economic context of health care provision. He discusses financial issues that are integral to working with CSHCN, including costs to health plans, practitioners, and families. Costs and types of services CSHCN receive are compared with those received by children without special health care needs. The final section of the finance chapter addresses the current fiscal realities that all states face, and demonstrates how an unraveling of support could have a major deleterious impact on families, practitioners, hospitals, and communities.

REFERENCES

Beers, N., Kemeny, A., Sherritt, L., & Palfrey, J. (2003). Variations in state-level definitions: Children with special health care needs. *Public Health Reports, 118*, 434–447.

Castaneda, C. (2002). *Figurations: Child, bodies, worlds.* Durham, NC: Duke University Press.

Cooley, W. (1999). Responding to the developmental consequences of genetic conditions: The importance of pediatric primary care. *American Journal of Medical Genetics, 89*, 75–80.

Forrest, C.B., Simpson, L., & Clancy, C. (1997). Child health services research. Challenges and opportunities. *Journal of American Medical Association, 277*(22), 1787–1793.

Good, M.J.D-V. (1998). *American medicine: The quest for competence (with a new preface).* Los Angeles: University of California Press.

Ireys, H.T., Anderson, G.F., Shaffer, T.J., & Neff, J.M. (1997). Expenditures for care of children with chronic illnesses enrolled in the Washington State Medicaid program, fiscal year 1993. *Pediatrics, 100*(2; Pt. 1), 197–204.

Mayall, B. (2002). *Towards a sociology for childhood: Thinking from children's lives.* Philadelphia: Open University Press.

McGlynn, E.A., Halfon, N., & Leibowitz, A. (1995). Assessing the quality of care for children. Prospects under health reform. *Archives of Pediatric & Adolescent Medicine, 149*(4), 359–368.

Newacheck, P.W., Strickland, B., Shonkoff, J.P., Perrin, J.M., McPherson, M., McManus, M., et al. (1998). An epidemiologic profile of children with special health care needs. *Pediatrics, 102*, 117–123.

Perrin, J.M. (2002). Health services research for children with disabilities. *Milbank Q, 80*(2), 303–324.

Perrin, J.M., Kuhlthau, K.A., Gortmaker, S.L., Beal, A.C., & Ferris, T.G. (2002). Generalist and subspecialist care for children with chronic conditions. *Ambulatory Pediatrics, 2*(6), 462–469.

U.S. Public Health Service. (2002). *Closing the gap: A national blueprint to improve the health of persons with mental retardation. Report of the Surgeon General's conference on health disparities and mental retardation.* Washington, DC: Author.

1

CHILDREN WITH SPECIAL HEALTH CARE NEEDS:

EVOLVING DEFINITIONS, EVOLVING ESTIMATES

Ruth E.K. Stein

W ho are children with special health care needs (CSHCN)? How many are there? How do we begin to assess their actual care and service needs?

The answers to these questions hinge on who is—and who is not—counted. This, in turn, depends on the way the term *population of interest* is defined. Definitions of the populations and the tools used to implement the definitions determine who can receive care, what kind of care can be received, when it can be received, who will be supplying the care and for how long, and, most important, who will pay for it. Defining the populations of interest also affects who is included in the research and how we interpret the research findings. The results of the research will determine what we do and do not know about children with health conditions.

This chapter introduces the reader to the most common definitions used to identify the population of children with special health care needs. Some were developed by researchers, some by the programs and agencies that determine eligibility, and some by policy makers. In more recent years, there has been an appreciation of the need to increase the consistency of the definitions employed and to find practical ways to put them to use. The chapter discusses that evolution and reviews various estimates and characterizations of the population in question. It also provides the reader with enough background to understand that how the population is specified depends on the method used and reflects the scope of the definition adopted. As a result, depending on the conceptualization of the definition and the techniques used to implement the definition, a different set of children will be included. The goal of this chapter is to help the reader appreciate the paramount importance of the terms that are used to define the children and their conditions and the tools to make them operational and how they affect the interpretation of information about the children's ongoing health-related experiences and outcomes. This chapter also provides the core justification for the noncategorical approach on which this book seeks to build.

HISTORY OF THE TERMINOLOGICAL DEBATE

The success of modern Western medicine has brought about a large increase in the number of children living with continuing health conditions and service needs. In earlier eras, far fewer children who developed impairments of their body systems survived for prolonged periods. The primary exceptions were children with mental retardation or neurological, sensory, or motor impairments or other non–life-threatening structural anomalies, but even those children were more subject than healthy children to early death from infections before the advent of effective immunizations and antibiotics. For example, children with Down syndrome often died from complications of their heart conditions or from pneumonia, children with mobility problems often succumbed to serious infections secondary to pressure ulcers, and children with eating difficulties had nutritional deficiencies that limited their life experience. It is not surprising that the early programs to provide assistance to children were designated the Crippled Children's Program (Hutchins, 1997). These programs originally served children with orthopedic, motor, and cognitive impairments and sensory deficits rather than children with other types of chronic illnesses or medical conditions.

Except in locations without access to biomedical intervention, large numbers of children now survive with myriad conditions to adulthood. Some conditions are rare congenital anomalies (birth defects) and inborn errors of metabolism. Others are more common conditions currently experiencing a high degree of public awareness such as asthma, diabetes mellitus, seizure disorders, sickle cell anemia, or hemophilia. Some children have autoimmune diseases such as systemic lupus erythematosis or juvenile rheumatoid arthritis. Others have sensory or motor problems or cognitive impairments with or without obvious causes. Large numbers of children also are surviving malignancies and end-stage organ disease (kidney, heart, or liver failure) that previously would have been fatal but now are being treated with organ or tissue transplantation (Gortmaker & Sappenfield, 1984).

During the second half of the 20th century, subgroups of children were classified by the clusters of diseases treated by various types of medical specialists. Advocacy organizations—Juvenile Diabetes Association, Epilepsy Foundation, Muscular Dystrophy Foundation—grew up around each category, resulting in the development of services, benefits, and research for each set of conditions. Such groups advocated for specific types of conditions such as polio, diabetes, renal conditions, malignancies, and mental retardation. In the more recent past, there has been similar advocacy to create special services for children living with HIV/AIDS.

However, in their classic monograph *Chronic Childhood Disorders,* Pless and Pinkerton (1975) clearly demonstrated large areas of commonality in the life experiences of these children and families and argued for a common approach to their conditions. Other people have confirmed their overall findings about the commonalities in terms of the psychosocial outcomes and life experiences of these children and their family members (Hobbs & Perrin,1985; Jessop & Stein, 1985; Stein & Jessop, 1989). Moreover, as the population of affected children and families has increased, parents and advocates have seen the potential benefits of banding together across disease boundaries and in so doing have found strength in numbers. A new type of more inclusive advocacy group has emerged with more political power.

Noncategorical Approach

The *noncategorical* or *generic* approach, set in motion by Pless and Pinkerton (1975), emphasizes the similarities rather than the differences across children with dissimilar conditions. It considers the commonalities among children with a wide range of ongoing health conditions and impairments, and it highlights dimensions of illnesses or conditions, such as whether they are congenital or acquired, stable or unstable, progressive or nonprogressive, and whether they involve visible or invisible conditions or motor or sensory impairment. There is considerable evidence that these characteristics often are more important in the daily lives of the children and their families than the specific diagnosis, which is the essential and primary feature in the selection of biomedical treatments.

During the early years of this paradigm, or approach, children typically were grouped together under the blanket designation *chronic illness.* However, many people found this term unsatisfactory because some children had exacerbations and remissions and did not always act or feel ill, and because many of the conditions, especially those of a more structural nature such as spina bifida, cleft palate, and cerebral palsy, were not thought of as illnesses at all. Some people solved this problem by using the term *children with a disability.* Still others called the children *handicapped* or referred to them as *children with chronic conditions.* These terms were considered stigmatizing by some people, and there was a general reluctance, especially on the part of parents, to accept these umbrella terms as appropriate descriptors of their children's health care issues. Other people were put off by the potential implication that the word *chronic* meant fatal or no hope for improvement. In 1981, the U.S. Maternal and Child Health Bureau (MCHB) convened a conference to establish research priorities for the coming decade. One of the conference priorities was to set the agenda for research of issues related to this vaguely defined population of children. In preparation for the conference and in recognition of the unsatisfactory nature of the existing terminology, the term *children with special needs* (CSN) was first introduced by the co-chairs of the committee assigned to consider research priorities for children with ongoing conditions and disorders (Nelson & Stein, 1982). The term was put forth as a substitute for all existing terms in the hope that it would be a more accurate and socially acceptable descriptor of the population of interest. It was introduced with the goal of helping researchers and advocates describe this population's need for health care and related services and as an inclusive umbrella term. It was meant to encompass the full range of different conditions, illnesses, and disabilities experienced by the population of children with many variations in health. It also was meant to reinforce the commonalities of the issues facing the children and their families, and because it did not include the word *chronic*, it was hoped that it would be less stigmatizing than previous terminology. Shortly thereafter, *children with special needs* evolved into *children with special health care needs*, also referred to as CSHCN.

At the time of its introduction and throughout the initial period of using *children with special needs* and *children with special health care needs*, the terms included only children who actually had chronic conditions and/or impairments. The issue of being at risk for such conditions or impairments, which is part of the more recent conceptualization, was not part of the original discussions. The inclusion of such children occurred in the mid-1990s, when there was a concerted effort to actually define who was included under these umbrella terms. Until then, there was no official specification, so that prior to the introduction of formal definitions, two people using the terms might have assumed that different groups of children were included.

The Need for Specificity: Noncategorical Definitions

To make clear who fit under the broad noncategorical terms *children with special needs* and *children with special health care needs*, a research group that included this author and that was based at the Albert Einstein College of Medicine, put forward a definition in an academic paper published in 1993 (Stein, Bauman, Westbrook, Coupey, & Ireys, 1993). The definition sought to provide a framework for implementing a noncategorical approach to research and services and, as such, it included only those children currently living with health conditions regardless of their origins or cause. The article did not refer to CSHCN; instead, it referred to children with serious ongoing health conditions. Shortly after its publication, a second group published another article also arguing strongly for a noncategorical approach to chronic health conditions in childhood, but stopping short of specifying a definition (Perrin et al., 1993).

The Einstein group's article proposed that a child who fits the designated classification is identified by 1) the presence of a biological, psychological, or cognitive condition; 2) the condition is of at least one year's duration (i.e., lasting or expected to last for 12 months); and 3) the condition is causing a *consequence* (Stein et al., 1993). The *duration* statement differed from Pless and Pinkerton's proposal of a 3-month criterion (1975). The Einstein group's proposal was intended to be certain that on the one hand a child with a temporary consequence (e.g., broken leg) was excluded, and on the other hand, even at the time of onset, a child with a new condition that was expected to endure would be counted. The Einstein group's paper defined three types of major condition-related consequences: functional limitations compared to that of age-mates, dependence on compensatory mechanisms or assistance, and use of services above those generally needed by age-mates (Stein et al., 1993). *Functional limitations* are restrictions that healthy children do not experience in ability to perform activities or tasks. *Dependence on compensatory mechanisms or assistance* includes the use of medications, treatments, devices, or help from another in performing activities or tasks. This assistance includes braces or technology as well as medications or dialysis that help a child to function. It is not always measured by other definitions but is viewed by the authors as critical to maximizing the functioning of children whose underlying conditions may not be eliminated. Increased use of services included those in the health, mental health, and special education systems. (See Table 1.1 for noncategorical, consequence-based definitions of children with special health care needs.)

The Rationale for the Noncategorical Approach

The Einstein article was the first to focus on the child rather than the condition, and it did so by explicitly examining the *consequences* that the condition has on a child's life (Stein et al., 1993). In that sense, the article broke new ground and has become a central feature of all current noncategorical definitions. One advantage of this approach is that it specifically allows for a child's identification as a child with a special

Table 1.1. Noncategorical, consequence-based definitions of children with special health care needs

Stein et al. (1993)	Maternal and Child Health Bureau (MCHB)
Children with special health care needs have disorders that • Have a biological, psychological, or cognitive basis • Have lasted or are virtually certain to last for at least 1 year • Produce any one, or more, of the following consequences: • Functional limitations • Dependency on compensatory mechanisms or assistance • Service needs or use above usual for age	Children with special health care needs are those • Who have or are at increased risk for a chronic physical, developmental, behavioral, or emotional condition • Who require health and related services of a type or amount beyond that required by children generally
Source: Stein et al. (1993). Framework for identifying children who have chronic conditions: The case for a new definition. *Journal of Pediatrics, 122,* 342–347.	*Source:* McPherson et al. (1998). A new definition for children with special health care needs. *Pediatrics, 102,* 137–140.

health care need irrespective of whether there is a named diagnosis. This is important for three reasons: 1) the epidemiology of childhood health conditions (including very rare conditions), 2) the inconsistencies in the terms used to identify conditions, and 3) the potentially long lists that would have to be included in surveys seeking data on children who have a full range of conditions. In addition, the article allowed for the inclusion of children who present diagnostic dilemmas or who have poor access to care, but who also have been experiencing significant consequences over a long period. Condition lists have been biased toward identifying children with access to care, because these children are seen by physicians and specialists and consequently are more likely to be diagnosed than children without access to care. Another advantage of counting children, not diagnoses, is that a high proportion of children with special needs (more than one third) have more than one diagnosis. And finally, the Einstein approach does not count children who had a diagnosis that is no longer causing consequences (Stein, 1996; Stein et al., 1993; Stein, Westbrook, & Bauman, 1997). However, because the approach does not differentiate among conditions or their biological bases, it has no immediate use in relation to biomedical therapies directed at controlling a given disorder or in biomedical research (Stein, 1996).

Maternal and Child Health Bureau Definition of CSHCN

Although the efforts described above were viewed by many as defining the group of CSHCN, and later work clearly builds on this foundation, by the 1990s, advocates were beginning to express concern that the term *special health care needs* should include the special needs of children who were at risk because of social vulnerabilities that might increase the likelihood that they would experience a chronic health condition. Such children included those in foster care, those living in poor housing with dangerous environmental exposures or physical risks, and those living in poverty who were known to have larger lifetime risks for ongoing health conditions.

As a response to this, the MCHB, which had been using the term *children with special health care needs* for some time, created a panel to adopt a formal definition. That panel decided to extend the definition of the population covered by the umbrella term *children with special health care needs* to include those *at risk* for special health care needs (McPherson et al., 1998). In doing so, the agency was responding to the very real perception that there were groups of children beyond those with chronic conditions or biological/anatomical impairments who also had special health care needs. The agency therefore decided that any definition of *children with special health care needs* should include children who are *at risk* as well.

While there is no doubt that children at risk also have special health care needs, and the inclusion opens an avenue for care and service provision (see Chapters 9 and 10), the result has been considerable confusion about the meaning of the term *children with special health care needs*. In some ways this is ironic because the change from *children with special needs* to *children with special health care needs* was made partly to avoid confusion about the term *special needs*, which some people thought included children who needed extra services because of social issues (e.g., living in poverty).

This confusion increased further when the MCHB adopted a formal definition of *children with special health care needs* in 1998 (McPherson et al., 1998; see Table 1.1). Not only was there ambiguity in the meaning of the term *children with special health care needs*, but there also were inconsistencies in the way people thought about risk factors. Consequently, it was difficult to arrive at a clear-cut or agreed-upon way to put into operation the at-risk component of the definition.

Another concern with the MCHB definition was that its two components (condition and services) were linked by the word *and*, but its implementation usually presumed that either component alone qualified a child to be included (cf. Newacheck et al., 1998).

In the intervening years, there has been a great deal of coalescence within the maternal and child health community about the usefulness of the noncategorical approach. Most believe that the differences between the MCHB and Einstein definitions are relatively minor compared with their similarities, especially because all of the tools used to implement the two definitions tend to have similar parameters. As a result, a great deal of progress has been made within the field using the two definitions, particularly in terms of gathering data about the population of CSHCN. Differences revolve principally around two issues: 1) whether it is important to distinguish between services on the one hand and compensatory mechanisms and assistance on the other (which are combined in the MCHB definition but distinguished by the Einstein group) and 2) whether to include at-risk children. However, it is acknowledged by virtually all involved in the care of or research regarding CSHCN that current ways in which the definitions are employed do not assess those at risk in any meaningful way. Several initiatives are now under way to put into place a definition and mechanism for identifying children at risk of developing ongoing health conditions, but to date that has not happened.

The discussion that follows includes a review of some of the primary tools for implementing the noncategorical approach. However, while this approach has been used for a variety of purposes, there continues to be considerable resistance to it among some medical specialists and those outside the field, especially those involved with biomedical sciences and the policy arena. The skeptics continue to question the utility of the noncategorical definition and to express discomfort with what they perceive to be a lack of clarity about which diagnostic categories are included. They continue to think that they know what individual diagnoses mean, despite the large amount of data showing that there is tremendous inconsistency in what parents mean when they say, for example, that their child has asthma, or in how consistently physicians code a diagnosis on a patient encounter form.

TOOLS TO IDENTIFY CHILDREN WITH SPECIAL HEALTH CARE NEEDS

Just as definitional criteria affect estimated numbers, so, too, do the methods used to identify which children meet this criteria. It is therefore important to think about the methods used and their implications. How important is it to identify everyone? Is it better to over- or under-identify children who might meet the definition? Should one look at the health care system, where it is possible to miss children who are not receiving care or who have been stabilized successfully, or should one look at the community? What is the accuracy of parent responses to questions or of coded billing information? Clearly the answers to these questions depend on the purpose of identification. Because no method is perfect, there is a powerful link between the match of the purpose and the technique employed. Within each method there must be consideration of what is a good enough net to use, who will be missed, and whether and under what circumstances it is acceptable to have missed people who meet the theoretical definition.

Several instruments or tools have been developed with the specific purpose of using the definitions of the noncategorical approach to find the target population, but in doing so the instruments have had differing purposes or goals. The tools fall into two categories. One type or approach uses a parental interview strategy focused on assessing the consequences of the conditions. The other employs a utilization-based approach for users of the medical care system and depends on clinical records and diagnostic related groupings, or DRGs (described below), to classify levels of illness or impairment. Each is described along with its strengths and shortcomings.

Consequence-Based Approach

The consequence-based approach depends on identifying children based on their functional limitations and the services and compensatory assistance they use. Unlike the traditional approach of identifying children by their diagnoses, this approach is independent of having or knowing a diagnosis or choosing among one of several to decide which is the most important. The source of the information is typically from a parent or caregiver.

Questionnaire for Identifying Children with Chronic Conditions (QuICCC)

The oldest instrument to use in the consequence-based approach is the Questionnaire for Identifying Children with Chronic Conditions (QuICCC; Stein et al., 1997). This is the only tool that began with a conceptual definition (the Einstein definition described in Stein et al., 1993) and that was specifically designed to implement that definition. The original purpose for designing the QuICCC was to screen children in households for a national survey with the specific purpose of assuring that children who might have relevant consequences will not be missed. Thus, this tool tried to be as comprehensive as possible in identifying consequences. The tool consists of 39 items, most of which have three parts. The first part asks about the presence of a specific consequence and, except for a few items that assume long duration or permanence (e.g., blindness), the question sequence asks whether the consequence is based on a health condition and whether it has the necessary duration (has lasted or is expected to last 1 year or more). This strategy was based on extensive field testing demonstrating that the majority of parents could not relate to general questions about whether their child has a chronic condition without the consequences being identified (e.g., taking medication prescribed by a doctor). The QuICCC has been validated against physician classifications of whether or not a child meets the specific definition, and very good concordance was demonstrated between the physicians' classification and the parents' answers on the instrument (Stein, Bauman, Epstein, Gardner, & Walker, 2000). Thus, it appears to have achieved its goals. It has a weakness, however, in that it is long, especially for children who have a lot of health consequences. For those without consequences it can be administered very efficiently.

Because the definition of children with special health care needs used in the QuICCC involved three different kinds of consequences, and the QuICCC operationalized or implemented each of these types of consequences separately, there has been an opportunity to assess how each element—functional limitations (16 items), compensatory mechanisms and assistance (12 items), and service use and need (11 items)—contributes to the identification of different segments of the CSHCN population. One thing has become clear: There are children with significant health challenges who are identified by only one of the three components. (This is true for each of the three types of consequences.) Any approach that did not include all the types of consequences would leave out substantial numbers of children (Westbrook, Silver, & Stein, 1998). Moreover, it appears that the more types of consequences identified by the respondent, the more severely impaired the child in question is likely to be and the higher the cost of care (Silver, Stein, Shenkman, Cruz, & Vogel, 2005; Stein, Silver, & Bauman, 2001a). This ability to discriminate types of consequences is one of the strengths of the instrument. Moreover, the QuICCC and related instruments are based on parent responses to questionnaires, and therefore tap low technology elements such as learning and mental health impairments that are not always known to or inventoried in databases collected by health care systems.

Most of the items of the QuICCC were incorporated into the 1994–1995 National Health Interview Survey on Disability, collected by the National Center for Health Statistics (Stein & Silver, 1999). These items together with a few substitute items were programmed to mimic the full content of the QuICCC (Stein & Silver, 1999), and that item set has been used for analyses of the national data by several investigators.

Questionnaire for Identifying Children with Chronic Conditions—Revised (QuICCC-R)

The length of the QuICCC posed a problem for some uses. Therefore, to reduce the number of questions, the developers of the QuICCC, funded by the MCHB, converted the original items into a shorter and more efficient tool. The revised QuICCC, QuICCC-R, uses only those 16 items from the original QuICCC that would identify the largest proportion of children (Stein et al., 2001b). In this case, the goal was to develop an instrument that would identify as many of the targeted children as possible using a markedly reduced item set. It is estimated that the 16 items in the QuICCC-R capture up to 98% of the children identified by the full QuICCC (Stein, Silver, & Bauman, 2001b). This instrument, however, does miss some children with severe but rare consequences, and because it inventories fewer consequences than the QuICCC, it also has a more limited ability to discriminate among levels of severity and cost. Notwithstanding these limitations, the instrument is useful as a means of screening a population more quickly and with only a very small amount of under identification. However, if it were being used to identify children for service eligibility, it would have to provide a fail-safe mechanism for those with rare but important consequences.

CSHCN Screener

The CSHCN screener was developed by a team based at the Foundation for Accountability that included one of the developers of the QuICCC and QuICCC-R (R.E.K. Stein), and it is heavily based on these earlier instruments (Bethell, Read, Stein, Blumberg, Wells, & Newacheck, 2002). The original purpose of designing the tool, now called the CSHCN screener, was to draw a sample of CSHCN within a health plan who had a wide range of different types of diagnoses, for quality improvement purposes only. Because the measures that were being used to assess quality relied on questionnaires from health care enrollees, the data were sought from the respondents for the children (the children's parents). The original idea was to develop a short questionnaire that would identify children who would reflect a range of diagnoses represented within a plan. The development group did not think it was important to identify all CSHCN but rather a sample that was sufficiently diverse that the health plans could not *play to the test* or focus on improving care only for children with one or two named conditions. Thus, diagnostic heterogeneity was a goal, but neither completeness nor comprehensiveness was a primary consideration. As a result, low frequency consequences were not as important in the selection of the item content, because children with rare conditions were not likely to be part of a sample of a few thousand children on whom quality studies are often done. The instrument was validated for its original purpose—to identify a diagnostically heterogeneous population of children with special needs within plans—but performed so well in identifying the large majority of the children that it was rapidly recommended for broader purposes (Bethell, Read, Neff et al., 2002; Bethell, Read, Stein et al., 2002).

In trying to make the questionnaire short, several questions were made more complex, leading to some concern about the meaning of a yes/no answer. However, its brevity and ability to identify many children with relatively few questions has made it a popular choice for a wide range of other uses for which it has not been as well studied. These include epidemiologic studies to ascertain prevalence—that is, to monitor how many children in the population have special health care needs—and to compare children with and without special health care needs on a wide range of issues. The questionnaire is now included in many U.S. surveys conducted by the National Center for Health Statistics—for example, the National Health Interview Survey, the Medical Expenditure Panel Survey, the National Survey on Children's Health, and the National Surveys of Children with Special Health Care Needs conducted in 2000–2001 and 2005–2006.

Diagnostic Related Grouping (DRG)-Based Systems

In contrast with the consequence-based approach, the Diagnostic Related Grouping (DRG)-Based Systems depend on coded medical information that is usually entered by a physician or other health services provider. In an indirect way it builds on diagnoses and groups them into categories.

National Association of Children's Hospitals and Related Institutions: Classification System for Congenital and Chronic Health Conditions

At about the same time that parental questionnaires were being developed, the National Association of Children's Hospitals and Related Institutions (NACHRI), an association concerned with the well-being and financial viability of children's hospitals and related facilities, developed an alternative approach that was based on mining the large and growing computerized patient billing systems. Their approach to identifying CSHCN was driven by cost concerns and the desire to predict accurately a child's future health care utilization and, hopefully, to use such a system to get tiered reimbursement from managed care plans. The principal outgrowth of this endeavor is the diagnostic related grouping (DRG) system based on diagnostic codes and their relationship to the cost of services (Muldoon, Neff, & Gay, 1997; Neff et al., 2001). The NACHRI DRG system seeks to identify conditions that would fit the two noncategorical definitions above. This system, owned and licensed by 3M Health Information System, classifies children by nine major categories, using administrative data from hospitals. The categories, ranging from acute minor conditions to severe life-threatening ones, are based on hospital coding of reason for visits, services rendered, and costs. They have since been collapsed by a number of investigators into five major categories that have been shown to be associated with different levels of expenditures within the health care system. It is somewhat less likely to include some of the mental health and learning impairments when these services generate expenditures in other systems, and it can only be applied to children for whom there are already data in the system—that is, for health care users.

Findings made using this system are highly predictive of health care costs in the future. However, the system is dependent on access to and extraction of several months of prior health service records and accurate coding of the primary and secondary conditions, which does not always happen. The system also cannot evaluate new enrollees in a plan or health care system or gather information on patients who are not active in the database such as those with poor access to care. Its accuracy also is dependent on computerized systems that can be mined efficiently and on an up-to-date assessment of the parameters used in grouping conditions. Thus, the validity of findings requires that the programs used for analyses be updated and validated as new therapies and standards for management that have major cost implications are added or substituted.

Diagnostic Algorithms

Other investigators have turned to DRG billing codes to identify groups of CSHCN using more informal and often pragmatic solutions. An example is the algorithm developed by Perrin et al. (1999), which uses a list of common diagnoses. This technique is helpful in examining children with high-prevalence conditions. Such schemes identify the majority of CSHCN but not all of them because the number of children who have types of rare conditions in any given population is relatively small compared with children who have more prevalent health conditions. Such techniques cannot be used for epidemiologic purposes (e.g., estimating the size of the population), but they do allow research to proceed on subgroups of children with several types of chronic conditions. Again, those with poorer access to health care are likely to be less well represented.

Limitation of Activities

Assessing the number of people with limitations of activities is a method often used only for adults because adult limitations of activities are related to work and activities of daily living, something young children do not do independently. A major shortfall of this approach with children is that activities are defined as limitations of play for younger children and of school or schoolwork for older children. As a result, overall rates of functional limitations are relatively low among children in general and especially among young children, and those that are measured, predominantly among older children, largely represent disabilities that interfere with education (Hobbes & Perrin, 1985). This conceptualization of *limitations* does not encompass the full range of consequences of health conditions intended in the noncategorical approach set forward by either the Einstein group or the MCHB definition and, as discussed below, includes only about half the children identified by other methods.

Despite these shortcomings, Newacheck, Budetti, and Halfon (1986) traced the trend in children with functional limitations over the past several decades, and the data they analyzed from a number of sources suggested that from 1960 to 1981 the percentage of children less than 17 years old with an activity-limiting chronic condition increased from 1.8% to 3.8%. They reported that some of the increase in rates reflected changes in methods and the wording of questions, but some of the increase appeared to occur in a period during which the method of data collection was stable. Subsequently, through the year 1994, the rate rose to 6.5%, representing an estimated 4.4 million noninstitutionalized children less than 18 years of age (Newacheck & Halfon, 1998). Among these children, the most common causes of activity limitation were respiratory or mental impairments. Almost 7% of children in the United States are reported to have activity-limiting conditions.

Thus, there has been more than a tripling of rates from less than 2% to 6%–7% in the last 40 years. In addition, some of the apparent differences in rates among White non-Hispanic and Black non-Hispanic children appear to be explained by differences in poverty levels (Newacheck, Stein, Bauman, & Hung, 2003).

Eligibility for Supplemental Security Income

Another gross indicator of the extent of the CSHCN population has been an examination of children receiving Supplemental Security Income (SSI). The number of eligible children rose from approximately 290,000 U.S. children in the early 1990s to more than 960,000 children in 2003 (Social Security Administration, 2003). This is due in part to the alteration in definition of *eligibility* as a result of the change in the implementation of eligibility subsequent to the Zebley decision (*Sullivan v. Zebley*, 1990) in which the Supreme Court found that children with multiple disabilities (no one of which met the threshold of disability) needed to be assessed in terms of the total effect of their disabilities on their functioning (Perrin & Stein, 1992). It is also due to the addition of a new mental health conditions list to the SSI qualifying criteria. Several other cautions should be used in considering the SSI data. The numbers represent only low-income children because of the requirement that the recipients meet both financial eligibility for SSI and the health criteria of having life-threatening conditions or substantial limitations in functioning. Thus, this method undercounts substantially the numbers of CSHCN, because of both the income restriction and the spectrum of severity required to qualify. (For more information on SSI, see Chapters 2 and 3.)

ESTIMATES OF THE CSHCN POPULATION

The size of the CSHCN population has been estimated in different ways over many decades. In older studies, estimates were derived from condition lists. Using this method, prevalence varied from 4% to 31% (Gortmaker & Sappenfield, 1984; Jessop & Stein, 1995; Newacheck & Taylor, 1992). The huge variation in estimates remained a problem for the field, although many experts originally thought that the true number was somewhere between these extremes. With the advent of noncategorical, consequence-based methods, the field began to obtain new estimates.

The first opportunities to assess the epidemiology and estimate the size of the population using these new methods and definitions were through surveys conducted in the mid-to-late 1990s. Original estimates using the QuICCC in a random digit-dialing phone survey of more than 700 households with children produced an estimate of 19% (Stein et al., 1997). The National Health Interview Survey on Disability, using a similar algorithm, produced an estimate of 14.8% to 15.3% when corrected for the full-item content of the QuICCC (Stein et al., 1993; Stein & Silver, 1999). The mechanism used by the National Health Interview Survey to determine childhood disability for a follow-up interview generated a 16% estimate, and analyses by Newacheck et al. (1998) calculated that 18% of children met the MCHB definition. While the definitions for CSHCN varied slightly, and may explain the differences between the estimates, a comparison of the varying algorithms showed consistency in the rates being higher among males, older children, children from homes without two parents or with less educated parents, and the poor (Newacheck et al., 1998; Stein & Silver, 1999, 2002).

Subsequently, a number of surveys have been conducted using

the CSHCN screener. Preliminary field-testing had indicated that the CSHCN screener produced lower estimates than the QuICCC-R to which it was compared (Bethell, Read, Neff, et al., 2002). This is not surprising given the purposes of the different measures. Nonetheless, the National Survey of Children with Special Health Care Needs, a telephone-based national survey of more than 35,000 children conducted using the CSHCN screener in 2000–2001, produced an estimate of 12.9% (Blumberg et al., 2001). The National Survey of Children's Health, a telephone survey of more than 100,000 U.S. children in which one child per household was surveyed, also using the CSHCN screener, yielded a figure of 12.8% (van Dyck, Kogan, McPherson, Weissman, & Newacheck, 2004). National estimates based on the ongoing Medical Expenditure Survey, a panel survey of household health expenditures using a subsample from the National Health Information Survey, suggested a prevalence of 17.6%. All of these surveys were conducted by the National Center for Health Statistics (Blumberg et al., 2001). It is unclear whether this increment across surveys represents a true increase in prevalence or is related to differences in implementation of the screener. The 2005–2006 National Survey of Children with Special Health Care Needs is currently in the field and again using the CSHCN screener.

Estimates using the NACHRI system have produced numbers in a similar range (Neff et al., 2001). It is unclear whether these multiple methods are identifying the same children. Most of the evidence suggests that there are similar overall rates, but there are differences in who is selected by each measure (Bethell, Read, Neff et al., 2002; Jessop & Stein, 1995; Ryan, Stein, Auinger et al., 2005).

Within this context, it is important to point out that only 49% to 66% of the children identified by any of the methods experienced functional limitations, which entailed the inability to participate in the usual play or school activities (Stein et al., 1997; Westbrook et al., 1998). Moreover, among children who did experience functional limitations, only a minority were severely affected; that is, only a minority were fully limited in their ability to play or attend school (Newacheck & Halfon, 1998; Newacheck et al., 1998).

Characteristics of the CSHCN Population

Virtually all methods used to estimate the size of the CSHCN population demonstrate some distinctive patterns relating to age, gender, income, and race–ethnicity.

Age of Child

All methods show that the number of identified children increases with age. Although it is clear that there is some acquisition of conditions as children age, there is a perception in the field that existing methods for identification of CSHCN are less adequate for detecting children who are younger than for older children, and that substantial numbers of infants, toddlers, and preschoolers who have special health care needs are not identified (Newacheck & Halfon, 1998; Newacheck et al., 1998; Stein & Silver, 2002).

Gender of Child

Data using almost all methods show a preponderance of males. The magnitude of this difference varies from trivial to as many as one and a half times more than females (Newacheck & Halfon, 1998; Newacheck et al., 1998; Stein & Silver, 2002).

Income of Family

It is quite clear that the rate of CSHCN is higher among those living at or near the poverty threshold (Newacheck & Halfon, 1998; Newacheck et al., 1998; Stein & Silver, 2002). One concern is that the methods used to identify children are not confounded by an income bias, although none of the methods of identification, except those that use SSI, involves income as a variable. The pattern of higher rates is found even in analyses that are controlled for levels of insurance. In these analyses, rates do not appear to equalize, despite the commonly held belief that access to insurance may improve health disparities (Bauman, Silver, & Stein, 2006). Insurance rates are actually higher among CSHCN than other children (Silver & Stein, 2001). A likely reason for this is that SSI and many state Medicaid plans provide easier access to Medicaid for children with high health care costs. One speculation is that the persistently higher rates of CSHCN among the poorer families may reflect the lack of access to preventive measures (Stein & Silver, 2005).

Race–Ethnicity[1] of Family

Hispanics are consistently underrepresented among counts of CSHCN compared with their proportion in the population as a whole. The rea-

---

[1] The designations in this section, while not in current use, are used here because they represent the way the data were collected and coded by the National Center for Health Statistics.

sons for this are probably complex and poorly elucidated by the studies to date. Some studies have suggested that this is part of the Hispanic paradox (Palloni & Morenoff, 2001) in which Hispanics are healthier than others on a number of measures. However, variation in the rate of underrepresentation across methods suggests that there may be methodological reasons for the finding as well. These might include differences in the meaning of some of the questions for people of different backgrounds. The pattern for "Other"—non-Hispanics who are neither White nor Black—also is one of consistent underrepresentation among CSHCN. These findings, again, seem to be independent of the method used for identification and warrant further exploration.

The relationship of racial differences among non-Hispanic Whites and non-Hispanic Blacks varies somewhat with methods, but non-Hispanic Blacks are somewhat more likely to be identified by some of the methods. Yet, when poverty is accounted for, Blacks and Whites seem equally represented among CSHCN (Newacheck & Halfon, 1998; Newacheck et al., 1998, 2003; Stein & Silver, 2002).

CONCLUSION

Our concepts of children's ongoing health conditions have evolved considerably over time. In the past 20 years, there has been a coalescence within the field about the current use of the term *children with special health care needs* and the various approaches used to identify children who fit this categorization. However, there is still considerable debate between those within and outside the field about the utility of these approaches, as well as a considerable amount of evolution of the definitions in vogue at different times. This diversity of approaches is sometimes useful, but it means that findings have to be compared carefully because, despite superficial resemblance, different reports of data may not actually refer to the same groups of children.

This problem is more than academic. Definitions determine not only who is counted and what the prevalence of condition is believed to be, but they also determine eligibility for services and hence the actual distribution of care. There is little consistency across programs under the jurisdiction of different divisions of federal, state, and local governments in the way they currently identify CSHCN and their families and the programs meant to help them (see Chapter 2). Educational systems have extensive criteria, based on a series of major pieces of federal legislation, that children need to meet to qualify for special needs programs, but the consistency with which these criteria are applied and the caveats added in different locales make it difficult to describe exactly who qualifies across the nation. There are similar inconsistencies in the qualifications around the block grants from the Title V program, which is suppose to have oversight responsibilities for CSHCN in each state, and the early intervention programs, which are designed by each state to provide early services to high-risk children. In each state, there is commonality in some aspects of the programs (e.g., the minimum standards set by the federal programs), but great diversity in what they include beyond that minimum. Although the issues raised in this chapter are now gaining attention and there is increased effort to consolidate, nearly every state has a unique method of deciding who qualifies for care or services under these policies.

Precise estimates of the size of the CSHCN population will depend on the purpose for which each estimate is being made as well as the method of identification employed. This variation may be useful in terms of the immediate goals of a program or agency, but it has major implications for the field because it reflects a lack of consistency or consensus on how the term *children with special health care needs* or any successor term is, or should be, used. The variation also impedes the acquisition of knowledge about the population of interest. The challenges this presents are reflected in the chapters that follow. These challenges are of paramount importance to the future of care and services for children with special health care needs and their families.

The definitions and approaches described above have the potential to affect an individual's ability to qualify for assistance. They also can affect advocacy work, often unnecessarily pitting advocates with different agendas against one another instead of helping to increase the number of coalition members to broaden advocacy for the needs of all children. Parents and other concerned individuals should therefore make every effort to familiarize themselves with relevant definitions and to work for equity in the services provided to children with differing conditions and consequences.

For policy makers and program planners, the various definitions and related survey findings may have an impact on the adequacy of planning efforts and the usefulness of products or outcomes. The definitions and survey findings should, therefore, be of paramount concern.

Finally, individual providers also can find important implications in this discussion. They need to know the definitions used in their particular region and by the insurers or payers with whom they work as well as the service agencies that provide programmatic support. Familiarity with these issues can help ensure that providers refer all appropriate children and families for the services to which they are entitled, and can help them target advocacy efforts on behalf of the children and families for whom they provide care.

REFERENCES

Bauman, L.J., Silver, E.J., & Stein, R.E.K. (2006). Cumulative social disadvantage and child health. *Pediatrics, 117*, 1321–1328.

Bethell, C., Read, D., Neff, J., Blumberg, S., Stein, R.E.K., Sharp, V., & Newacheck, P.W. (2002). Comparison of the children with special health care needs screener to the questionnaire for identifying children with chronic conditions—Revised. *Ambulatory Pediatrics, 2,* 49–57.

Bethell, C., Read, D., Stein, R.E.K., Blumberg, S.J., Wells, N., & Newacheck, P.W. (2002). Identifying children with special health care needs: Development and evaluation of a short screening instrument. *Ambulatory Pediatrics, 2,* 38–48.

Blumberg, S.J., Olson, L., Frankel, M., Osborn, L., Becker, C.J., Srinath, K.P., & Giambo, P. (2001). *Design and operation of the national survey of children with special health care needs* (Health Statistics Series 1, Number 14). Washington, DC: National Center for Health Statistics. Centers for Disease Control and Prevention.

Gortmaker, S., & Sappenfield, W. (1984) Chronic childhood disorders: Prevalence and impact. *Pediatric Clinics of North America, 31,* 3–18.

Hobbs, N., & Perrin, J.M. (1985). *Issues in the care of children with chronic illness: A sourcebook on problems, services, and policies.* San Francisco: Jossey-Bassy. Retrieved June 21, 2005, from http://www.childtrendsdatabank.org/status.cfm

Hutchins, V.L. (1997). A history of child health and pediatrics in the United States. In R.E.K. Stein (Ed.), *Health care for children: What's right, What's wrong, What's next* (pp. 79–106). New York: United Hospital Fund.

Jessop, D.J., & Stein, R.E.K. (1985). Uncertainty and its relation to psychological and social correlates of chronic illness in children. *Social Science and Medicine, 20,* 993–997.

Jessop, D.J., & Stein, R.E.K. (1995). Consistent but not the same: Effects of method on chronic conditions rates. *Archives of Pediatrics and Adolescent Medicine, 149,* 1105–1110.

McPherson, M., Arango, P., Fox, H., Lauver, C., McManus, M., Newacheck, P.W., et al. (1998). A new definition of children with special health care needs. *Pediatrics, 102,* 137–140.

Muldoon, J.H., Neff, J.M., & Gay, J.C. (1997). Profiling the health service needs of populations using diagnosis-based classification systems. *Journal of Ambulatory Care Management, 20,* 1–18.

Neff, J.M., Sharp, V., Muldoon, J., Graham, J., Popalisky, J., & Gay, J. (2001). Identifying and classifying children with chronic conditions using administrative data with the clinical risk group classification system. *Journal of Ambulatory Pediatrics, 2,* 72–79.

Nelson, R., & Stein, R.E.K. (1982). Children with special needs: Recommendations and rationale. In L. Klerman. (Ed.), *Research priorities in Maternal and Child Health* (pp. 37–43). Washington, DC: The Office for Maternal and Child Health, Health Services Administration, Public Health Service, U.S. Department of Health and Human Services.

Newacheck, P.W., Budetti, P.P., & Halfon, N. (1986). Trends in activity-limiting chronic conditions among children. *American Journal of Public Health, 76,* 178–184.

Newacheck, P.W., & Halfon, N. (1998). Prevalence and impact of disabling chronic conditions in childhood. *American Journal of Public Health, 88,* 610–617.

Newacheck, P.W., Stein, R.E.K., Bauman, L.J., & Hung, Y.Y. (2003). Are their disparities between white and black children in disability prevalence? *Archives of Pediatrics and Adolescent Medicine, 157,* 244–248.

Newacheck, P.W., Strickland, B., Shonkoff, J.P., Perrin, J.M., McPherson, M., McManus, M., et al. (1998). An epidemiologic profile of children with special health care needs. *Pediatrics, 102,* 117–123.

Newacheck, P.W., & Taylor, W.R. (1992). Childhood chronic illness: Prevalence, severity, and impact. *American Journal of Public Health, 82,* 364–337.

Palloni, A., &. Morenoff, J.D. (2001). Interpreting the paradoxical in the Hispanic paradox: Demographic and epidemiologic approaches. *Annals of the New York Academy of Sciences, 954,* 140–174.

Perrin, E.C., Newacheck, P., Pless, I.B., Drotar, D., Gortmaker, S.L., Leventhal, J., et al. (1993). Issues involved in the definition and classification of chronic health conditions. *Pediatrics, 9,* 787–793.

Perrin, J.M., Kuhlthau, K., McLaughlin, T.J., Etner, S.L., & Gortmaker, S.L. (1999). Changing patterns of conditions among children receiving Supplemental Security Income disability benefits. *Archives of Pediatric and Adolescent Medicine, 153,* 80–84.

Perrin, J.M., & Stein, R.E.K. (1992). Reinterpreting disability: Changes in SSI for children. *Pediatrics, 88,* 1047–1051.

Pless I.B., & Pinkerton P. (1975). *Chronic childhood disorder: Promoting patterns of adjustment.* Chicago: Year Book Medical Publishers.

Ryan, S.A., Stein, R.E.K., Auinger, P., et al. (2005, May). *Utilization and expenditure profiles for CSHCN differ by identification methods.* Poster presentation at the annual meeting of the Pediatric Academic Societies, Washington, DC.

Silver, E.J., & Stein, R.E.K. (2001). Access to care, unmet health needs and poverty status among children with and without chronic conditions. *Ambulatory Pediatrics, 1,* 314–320.

Silver, E.J., Stein, R.E.K., Shenkman, E., Cruz, V., & Vogel, B. (2005, May). *Can the questionnaire for identifying children with chronic conditions predict service use and expenditures in SCHIP?* Poster presentation at the annual meeting of the Pediatric Academic Societies, Washington, DC.

Social Security Administration. (2005). *Children Receiving SSI, December 2003* (SSA Publication No. 13-11830). Washington, DC: Office of Policy, Office of Research, Evaluation, and Statistics.

Stein, R.E.K. (1996). To be or not to be . . . non-categorical. *Journal of Developmental and Behavioral Pediatrics, 17,* 36–37.

Stein, R.E.K., & Jessop, D.J. (1989). What diagnosis does not tell? The case for a non-categorical approach to chronic illness in childhood. *Social Science and Medicine, 29,* 769–778.

Stein, R.E.K., & Silver, E.J. (1999). Operationalizing a conceptually based non-categorical definition: A first look at U.S. children with chronic conditions. *Archives of Pediatrics and Adolescent Medicine, 153,* 68–74.

Stein, R.E.K., & Silver, E.J. (2002). Comparing different definitions of children with chronic conditions in a national data set. *Ambulatory Pediatrics, 2,* 63–70.

Stein, R.E.K., & Silver, E.J. (2005). Are rates of functional limitations associated with access to care? A state-level analysis of the National Survey of Children with Special Health Care Needs. *Maternal and Child Health Journal 9* (Supp. 2), S33–39.

Stein, R.E.K., Bauman, L.J., Epstein, S.G., Gardner, J.D., & Walker, D. (2000). How well does the QuICCC identify individual children who have chronic conditions? *Archives of Pediatric Adolescent Medicine, 154,* 447–452.

Stein, R.E.K., Bauman, L.J., Westbrook, L.E., Coupey, S.M., & Ireys, H.T. (1993). Framework for identifying children who have chronic conditions: The case for a new definition. *Journal of Pediatrics, 122,* 342–347.

Stein, R.E.K., Silver, E.J., & Bauman, L.J. (2001a). *How well does the number of QuICCC domains measure severity?* Poster presentation at the annual meeting of Pediatric Academic Societies, Baltimore, MD.

Stein, R.E.K., Silver, E.J., & Bauman, L.J. (2001b). Shortening the Questionnaire for Identifying Children with Chronic Conditions (QuICCC): What is the consequence? *Pediatrics, 107,* pe61.

Stein, R.E.K., Westbrook, L.E., & Bauman, L.J. (1997). The Questionnaire for Identifying Children with Chronic Conditions (QuICCC): A measure based on a noncategorical approach. *Pediatrics, 99,* 513–521.

Sullivan v. Zebley, 493 S. CT. 521, 525 (1990).

van Dyck, P.C., Kogan, M.D., McPherson, M.G., Weissman, G.R., & Newacheck, P.W. (2004). Prevalence and characteristics of children with special health care needs. *Archives of Pediatrics and Adolescent Medicine, 158,* 884–890.

Westbrook, L.E., Silver, E.J., & Stein, R.E.K. (1998). Implications for estimates of disability in children: A comparison of definitional components. *Pediatrics, 101,* 1025–1030.

2

Policies and Programs Relevant to Children with Special Health Care Needs

Karen Kuhlthau, Sheila Bloom, Monica Marthell, and Hodon Mohamed

Numerous state and federal government-backed policies and programs address the needs of U.S. children with chronic conditions, special health care needs, and disabilities, along with their
families. This chapter provides an overview of relevant policies and
programs in the hope of demystifying the options. In doing so, it seeks
to promote smoother sailing for both parents and providers as they
make their way through the sometimes murky sea of programs and
policies.

Major relevant policies include those related to education services, direct services, social welfare or cash benefits, and insurance
systems. Note that policies and programs often serve multiple purposes or provide multiple services; where possible, we try to reflect
this diversity. We also try to represent the diversity of the children
and families served.

For simplicity's sake, we will refer to the group of children addressed by the policies or programs under discussion as children with
special health care needs, or CSHCN, unless the program or policy specifically uses different terms. Although we focus on programs that target
CSHCN, we also include major programs that serve all children if the
programs are particularly relevant to CSHCN and their families. For
example, some of the income-support programs are available to all
families but may be of special interest to families with CSHCN. We
address the crosscutting needs of CSHCN and provide advice that is
relevant to parents and providers involved in CSHCN care.

This overview focuses on federal and state programs with some
mention of other relevant programs. We try to note both federal and
state policies (public laws or state and federal regulations) that are primarily responsible for enacting the programs. (*Note:* There is some un-
avoidable overlap of financial information in Chapters 2 and 3.)

EDUCATION PROGRAMS

The educational system plays a major role in most children's lives. Relevant educational programs include special services and programs for CSHCN that seek to ensure that children are appropriately served in the educational system.

Individuals with Disabilities Education Act

The Individuals with Disabilities Education Act of 1990 (IDEA), formerly called the Education for all Handicapped Children Act of 1975 (EAHCA), was enacted "to assure that all children with disabilities have available to them a free appropriate public education which emphasizes special education and related services designed to meet their unique needs" (Individuals with Disabilities Education Act, 1990). Although this important piece of legislation may seem, on the face of it, irrelevant for young children not yet in school, services provided under IDEA can start at birth. IDEA occupies a place of primary importance for parents of CSHCN, especially those who place a high value on education and school readiness.

Infants and Toddlers with Disabilities Program

Part C of IDEA, the Infants and Toddlers with Disabilities Program (ITDP), was originally established as Part H of the Education for all Handicapped Children Act. The program provides financial assistance to states to develop coordinated, statewide service systems for children with disabilities or, in some states, at risk to develop disabilities, up to 3 years of age and their families. Each state chooses an agency (e.g., education or public health department) to provide Part C early intervention (EI) services to this age group. For information on a particular state, please see the links to state resources on the National Dissemination Center for Children with Disabilities web site (National Dissemination Center for Children with Disabilities, 2006; see http://www.nichcy.org/states.htm for information on a particular state).

Eligible children include those who have developmental delays in cognitive, physical, communication, socioemotional, and adaptive development. Early intervention services are provided for about 200,000 children in the United States (U.S. Department of Education, Office of Special Education Programs [USDE OSEP, 2005]) and can be critically important both for providing children with developmentally appropriate services early in life and for linking children and families with relevant community services. Children with conditions having a high probability of developmental delay may be eligible for early inter-vention services.

Every child receiving Part C services must have an individualized family service plan (IFSP), which provides a broad picture of the ser-vices the child and family will need and who will provide those services. Examples of the services, which are offered at no fee or on a sliding scale, include speech–language and audiology support, family training, home visits, occupational and physical therapies, and psychological counseling. States must follow predefined procedures to assure parental and child rights. Children are transitioned from Part C to Part B services as they near the age of 3. It is important to plan ahead to understand the timing of the transition and the impact it may have on services provided.

Part B of IDEA

Special educational services provided under Part B of IDEA require public school systems to develop free and appropriate educational ser-vices for children with disabilities starting at age 3. A student is eligible for services if she or he has a disability and needs special educational assistance. Children with disabilities include those with mental retarda-tion; hearing, speech–language, or visual impairments; and serious emotional disturbances (U.S. Department of Education, Office of Spe-cial Education Services [USDE OSEP], 2005).

Each child in special education also needs an individualized educa-tion program (IEP). The IEP, which delineates the delivery of special educational supports and services, is created by a team that includes parents, teachers, and students or school staff. IDEA established the procedures to develop an IEP, although states and schools have some flexibility in determining the process (U.S. Department of Education, Office of Special Education and Rehabilitative Services [USDE OSERS], 2000). IEPs are regularly reviewed and modified to reflect a child's changing needs. Services should, to the extent possible, be provided in the least restrictive environment.

Rehabilitation Act of 1973

Section 504 of the Rehabilitation Act of 1973 prohibits discrimination against children with disabilities in the public education system. Stu-dents protected under this section are determined to have physical or mental impairments that limit at least one major life activity. The law requires schools to provide these students with appropriate accommo-dations or educational services designed to meet their needs to the same extent as the needs of students without disabilities are met (U.S.

Department of Education, Office for Civil Rights [USDE OCR], 2005). Like the Americans with Disabilities Act (ADA), Section 504 is civil rights legislation, not a source of funding for programs. To receive a Section 504 plan, a student follows a process similar to receiving an IEP through IDEA.

No Child Left Behind Act

The No Child Left Behind Act (NCLB) of 2001, a revision of the Elementary and Secondary Education Act (ESEA) of 1965, is the main federal law affecting education from kindergarten through high school. One of its principles is to hold schools and teachers or interventionists accountable for results. This emphasis on accountability, often effected through comparison of standardized test scores, has a potentially positive impact for CSHCN who are included in the testing process and therefore in a school's ratings. As such, it may encourage schools to place a newfound emphasis on teaching CSHCN. CSHCN, including children with IEPs, must be included in the accountability system of NCLB, and test results for children served by IEPs are reported separately if the group of children is sufficiently large to meet the state's statistical standards. Of note, CSHCN may be eligible for accommodations during testing (for a discussion of the alternate achievement standards for students with disabilities, see U.S. Department of Education, 2005).

SERVICES AND PROGRAMS

Some services are provided through programs that serve all children and others are provided through programs that are designed to serve CSHCN. Parents should note that children may be eligible to receive services through more than one of these programs.

Maternal and Child Health Title V Services

The federal Maternal and Child Health Bureau (MCHB) Division of Services for Children with Special Needs provides leadership in programs for CSHCN and their families. Its Integrated Services Branch promotes models of community-based care in six areas:

- Medical home

- Financing/managed care

- Family participation/cultural competence

- Healthy and ready to work

- Community integrated services
- Universal screening of newborn hearing

MCHB also provides discretionary grants for special projects of regional and national significance (SPRANS) and for community integrated service systems (CISS). These projects include training programs, innovative service delivery, treatment centers, and prevention programs.

States provide maternal and child health (MCH) services with support from federal block grants under Title V of the Social Security Act of 1935. (See Chapter 3 for more on Title V block grants.) Title V was authorized to improve the health of all women, children, youth, and families, including children with disabilities; it was critical to the formulation of health departments in some states. Programs and services differ state to state, but at least 30% of the block grant funding must be used to serve children with special health care needs (U.S. Department of Health and Human Services, 2004; see https://performance.hrsa.gov/mchb/mchreports/link/state_links.asp for information on state MCH programs).

Foster Care Program

Funded by federal reimbursements to the states, the foster care program was established in 1980 under Title IV of the Social Security Act of 1935. Under this law and its revisions (especially the Adoption and Safe Families Act in 1997), children are placed voluntarily or through court order in foster care with a state-approved family (related or not related), or in an institutional setting such as a licensed family home or group home. Subject to specific eligibility requirements (related to the type of placement and the child's resources), children in foster care are eligible for Medicaid (U.S. House of Representatives, 2000). Foster care programs can pay larger stipends to families hosting children with special health care needs.

Private Sector Initiatives

Although health-related benefits through employment often appear to be limited to health insurance, many other private sector benefits may be relevant to CSHCN. For example, some employers may provide on- or off-site child care (sometimes including special accommodations for CSHCN). Employers also may provide flexible work arrangements, information and referral to community services, and counseling (Center for Child and Adolescent Health Policy, 2004). Because a majority of parents of CSHCN are employed, these social and health-related services are important, if under appreciated, services relevant to children and their families.

Many companies, especially large companies, provide employee-assistance programs (EAPs) or work-life programs to manage information and referral services—for example, information about child care services in the neighborhood equipped to serve a child in a wheelchair. Some companies provide legal services, which can be important when setting up trusts or when litigation is necessary. Disability-related support groups at some companies may offer peer support to parents, and companies often provide confidential mental health counseling through their EAP or a related program. These services can be especially helpful at times of transition, or during a child's acute episodes; parents can take advantage of the services where they exist. Although civil rights laws should provide protection against discrimination, use of these services may require some disclosure of the child's special needs, and therefore parents may wish to determine the level of confidentiality in the program and consider the pros and cons of disclosure before they seek services.

Family and Medical Leave Act

Another important entitlement that parents should become familiar with is the Family and Medical Leave Act of 1993. This act provides eligible employees (in companies with at least 50 employees) up to 12 weeks of unpaid leave yearly for the care of a family member. This leave can be taken in one large chunk (e.g., to cover care after a hospitalization) or in smaller segments (to cover meetings with school personnel or health care providers). The employee's job is protected during the leave and health insurance is maintained. The federal Department of Labor's web site contains information about the act (Compliance Assistance—Family and Medical Leave Act [FMLA]; http://www.dol.gov/esa/whd/fmla/).

Americans with Disabilities Act

The Americans with Disabilities Act (ADA) of 1990 enhances the civil rights of children (and adults) with disabilities. It prohibits discrimination on the basis of disability in employment in the private sector, in state and local governments, in public accommodations, at commercial facilities, in transportation, and in telecommunications. Of particular importance to CSHCN are equal access requirements in schools, in the community, and at workplaces as children transition into adulthood.

Clinical Services and Programs

Efforts to include children in clinical trials have resulted in stricter federal policies concerning these efforts; for example, the Federal Drug Administration (FDA) recently crafted regulations regarding the inclusion of children in clinical trials (see the Food and Drug Administration Modernization Act of 1997 [FDAMA] and the Best Pharmaceuticals for Children Act of 2002). These regulations are highly relevant to CSHCN, especially children with rare conditions who are frequently enrolled in clinical trials and who would benefit from new drugs coming into the market.

Parent Support Groups

Parents can obtain substantial support from other parents. Family groups can provide information on federal, state, and local services as well as direct emotional support. Family support groups for CSHCN include Family Voices (http://www.familyvoices.org/), the Federation of Families for Children's Mental Health (http://www.ffcmh.org), Parent-to-Parent programs (for example, the Beach Center has a parent to parent map at http://www.beachcenter.org), and National Fiesta Educativa Inc. (http://www.fiestaeducativa.org/). Other support can be found that is specific to a particular condition or set of conditions (e.g., Learning Disabilities Association of America [http://www.ldanatl.org/], The Arc (http://www.thearc.org/, and Genetic Alliance (http://www.geneticalliance.org/).

New Freedom Initiative

Proposed by President George W. Bush in 2001, the New Freedom Initiative is designed to 1) increase access to assistive and universally designed technologies, 2) expand educational opportunities for Americans with disabilities, and 3) promote full access to community life (White House Domestic Policy Council, 2004). Among the initiative's important proposals for children are increased funding for IDEA and other education programs, improved access to technology, and promotion of employment. See www.disability.gov for the federal source of disability-related information and resources relevant to the New Freedom Initiative.

CASH BENEFITS PROGRAMS

One key concern for those who care for CSHCN is the financial burden entailed (Kuhlthau, Hill, Yuecl, & Perrin, 2005). Social welfare programs traditionally provide cash benefits and insurance to poor children and their families. In the past, children and families who obtained welfare benefits automatically obtained Medicaid insurance coverage. In recent years the provision of cash benefits and insurance has been delinked to some extent. This means that families may need to apply separately for Medicaid and cash benefits. Here we focus on cash benefit programs with some note of the links to insurance provision.

Supplemental Security Income

The Supplemental Security Income (SSI) program provides monthly payments for individuals with blindness and other disabilities who meet income and asset criteria. This program has become an important safety net for children and their families, although it covers only poor and near-poor children and children with relatively severe disabilities. Even so, the program provides consistent insurance coverage and supplemental income for eligible families. (Families who think they may be eligible can consult the U.S. Social Security Administration [SSA; http://www.ssa.gov/pubs/10026.html].) The program covers children who meet the criteria and who are under age 18. As of December 2003, nearly a million (960,000) children received SSI payments, representing 13.9% of the total SSI recipient population (Social Security Administration Policy Office, 2003). Overall, 2.35% of the U.S. population receives SSI (U.S. House of Representatives, 2000).

The Supplemental Security Income (SSI) program established in 1972 through the Social Security Act and amendments provides income for persons who had a disability and could no longer work, an adult conceptualization of *disability.* The act grants children with disabilities access to the funds, and recipients of the funds must meet eligibility requirements. The first payments under the act were made in 1974 (U.S. House of Representatives, 2000).

Eligibility (Physical and Financial)

The Personal Responsibility and Work Opportunity Reconciliation Act (PRWORA) of 1996 established the current definition of *disability.* Children are eligible if they have "a medically determinable physical or mental impairment which results in marked and severe functional limitations, and which can be expected to result in death or which has lasted or can be expected to last for a continuous period of not less than 12 months" (Personal Responsibility and Work Opportunity Reconciliation Act, 1996). A determination of a child's disability is made by the state's disability determination services office based on information received from medical and school sources as well as from individuals who have knowledge of the child. Of note, the 1996 welfare reforms barred most non-citizens from receiving SSI; subsequent legislation allowed some legal immigrants access to the program.

Families also must meet income and resource requirements. In general, when children live with their parents, most of the parents' income is *deemed*, or attributed, to the child. The deeming regulations and the asset limits for eligibility are somewhat complex. In general, children may receive SSI benefits with incomes at about double the poverty level and assets of less then $3,000 if the child lives with two parents (some assets and income may be excluded from the calculation). If the child lives with one parent, the asset limitation could drop to less than $2,000. *Deeming* rules change for children who live in institutions or who are at risk for living in an institution. For these families, more generous income levels are available (Social Security Administration, 2006).

Families may apply for SSI through their local Social Security offices. There is an appeals process if a family disagrees with a decision. For more information, see www.socialsecurity.gov/disability/

SSI and Medicaid

One of the major benefits of SSI receipt is that it confers Medicaid eligibility in most states. For children with substantial health issues, the insurance coverage through Medicaid can be as or more important than the cash benefit. Families may have private insurance and obtain Medicaid through SSI eligibility. This may be important when a child's needs are substantial or when private coverage is not complete.

In 32 states, SSI comes with automatic Medicaid eligibility, and in seven states, children need to submit a separate application for Medicaid. Eleven states, called the 209(b) states, have more restrictive criteria for Medicaid eligibility than for SSI.

SSI and Employment

In 1986, Congress added section 1619 to the Social Security Act, which allows recipients to work and receive Medicaid if there is no change in their disability (42 U.S.C. § 1382h). To further encourage older children with SSI to join the labor force, SSA created the Ticket to Work and Self Sufficiency Program in 1999. The Ticket to Work program provides vouchers for employment services, case management, vocational rehabilitation, and support services to help youth and young adults initiate and maintain employment without jeopardizing their benefits. While not directly relevant to children from birth to age 5, this information is important for planning purposes. It frees parents and providers to help children reach their full potential without concern about cancellation of SSI funds. This developmental encouragement can and should begin before the age of 5.

Temporary Assistance for Needy Families

Temporary Assistance for Needy families (TANF) is a state-run program based on federal guidelines that provides cash assistance for families living in poverty. TANF is not specific to CSHCN, but it has the potential to help these children. Generally speaking, however, if a child meets the income and disability criteria for SSI, that program is usually a more attractive option than TANF.

Eligibility

States consider family income levels, financial assets, and vehicle valuations when determining eligibility for TANF. For instance, in 2002, the maximum monthly income for application by a family of one adult and two children was $204 in Alabama, $923 in Alaska, $679 in California, $577 in New York, and $673 in Wisconsin (U.S. Department of Health and Human Services, Office of Family Assistance, 2004). These amounts equal the maximum cash benefits that families can receive in their TANF payouts. Even with TANF benefits, most eligible families remain in poverty. Eligibility is not for an unlimited time, and once a family is enrolled, benefits generally do not increase with the births of additional children.

TANF and Employment

To remain eligible for TANF, adults are required to work, although in some states, the parent of a very young child is exempt from the work requirement. Unsubsidized or subsidized employment in the private or public sectors, on-the-job training, searching for work, community service programs, and vocational educational training are among the activities that count toward fulfilling the work requirements. School attendance for high school dropouts also is accepted as work (U.S. House of Representatives, 2004). If work requirements are not met, sanctions are imposed and benefits are withdrawn from the household's adults.

TANF's work requirements can create substantial barriers for families with CSHCN who may find it especially difficult to obtain appropriate child care or medical support for their child while they are at work. Such care also can be prohibitively expensive (Perrin, Shayne, & Bloom, 1993). Further, TANF-enrolled parents of children with chronic conditions often report missing work due to a child's illness or missing medical appointments because they could not get time off from work (Smith, Wise, & Wampler, 2002). Thus, although TANF can provide much needed income for families living in poverty, it may fall short in meeting the needs of families with CSHCN.

TANF and Medicaid

Under Aid to Families with Dependent Children (AFDC), people receiving welfare benefits were automatically enrolled in Medicaid, the payer of health care for poor families and financed jointly by the federal and state governments. However, with the implementation of TANF in 1996, Medicaid and welfare were separated. Notwithstanding that, Medicaid rules indicate that anyone who would have been eligible for AFDC in 1996 is eligible for Medicaid. In addition, the current TANF income levels are so low that for the most part all TANF-eligible families are also eligible for Medicaid. The difference now is that separate applications must be made.

State Requirement Variability

Lifetime eligibility for TANF is limited to a maximum of 60 months for adults (not necessarily consecutive), although some states have opted for shorter durations. States are now experiencing adults reaching maximum TANF benefit time limits. After benefits for adults expire, some states continue benefits only for the children. In fact, child-only cases have increased as a percentage of states' caseloads from 18.9% in 1995 to 36.6% in 2002. To further support families, some states use state-only funds to extend benefits beyond the specified limits (USDHHS, OFA, 2004), and some states offer exemptions to the 60-month limit for benefits.

With limited lifetime benefits, other states have created programs to support families without having the time count against the maximum. For instance, *diversion programs* operating in Alaska, California, and Maryland offer short-term benefits to families without enrolling them in TANF; in exchange, families agree not to apply for TANF for a specified time frame. In this way, families receive support without exhausting the limited months of TANF benefits.

A potential problem is the fact that there are substantial state-to-state differences in the program. Providers should consider referring families living in poverty who are new to a state to the local welfare agency to determine eligibility even if the family was not qualified in another state. Also, providers should consider referring families to local welfare agencies when the home situation changes.

HEALTH INSURANCE COVERAGE

Health insurance is of great importance to CSHCN and their families. This section reviews the major mechanisms for obtaining health insurance and notes mechanisms that are unique for CSHCN.

Private Health Insurance

Two thirds (64%) of CSHCN are covered by private insurance (U.S. Department of Health and Human Services, Maternal and Child Health Bureau, 2004). Generally speaking, private insurance for children is obtained through a parent's employer, although it can be bought directly by individuals. Employers may purchase care through a fee-for-service plan where providers are paid for each visit, or they may purchase care through a health maintenance organization (HMO) where providers or insurers are paid on a per-member basis. Companies also may choose to self-insure, assuming the risk of health care costs. In self-insured companies, the employer essentially acts as its own insurance company and bears the financial risk of making payments to providers (some employers self-insure but have another company administer the insurance system).

Whether provided through self-insurance, fee-for-service organizations, or HMOs, employer-based private insurance varies substantially regarding costs to employees. Employers may pay all (or none) of the premium, and services covered by the insurance plan may differ among plans offered by the same company. Employees and private purchasers share the costs of care through copayments—nominal fees rendered at the time of service—and sometimes deductibles—specified amounts of medical costs that the insured party pays. Coinsurance plans require the employee to pay for a specified proportion of the care. These various forms of cost sharing can become a burden for families who need a substantial amount of care for their children. In addition, annual or lifetime maximum payments imposed by an insurer can be a problem for families of children with very high health care costs where these thresholds may be breached.

Self-insured companies may have more flexibility in providing alternative types of care than companies that purchase insurance, and, in some cases, employers can act as advocates to assure that their employees and dependents obtain covered health care. In other cases, employers may consider modifying their contracts with insurers to provide different coverage in the future, sometimes in response to the concerns of an employee.

Federal Regulations Protecting Private Insurance

Several federal regulations protect families' private insurance coverage when the primary named insurance holder loses or changes jobs. These protections are especially important for families of CSHCN because purchasing private insurance coverage can be prohibitively expensive. In addition, families may want to maintain coverage so that they can continue to see a particular set of providers, or they may want to change jobs with less anxiety about losing insurance coverage.

The Consolidated Omnibus Budget Reconciliation Act of 1985 (COBRA) requires employers with health insurance who have at least 20 employees to offer continued access to group health insurance to employees and their dependents (typically for 18 months) if an employee loses his or her job or if a reduction in hours eliminates health insurance eligibility (Employee Benefit Research Institute, 1997). Although COBRA is potentially a substantial benefit to CSHCN and their families, it comes with a cost: Employees may be required to pay as much as 102% of the premium out of their own pockets.

The Health Insurance Portability and Accountability Act of 1996 (HIPAA) provides additional protection for families of dependents with preexisting conditions. Specifically, the act

1. Places limits on group health plans denying coverage or charging extra for coverage based on a family member's past or present poor health

2. Helps to guarantee individuals who lose job-related coverage the right to purchase health insurance

3. Helps to guarantee the right to renew insurance regardless of health status

HIPAA does not limit the amount that can be charged for a policy. Providers may be more familiar with the parts of HIPAA that regulate the privacy of patient information, yet these coverage protections can be of vital importance to parents of CSHCN who wish to switch jobs.

Other regulations are relevant to the coverage of certain types of benefits. The Mental Health Parity Act of 1996 (MHPA, PL 104-204) prevents employers with more than 50 employees in group health plans from placing annual or lifetime dollar limits on mental health benefits that are lower than the limits for medical and surgical benefits. However, although the act provides some protection for families of children with mental health conditions, it does not require group health plans to include mental health services in the benefits package. Instead, it applies only to those plans that already have mental health coverage, and for those plans, it does not place limits on increases in copayments, on the number of visits, or on cost-sharing arrangements for mental health benefits (Centers for Medicare & Medicaid Services [CMMS], 2005a). Although enactment of the MHPA indicates that there is some awareness of the importance of mental health issues, its limited protection suggests that mental health issues will remain a challenge for families and providers.

Government Health Insurance

The government is an important source of insurance coverage for all children but especially for poor and near-poor children. Government health insurance can serve as the primary source of insurance or can provide additional coverage.

Medicaid

Medicaid, the primary source of government health insurance coverage for children in this country, was established in 1965 under the Social Security Act. Medicaid is managed at the federal level by the CMMS, but each state operates a Medicaid program with some discretion over whom the program covers and what services it provides.

Eligibility

More than 50 different groups are eligible for Medicaid, depending on each state's eligibility criteria. States have requirements and options for extending Medicaid coverage for children if family income exceeds Medicaid eligibility levels for up to 12 months, although regulations vary depending on different groups of children. Parents and providers are advised to check their local government web sites or www.insurekidsnow.gov for specifics. As with other programs, the rules are complex, but it is probably worth exploring eligibility if a family or child is potentially eligible.

Most important to CSHCN are provisions to provide Medicaid coverage for children who are at risk of being institutionalized or for whom medical costs are large enough to make the children eligible for Medicaid once medical costs are subtracted from family income. These provisions, called the *1915 waivers*, permit states to file waivers to obtain exceptions to Medicaid rules. Specifically, the 1915 waivers allow families to receive Medicaid funds so that their children can live at home rather than in an institution.

Other Medicaid-related legislation includes the Tax Equity and Fiscal Responsibility Act of 1982, which allows for different rules concerning how parent income is deemed to the child if the child could live in an institution but the family chooses to keep him or her at home. In some cases, regulations also allow for an enhancement of the Medicaid benefits to children eligible through this mechanism.

Provisions called the *1115 waivers* allow states to sponsor pilot programs such as the provision of Medicaid through managed care. In some cases, these programs are applied to all children who obtain services through Medicaid, and in other cases, some populations are *carved out* (excluded) from the 1115 programs.

An option for the medically needy allows states to extend Medicaid eligibility to persons who would be eligible for Medicaid under one of the existing groups except that their income or resources, or both, are above the state eligibility levels. Persons may qualify immediately or they may *spend down* by incurring medical expenses that reduce their income to their state's medically needy income level or below.

See Table 2.1 for some of the major Medicaid beneficiary groups. If parents suspect that they may be eligible, or a provider suspects that a family they service may be eligible, they should investigate applying to the program. Even for families with private insurance, if a child has

Table 2.1. Medicaid beneficiary groups

Mandatory populations	Optional populations
• Children age 6 and older below 100% FPL ($15,670 a year for a family of 3)	• Low-income children above 100% FPL who are not mandatory by age (see column on left)
• Children under age 6 below 133% FPL ($20,841 a year for a family of 3)	• Low-income parents with income above state's 1996 AFDC level
• Parents below state's AFDC cutoffs from July 1996 (median = 42% FPL)	• Pregnant women >133% FPL
• Pregnant women <133% FPL	• Disabled and elderly below 100% FPL ($9,310 a year for an individual), but above SSI level
• Elderly and disabled SSI beneficiaries with income <74% FPL ($6,768 a year for an individual)	• Nursing home residents above SSI levels, but below 300% of SSI ($1,692 a month)
• Certain working disabled	• Individuals at risk of needing a nursing facility or ICF-MR care (under HCBS waiver)
• Medicare Buy-In groups (QMB, SLMB, QI)	• Certain working people with disabilities (>SSI levels)
	• Medically needy

Reprinted from "Medicaid: An overview of spending on 'mandatory' versus 'optional' populations and services." (2005). *The Kaiser Commission on Medicaid and the Uninsured.* This information was reprinted with permission from the Henry J. Kaiser Family Foundation. The Kaiser Family Foundation, based in Menlo Park, California, is a nonprofit, private operating foundation focusing on the major health care issues facing the nation and is not associated with Kaiser Permanente or Kaiser Industries.

special health care needs and meets the income eligibility criteria, it may be worth obtaining Medicaid coverage in addition to private insurance to have access to the often-broader array of services (including services that are often important to CSHCN). As for many other programs, a family may be eligible in one state but not another. In some cases, children are eligible for Medicaid but parents are not; in other cases, only one child is eligible for Medicaid. This may be a deterrent to enrollment for some families.

Services Provided

Tables 2.3 shows the mandatory and optional services covered by Medicaid. In general, Medicaid benefits cover a wide variety of relevant special health care services. Yet, some providers do not accept Medicaid payments (reimbursements are generally quite low), which can limit access to children covered by Medicaid.

Early & Periodic Screening, Diagnosis, & Treatment (EPSDT) services have been mandated by Medicaid for all children since 1967. Children obtain the screening to ensure that their health and development meet certain predefined milestones. For children who do not meet developmental goals, states must provide medically necessary services

Table 2.2.   Medicaid acute care benefit

"Mandatory" items and services	"Optional" items and services*
• Physician's services	• Prescription drugs
• Laboratory and x-ray services	• Medical care or remedial care furnished by other licensed practitioners
• Inpatient hospital services	
• Outpatient hospital services	• Rehabilitation and other therapies
• Early and periodic screening, diagnostic, and treatment (EPSDT) services for individuals under 21	• Clinic services
	• Dental services, dentures
• Family planning and supplies	• Prosthetic devices, eyeglasses, durable medical equipment
• Federally qualified health center (FQHC) services	• Primary care case management
	• TB-related services
• Rural health clinic services	• Other specialist medical or remedial care
• Nurse midwife services	
• Certified pediatric and family nurse practitioner services	

*These benefits are treated as mandatory for children under 21 through EPSDT in this analysis.

Reprinted from "Medicaid: An overview of spending on 'mandatory' versus 'optional' populations and services." (2005). *The Kaiser Commission on Medicaid and the Uninsured.* This information was reprinted with permission from the Henry J. Kaiser Family Foundation. The Kaiser Family Foundation, based in Menlo Park, California, is a nonprofit, private operating foundation focusing on the major health care issues facing the nation and is not associated with Kaiser Permanente or Kaiser Industries.

Table 2.3. Medicaid long-term care benefits

"Mandatory" items and services	"Optional" items and services*
Institutional services	
• Nursing facility (NF) services for individuals 21 or over	• Intermediate care facility services for the mentally retarded (ICF/MR)
	• Inpatient/nursing facility services for individuals 65 and over in an institution for mental diseases (IMD)
	• Inpatient psychiatric hospital services for individuals under age 21
Home & community-based services	
• Home health care services (for individuals entitled to nursing facility care)	• Home- & community-based waiver services
	• Other home health care
	• Targeted case management
	• Respiratory care services for ventilator-dependent individuals
	• Personal care services
	• Hospice services
	• Services furnished under a PACE program

*These benefits are treated as mandatory for children under 21 through EPSDT in this analysis, with the exception of Home and community-based waiver services.

Reprinted from "Medicaid: An overview of spending on 'mandatory' versus 'optional' populations and services." (2005). *The Kaiser Commission on Medicaid and the Uninsured.* This information was reprinted with permission from the Henry J. Kaiser Family Foundation. The Kaiser Family Foundation, based in Menlo Park, California, is a nonprofit, private operating foundation focusing on the major health care issues facing the nation and is not associated with Kaiser Permanente or Kaiser Industries.

including some that the state may not typically cover. This essentially functions as a back door for children to obtain services through the Medicaid system. Because many CSHCN do not meet developmental goals, EPSDT can be an important pathway for them to obtain additional services.

Administration of Services

Medicaid is funded by a variable matching formula that is inversely related to a state's per-capita income and ranges from a 50% to an 85% match from the federal government to state expenditures (U.S. House of Representatives, 2000). State welfare or health agencies generally administer the Medicaid program, and states determine which optional populations and services to cover and provide. They must provide federally mandated services and may choose to cover optional services based on their resources, the needs of their state's population, and their commitment to the Medicaid package.

State Children's Health Insurance Program

Congress established the State Children's Health Insurance Program (SCHIP) in 1997 under Title XXI of the Balanced Budget Act of 1997. SCHIP sought to improve insurance coverage for children who exceed Medicaid's income eligibility limits but do not have enough money to purchase private health insurance. SCHIP covers about 4 million children nationwide (Centers for Medicare & Medicaid Services [CMMS], 2005b).

Eligibility

To be eligible for SCHIP, children must not be eligible to receive any other insurance including Medicaid. This provision was built into SCHIP to ensure that the program covers only those children who had no other public or private coverage options. SCHIP-eligible children must be under 19 years of age and below 200% of the federal poverty level (FPL), with some exceptions to expand to higher-income levels. Eligibility differs by age and state.

Program Design

SCHIP programs have three options for providing insurance coverage: expanding Medicaid eligibility levels, designing a separate children's health insurance program, or both. These three options mean that in some states SCHIP programs are not easily distinguishable from Medicaid coverage, and in other states, SCHIP programs are totally separate. Also, each state may choose to give its program a different name; therefore, it may not always be easy for consumers to know that a particular program is the state's SCHIP program.

Just as they have three options for determining how to provide coverage, states have options for determining which services to cover that relate SCHIP coverage to other types of coverage. Within each state's plan, coverage for well-baby and well-child care along with immunizations and emergency services must be included. In general, states seem to create plans for *typical* children, not for children with special needs; however, a handful of states have special provisions for children with special needs built into their SCHIP programs. States may impose cost-sharing requirements, although the federal guidelines impose limits on the cost sharing allowed (e.g., cost sharing for families above 150% of FPL cannot exceed 5% of the family's income).

Indian Health Service

Children with special health care needs who are Native Americans have one more source of services and insurance coverage available: the Indian Health Service (IHS). IHS is responsible for the delivery of health services to more than 1.6 million federally recognized American Indians and Alaskan Natives (U.S. Department of Health and Human Services, 2005). IHS provides direct services to residents of reservations located within a contract health service delivery area or to Native Americans residing in the United States who are members of a tribe. Coverage is based on IHS guidelines and the availability of funding. IHS is the payer of last resort and provides coverage for services not covered elsewhere or payments for services that are only partially covered (for more information, see http://www.ihs.gov/PublicInfo/PublicAffairs/ Welcome_Info/ThisFacts.asp).

CONCLUSION

Policies and programs relevant to CSHCN and their families are numerous. However, parents and providers must educate themselves about the policies and programs or they will not be able to take full advantage of the assistance and support to which they and the children they care for are entitled. As the chapter has shown, families may have policy-mandated access to programs that provide income support or health insurance. Increasingly, the legal rights of children and their parents are protected. There also is a movement afoot to create even more supportive polices and programs.

Yet, despite this progress, the arena of policies and programs is difficult to navigate. Nearly all programs have substantial variation from state to state. Eligibility in one state may mean nothing if a family moves to another state. On one hand, the substantial state-to-state variations may mean that programs are designed to best suit the needs of that state's population. On the other hand, the substantial variation means that it is difficult to advocate for these programs at the national level, and determining eligibility has an additional layer of complexity.

Further, even within any one state, eligibility for the programs is complicated. The income levels that confer eligibility are generally quite low for income support and government insurance coverage. Employment-based benefits are often available at the discretion of the employer, and relevant programs and regulations sometimes only pertain to large employers.

Another challenge is the gap between policy and practice, especially when mandates are unfounded. Legislation such as the Americans with Disabilities Act or the Family and Medical Leave Act can be difficult to put into practice even where the law is clear because enforcement can require legal action. On a more optimistic note, laws related to disability are getting stronger and family participation is gaining momentum. Also, the Internet provides families with increased access to information and referral in an easily accessible format.

REFERENCES

Americans with Disabilities Act. (1990). PL 101-336, 42 U.S.C. §§ 12101 *et seq.*

Balanced Budget Act of 1997, PL 105-33, 111 Stat. 251.

Best Pharmaceuticals for Children Act of 2002, PL 107-109 http://www.fda.gov/opacom/laws/pharmkids/contents.html

Center for Child and Adolescent Health Policy, (2004). *Children with special needs and the workplace: A guide for employers.* Retrieved June 2005, from www.massgeneral.org/ebs

Centers for Medicare & Medicaid Services. (CMM; 2005a). *The mental health parity act.* Retrieved June 29, 2005, from http://www.cms.hhs.gov/hipaa/hipaa1/content/mhpa.asp

Centers for Medicare & Medicaid Services. (CMM; 2005b). *SCHIP enrollment reports. Point in time enrollment for FY 2005.* Retrieved June 2005, from http://www.cms.hhs.gov/NationalSCHIPPolicy/SCHIPER/list.asp

Compliance Assistance—Family and Medical Leave Act (FMLA) http://www.dol.gov/esa/whd/fmla/

Consolidated Ommibus Budget Reconciliation Act (COBRA) of 1985, PL 99-272, 42 U.S.C. §§ 300 *et seq.*

Education for All Handicapped Children Act of 1975, PL 94-142, 10 U.S.C. §§ 1400 *et seq.*

Elementary and Secondary Education Act of 1965, PL 89-10, 20 U.S.C. §§ 241 *et seq.*

Employee Benefit Research Institute. (1997). *Education and Research Fund.* (5th ed.). Washington, DC; http://www.ebri.org/publications/books/index.cfm?fa = databook

Family and Medical Leave Act (FMLA) of 1993, PL 103-3, 5 U.S.C. §§ 6381 *et seq., 29 U.S.C. §§ 2601 *et seq.*

Food and Drug Administration Modernization Act (FDAM) of 1997, PL 105-115; 21 U.S.C. 301, *et seq.*

Health Insurance Portability and Accountability Act (HIPAA) of 1996, PL 104-191, 42 U.S.C. §§ 201 *et seq.*

Individuals with Disabilities Education Act (IDEA) of 1990, PL 101-476, 20 U.S.C. §§ 1400 *et seq.*

Kuhlthau K., Hill, K.S., Yucel, R., & Perrin, J.M. (2005). Financial burden for families of children with special health care needs. *Maternal and Child Health Journal, 9,* 207–218.

The Mental Health Parity Act of 1996, PL 104-204, 110 Stat. 2944.

National Dissemination Center for Children with Disabilities. Retrieved September 27, 2006, from http://www.nichcy.org/states.htm

No Child Left Behind Act of 2001, PL 107-110, 115 Stat. 1425, 20 U.S.C. §§ 6301 *et seq.*

Personal Responsibility and Work Opportunity Reconciliation Act of 1996, PL 104-193, 42 U.S.C. §§ 1305 *et seq.*

Rehabilitation Act of 1973, PL 93-112, 29 U.S.C. §§ 701 *et seq.*

Smith, L., Wise, P., & Wampler, N. (2002). Knowledge of welfare reform program provisions among families of children with chronic conditions. *American Journal of Public Health, 92,* 228–230.

Social Security Act of 1935, PL 74-271, 42 U.S.C. §§ 301 *et seq.*

Social Security Administration, Understanding Supplemental Security Income Spotlight on Deeming Parental Income and Resources, 2006 Edition http://www.socialsecurity.gov/notices/supplemental-security-income/spotlights/spot-deeming.htm

Tax Equity and Fiscal Responsibility Act of 1982, PL 97-248.

U.S. Department of Education. *Alternate achievement standards for students with the most significant cognitive disabilities: Non-regulatory guidance.* Retrieved August 2005 from http://www.ed.gov/policy/elsec/guid/altguidance.doc

U.S. Department of Education, Office for Civil Rights, Special Education and Rehabilitative Services. (2005). *Protecting students with disabilities.* Washington, DC: Author. Retrieved October 20, 2005, from http://www.ed.gov/about/offices/list/ocr/504faq.html)

U.S. Department of Education. Office of Special Education Programs (USDE OSEP, 2005). *History: Twenty-five years of progress in educating children with disabilities through IDEA.* Washington, DC: Author. Retrieved October 20, 2005, from http://www.ed.gov/policy/speced/leg/idea/history.html

U.S. Department of Education, Office of Special Education and Rehabilitative Services (USDE OSERS, 2000). *A guide to individualized education programs.* Washington, DC: Author. Retrieved October 20, 2005, from http://www.ed.gov/parents/needs/speced/iepguide/index.html

U.S. Department of Health and Human Services. (2004). *Understanding Title V of the Social Security Act: A guide to the provisions of the federal maternal and child health block grant.* Retrieved June 2004, from ftp://ftp.hrsa.gov/mchb/titlevtoday/UnderstandingTitleV.pdf

U.S. Department of Health and Human Services. FY 2005, Budget in Brief. Retrieved July 2006 from www.acces.us/PDF/fy2005bibfinal.pdf

U.S. Department of Health and Human Services, Maternal and Child Health Bureau (USDHHS MCHB; 2004). *The National Survey of Children with Special Health Care Needs Chartbook 2001.* Rockville, MD: Author.

U.S. Department of Health and Human Services, Office of the Assistant Secretary for Planning and Evaluation (USDHHS, 2002). *The 2002 HHS poverty guidelines.* Washington, DC: Author. Retrieved July 21, 2005, from http://aspe.hhs.gov/poverty/02poverty.htm

U.S. Department of Health and Human Services, Office of Family Assistance (USDHHS OFA, November 2004). *Temporary Assistance for Needy Families [TANF]: Sixth annual report to Congress.* Washington, DC: Author. Retrieved July 20, 2005, from http://www.acf.hhs.gov/programs/ofa/annualreport6/

U.S. House of Representatives, Committee on Ways and Means. (2000) *The 2000 Green Book background material and data on programs within the jurisdiction of the Committee on Ways and Means.* Retrieved June 14, 2005, from http://www.aspe.hhs.gov/2000gb

U.S. House of Representatives, Committee on Ways and Means. (2004). *The 2004 Green Book background material and data on programs within the jurisdiction of the Committee on Ways and Means, Section 7—Temporary Assistance for Needy Families [TANF].* Retrieved July 21, 2005, from http://www.gpoaccess.gov/wmprints/green/2004.html

U.S. Social Security Administration Office of Policy, Office of Research, Evaluation and Statistics. (December 2003). *Children receiving SSI.* SSA Publication No. 13-11830.

White House Domestic Policy Council. (2004). *New Freedom Initiative: A progress report.* Retrieved June 2005, from http://www.whitehouse.gov/infocus/newfreedom/toc-2004.html

3

MATTERS OF FINANCE:

How Do We Pay for the Care of Children with Special Health Care Needs?

John M. Neff

C hronic conditions in childhood often occur unexpectedly and generally could not have been prevented by a family or health professional's intervention. This is certainly true of almost all birth defects, malignancies, and a large group of disorders that occur individually and rarely, such as collagen vascular conditions, many genetic conditions, cerebral palsy, and spinal cord defects. Parents are usually unprepared, from the standpoint of personal resources and insurance coverage, to manage the financial realities they certainly will face. These include short-term costs, long-term financial needs, and support of the child's transition into adulthood.

When a child is first diagnosed with a chronic condition, among the immediate issues families face are the cost of any direct care not covered by insurance, potential copayments for inpatient and outpatient services, and long- or short-term limits of insurance coverage. These costs are difficult for any family to pay and will vary considerably according to the specific condition the child has, the long-term outcome of that condition, and the family's income and insurance status.

Experts knowledgeable about health care financing have known for several years that children as a group consume only a modest portion of national health care expenses. For example, the health care charges for an average child in the state of Washington total less than $1,000 a year (Neff, Sharp, Muldoon, Graham, & Myers, 2004). Yet there has been little information on how these expenses are distributed to children based on chronic conditions or special health care needs. Of all government sources, Medicaid is the principal support for children, and from this source, less than 25% goes to children. How much of this 25% goes to the healthy child and how much to the child with chronic conditions? What are the costs of care, how well are children with special health care needs supported, and what are the financial vulnerabilities of these children and their families? These are some of the issues covered in this chapter.

Until relatively recently, there have been very few reasonably accurate estimates of the financial impact of children with chronic conditions either on society as a whole or on individual families of these children. With the advent of new measurement tools, population surveys, and a renewed focus on this population, knowledge in this area has increased considerably in the United States.

It is now possible to identify some of the very real costs, and the amount of insurance coverage, associated with caring for these children. Families with children who have chronic conditions and special health care needs bear a disproportionately heavy financial burden of health care costs compared with families of healthy children. This chapter summarizes some of the research that has identified this disparity, emphasizes the importance of families of children with special health care needs (CSHCN) having comprehensive and continuous health insurance for their children, and analyzes the consequences of failures in the system. The first section of the chapter discusses the various methods used to identify CSHCN and measure costs. This is followed by sections on

- The distribution of costs to CSHCN compared with children without special health care needs

- The impact of mental health conditions on overall costs of care

- The out-of-pocket expenses (costs not covered by insurance) that families bear

- The growing cost of medications

- The added cost to practitioners for caring for CSHCN

- The convoluted, fragmented, and, to a large degree, inadequate systems of insurance support available to families with CSHCN

Finally, the chapter addresses the deterioration of what is a very inadequate and basically unfair system of care, and summarizes the steps that families should take now to prepare themselves and what all must do to work toward building a better system of care in the future.

METHODS TO IDENTIFY CHILDREN WITH SPECIAL HEALTH CARE NEEDS AND TO MEASURE COSTS

Although there has been some understanding of the health care costs for children with very specific categorical conditions, such as asthma and attention-deficit/hyperactivity disorders (ADHD), it has been difficult to determine the health care costs for children with chronic conditions as a group apart from healthy children. This was primarily because no uniform definition for these children was available to health services investigators. In 1998, the federal Maternal Child Health Bureau's (MCHB) Division of Services for Children With Special Health Care Needs established a work group to develop a definition that described, noncategorically, children with chronic conditions. The term *children with special health care needs,* or *CSHCN,* was used and defined "as those children who have or are at increased risk for a chronic physical, developmental, behavioral, or emotional condition and who also require health and related services of a type or amount beyond that required by children generally" (McPherson et al., 1998). Since 1998, this definition, with some modifications, has been used to develop instruments that can identify CSHCN and measure their health care costs. A principal modification of this definition was to eliminate measurements for children *at increased risk.* At-risk populations include, among others, children who are poor, homeless, and abused. These children, while certainly at risk for having a special health care need, are difficult to identify, stratify by severity of risk factors, or quantify consistently in large population groups. Therefore, analyses of costs focus on children who actually have a chronic condition that is expected to last at least a year and that requires services that are of a type or amount beyond that required by children generally.

Three basic methods have been used to identify these children and to measure their associated health care costs: the CSHCN Screener, CRG data, and MEPS data.

CSHCN Screener

The first method entails a survey instrument called the CSHCN screener (Bethell et al., 2002). The CSHCN screener was developed in 2001 to identify children with special health care needs as opposed to other (healthy) children, to measure health care consumer satisfaction, and to provide a means of quality assurance. It has been used by the MCHB in conjunction with the National Center for Health Statistics in the national survey of families in the United States to assess for the first time the prevalence and characteristics of children with special health care needs (van Dyck, Kogan, McPherson, Weissman, & Newacheck, 2004). This assessment has enabled state and federal governments, as well as advocacy groups, to understand the magnitude of the problems that such children face, to determine how well CSHCN families' needs in the United States are being met, and to identify gaps in the health care delivery system for this population. This survey was administered using a list-assisted, random-digit, dial-telephone-survey method built into the existing State and Local Area Integrated Telephone survey (van

Dyck et al., 2004). It was administered to a representative sample from each of the 50 states and the District of Columbia. This type of survey data should be interpreted with caution because the information comes from parental surveys. Parental impressions may under- or over-report the quality of services. The extent of a child's special needs also may vary according to parental information and individual impressions of their own child's health status.

CRG Data

3M Health Information Systems (3M HIS), in collaboration with the National Association of Children's Hospitals and Related Institutions, has developed software called Clinical Risk Groups (CRG) to identify children as well as adults with chronic conditions. CRG uses health care claims data, collected for billing purposes, that contain valuable information on specific conditions and health-related charges. This software tool groups diseases into several condition categories and severity levels (Hughes et al., 2004) and defines conditions that can be expected to last at least a year and require additional services. CRG was initially developed as a risk adjustment tool to predict populations with high-risk and high-cost conditions and to adjust payments accordingly. There are several such instruments available, but CRG has been used to identify cost patterns and health services utilization specifically for CSHCN and was developed using the CSHCN definition for children. Studies using this tool have provided comparative analysis for CSHCN from several states and different types of health care plans. This method has been used in Washington State in a commercial health care plan, nationally in a large managed-care commercial health plan, and in Medicaid data sets from several states. (Ireys, Humensky, Peterson, Wickstrom, Manda, & Rheault, 2002; Neff et al., 2002, 2004; Shenkman et al., 2004). Health plan data, however, need to be interpreted with caution because expenses often are reported as charges and not as reimbursement to families or providers to cover actual expenses of care. In addition, health plan administrative data records information only on those children who are enrolled in the plan and who interact with the health care system. This type of data does not record the family expenses relating to CSHCN that are not covered by insurance. Ultimately, the information depends on the accuracy of the specific coding practices of the provider and the health plan.

MEPS Data

The third method for identifying CSHCN uses the Medical Expenditure Panel Survey (MEPS). This is a nationally representative longitudinal survey that collects detailed information about health care utilization and expenditures, health insurance and health status, and considerable socioeconomic data. MEPS links this survey data to administrative data sources (Medical Expenditure Panel Survey [MEPS], 2000).

Using MEPS has made it possible to identify not only the charges to health care plans for medical expenses, but also other real expenses incurred by families, such as costs not covered by insurance and expenses necessary for the support of the child. These are termed *out-of-pocket* expenses. Through MEPS, it also is possible to correlate the costs of health care with the families' economic status. Before these specific surveys, data sets, and software tools were available, there was little or no information on overall medical care costs or quality of care for families of CSHCN.

DISTRIBUTION OF COSTS

As noted, the percentage of children with special health care needs estimated to be in the U.S. childhood population varies somewhat depending on the survey methodology: 9.5% by CRG estimates (Neff et al., 2004), 12.8% from the CSHCN survey (van Dyck et al., 2004), and 16.2% from MEPS (Newacheck & Kim, 2005; see Figure 3.1). In reality, these children have conditions with a wide range of severity and complexity, and much of this variability depends on the sensitivity of the methods used for identifying certain conditions and severity levels (see Chapter 1 for a more detailed discussion on identifying CSHCN). Information from administrative data also records only those children who

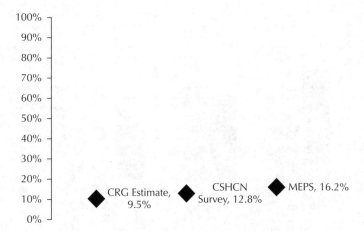

Figure 3.1. Estimates of CSHCN in the U.S. population versus services consumed. *Sources:* Neff et al., 2004; Newacheck & Kim, 2005; van Dyck et al., 2004.

interact with the health care system and are coded appropriately. Despite the differences in methodology, all of the surveys agree that CSHCN, while representing between 10% and 16% of the childhood population, account for 40% to 60% of total health care costs for children, and, on average, CSHCN have expenditures per child of more than three times that of non-CSHCN (Neff et al., 2004; Newacheck & Kim, 2005). However, the pattern of expenditures varies considerably. CSHCN, in comparison with non-CSHCN, account for more than five times higher hospital care expenses, more than twice the amount of physician services, seven times the amount of nonphysician expenses and five times the number of prescribed medications (Neff et al., 2004; Newacheck & Kim, 2005). The distribution of these expenses also is strikingly different for CSHCN compared with non-CSHCN (see Figure 3.2). While inpatient hospital charges account for about 20% of the total charges for non-CSHCN, they account for between 36% and 67% of total charges for children with chronic conditions, increasing with the severity and complexity of the condition (Neff et al., 2004). From another perspective, CSHCN account for 52.5% of all children's hospital days (Newacheck & Kim, 2005). Prescription medications and home health care together account for one third of health care expenses for CSHCN compared with one twentieth of the expenses for non-CSHCN (Newacheck & Kim, 2005).

These differences become even more pronounced when analyzed according to the severity of the conditions (Neff et al., 2004); for example:

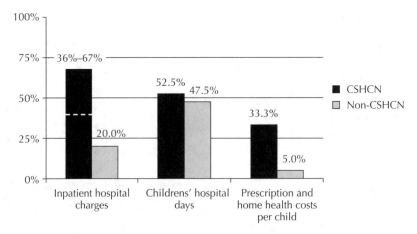

Figure 3.2. Distribution of health care expenses for CSHCN and non-CSHCN. *Sources:* Neff et al., 2004; Newacheck & Kim, 2005.

- Children with metastatic malignancies and catastrophic chronic conditions—less than 1% of children—account for approximately 15% of all children's health charges (Neff et al., 2004). The annual median charge per typical non-CSHCN is under $200 but is more than five to nearly 40 times higher in CSHCN, depending on the specific condition and severity of that condition (see Figure 3.3).

- When analyzed by hospitals that admit children in the state of Washington during the 1990s—a period of considerable health care reform—the hospitalization of children with non-chronic conditions decreased at a greater rate than the rate of hospitalization of children with chronic conditions. By the end of the decade, more than 40% of all children hospitalized in Washington State had chronic conditions (Neff, Valentine et al., 2002).

- When analyzed by referral status, 60% of all children discharged from pediatric referral centers were those with chronic conditions (Neff, 2002).

The overall picture from all of these data sources is one showing that CSHCN consume considerable resources and are the major consumers of child health care costs compared with children who do not have a chronic condition. Hospitalizations represent the major source of these

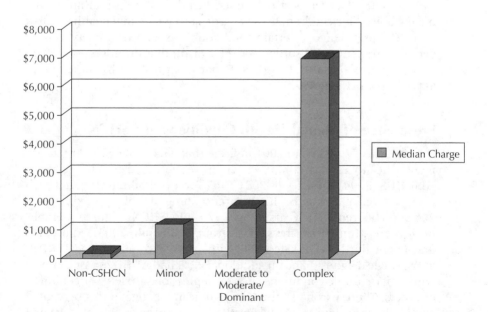

Figure 3.3.   Annual median charges for non-CSHCN and for CSHCN according to severity of condition. *Source:* Neff et al., 2004.

costs, and these hospitalizations are distributed unevenly among hospitals depending on their specialty designations (e.g., children's hospitals).

THE COSTS ASSOCIATED WITH MENTAL HEALTH CONDITIONS

Among other issues that are important when considering the high cost of caring for children with chronic conditions is the impact of mental health conditions, occurring either as single entities or as co-morbid conditions in children who have other primary or secondary non-mental health chronic conditions. Critically important is the fact that if children have mental health conditions and if for some reason appropriate mental health services are not available, the children's families will interact with hospital emergency departments as their only source of care. This will certainly result in an inappropriate and generally ineffective and expensive use of health care services.

Prevalence of Mental Health Conditions in Children

To understand the magnitude of this issue, the Surgeon General of the United States' latest report on mental health indicated that approximately one in five children 9–17 years of age have mental health conditions. The prevalence of certain conditions is as follows: anxiety disorders—13.0%, mood disorders—6.2%, disruptive disorders—10.3%, and substance abuse—2.0% (U.S. Department of Health and Human Services [USDHHS], 1999).

Prevalence of Mental Health Conditions in CSHCN

National survey data from 2001 indicate that 25.4% of CSHCN require mental health care, and 4.5% have an unmet need for this service (USDHHS, 2004). In a 1999–2001 CRG survey of administrative data from a large national health insurance program of approximately 240,000 children 5–18 years of age, 37% of CSHCN required mental health care (Humensky, Ireys, Wickstrom, & Rheault, 2004). Approximately one third of those identified with a mental condition had ADHD as the single diagnosis, and an additional 22% had ADHD in association with other chronic conditions such as depression, anxiety, or conduct disorders. There was no statistically significant change in this percentage of children with a mental health condition over the three years surveyed.

Effect of Mental Health Conditions on Medical Expenses

The families of the children with special health care needs who had emotional or behavioral disorders paid 12% more in copayments and deductibles than families of children with special needs without emotional disorders. The distribution of costs across services was different from costs for those without mental health disorders. Mental health services accounted for 22.2% of the payments of families with a child who has a mental health condition, and only 0.6% of the payments of families who had a special needs child without a mental health condition. For prescription drugs, the difference was 36.9% compared with 30.8% (see Figure 3.4). In addition, the average payment per member per month (PMPM) by families of CSHCN and emotional or behavioral disorders increased by 35.4% from 1999 to 2001. This increase was largely driven by increases in the cost of prescription drugs and emergency services, which increased by 69.2% and 52.3%, respectively (Humensky et al., 2004).

There is very little data on the cost of coexisting mental health and chronic physical conditions, but what there is suggest that coexisting mental health conditions increase the cost of care of children with other chronic conditions. In one study in Alberta, Canada, using analysis of administrative data of 6- to 17-year-old children, the prevalence of mental health disorders was 9.5% in boys and 12.0% in girls, increasing by age and strongly associated with socioeconomic status. Children on welfare, perhaps because of the stress of poverty on families or the presence of depression in parents, were nearly twice as likely to have an

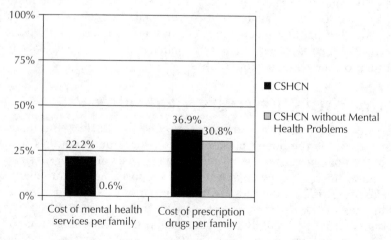

Figure 3.4. Cost of services and prescription drugs for CSHCN with and without mental health problems. *Source:* Humensky, Ireys, Wickstrom, & Rheault, 2004.

associated mental health condition (Spady, Schopflocher, Svenson, & Thompson, 2001). In this same population, the authors studied the association of psychiatric disorders coexisting with other medical and or psychiatric conditions and observed that children with a co-morbid mental health condition had 1.4 (boys) to 5.2 (girls) times greater use of health services over those without a mental health co-morbid condition (Spady, Schopflocher, Svenson, & Thompson, 2005). In one study of children from birth to age 17 supported by Supplemental Security Income (SSI) in the state of Washington in 1992 and 1993, the total annual Medicaid charges for children with physical and coexisting mental health conditions was $16,300. This compared with $12,600 for those with only physical conditions and $7,300 for those with only mental health conditions (Neff, Muldoon, Gay, & Anderson, 2001).

It is not surprising that a child with a chronic medical condition and a coexisting mental health condition such as depression or conduct disorder, if untreated, will interact with the health system more frequently than a child without such a condition, and that this interaction will most likely be in the emergency department or as an unplanned hospitalization (Stewart, Rao, Emslie, Klein, & White, 2005).

The implications of this study are that the availability, access, and support of mental health services for children and the way that these services are organized with other components of health care delivery systems have a great impact on families with CSHCN. When mental health services are unavailable, the expense of caring for CSHCN who have an associated mental illness will certainly increase and be borne disproportionately by families.

Two questions remain: 1) How can we be sure that these mental health services are available and coordinated with the other services in a fashion that best meets the needs of these families and their children? 2) Will our society rise to this challenge or continue to leave this burden on the shoulders of families?

OUT-OF-POCKET EXPENSES FOR FAMILIES

The next section discusses insurance coverage for CSHCN. But first we must examine the out-of-pocket expenses for families with a CSHCN that are not covered by insurance. These expenses often are considerable and underestimated from claims data reports. Health care plans or claims data information can provide information on copayments or the differences between charges and actual reimbursements, but not the costs incurred by a family for added supportive services for the child or home and transportation expenses to meet certain disabilities requirements.

There are two important considerations that must be recognized in any discussion of out-of-pocket costs to families, and they are directly related to the severity of the child's condition and the child's functional impairment. The first consideration is the financial impact of a child with a chronic condition on the family's current income, and the second is the fact that support for conditions, such as mental health care and dental care, are poorly covered by all insurance programs.

Impact on Family Income

When a family in which both adults are employed has a child with special health care needs, the parents' employment patterns may change dramatically, depending on the child's condition and the long-term complexity of the condition. Additional home care and supervision needs often require one adult member of the family to limit employment or require the family to find a source of additional income to pay for the necessary care. Decisions have to be made concerning which family member is the most appropriate caregiver and which has the income and insurance package that best meets the medical needs of the child.

When a single parent has a child with special needs, he or she will in all probability need to stay employed and may also have to obtain additional resources to meet the added costs for home care or supervision of the child. If the parent finds that there are no other resources available, the remaining option may be to rely on Temporary Assistance for Needy Families (TANF), known as welfare, and/or Medicaid support. Families may be faced with unexpected expenses, such as home remodeling to accommodate limitations in mobility, and additional service needs for their child. Transportation methods may need to change, and there may be a need to pay for certain special equipment and nutritional requirements. Insurance may not cover these specific expenses, forcing the family to make even more difficult employment and financial decisions (Heck & Makuc, 2000).

Kuhlthau and colleagues have confirmed these financial challenges. After analyzing the 2001 National Survey of Children with Special Health Care Needs, they reported that a little more than 40% of CSHCN families have one or more financial problems associated with having a CSHCN. A little more than 10% of the CSHCN families spent more than $1,000 in the year just prior to the survey on their child's medical care, and for 20% of CSHCN families, the added expense created financial problems directly related to this care. Eighteen percent of the overall sample of CSHCN families needed additional income, yet more than 25% reduced their work hours and 13% had a family member stop work completely to be able to take care of their child. The range of those who reported one or more financial problems related to CSHCN was wide, from 18% of families with the least severe CSHCN to more than 72% of families with the most severe CSHCN (Kuhlthau, Hill, Yucel, & Perrin, 2005).

If a child is not covered sufficiently by employment-based insurance, and family income is insufficient to meet the child's basic needs, the principal safety net payer is Medicaid, but this program is available only to families who meet certain minimal income standards, which vary from state to state. In such situations, families will have to expend savings and other personal resources until they meet the income levels of that state's Medicaid requirement.

Inadequate Insurance Coverage

Approximately 65% of children with special health care needs are insured through private, employer-based health insurance plans. Nyman and colleagues at Mathematica Policy Research, Inc., have undertaken one of the few studies in claims data that examine the extent of family cost sharing (Nyman, Ireys, Wickstrom, & Rheault, 2004). They analyzed administrative claims data, using CRGs for more than 200,000 children younger than 19 years covered by a large employer-based managed care plan, from 1999 through 2001. They found that a family with a child with special health care needs pays 10.4% of insurance costs in the form of copayments and deductibles, and that this cost increased over the 3 years of the analysis. Average monthly family copayment costs increased in those 3 years from $24.60 per member per month (PMPM) in 1999 to $34.00 in 2001, an increase of 38.2%. This copayment increase was higher and more pronounced for families of children with complex and catastrophic conditions; the average PMPM copayment for them increased 51% over 3 years from $68.30 to $103.23 in 2001. In contrast, families of children with minor chronic conditions increased by 35.3% from only $18.17 PMPM copayments in 1999, to $24.59 in 2001 (see Table 3.1). The categories of services that accounted for the highest proportion of costs included mental health

Table 3.1. Monthly share of insurance costs per family

	Avg PMPM [*] 1999	Avg PMPM [*] 2001	Percent 3-year increase
All CSHCN	$24.60	$34.00	38.2%
Complex CSHCN	$68.30	$103.23	51.0%
Minor CSHCN	$18.17	$24.50	35.3%

Source: Nyman, Ireys, Wickstrom, & Rheault, 2004.
* PMPM: payment per member per month

Table 3.2.   Cost sharing for family by service

Category of service	Proportion of copays
Mental health	30.8%
Prescription drugs	25.5%
Primary care visits	17.4%

Source: Nyman, Ireys, Wickstrom, & Rheault, 2004.

services, 30.8%; prescription drugs, 25.5%; and primary care visits, 17.4% (see Table 3.2). The expenses outlined in this study related only to those expenses covered by the insurance plan and not other uncovered health care related expenses. Another study from the 2000 MEPS data, using the CSHCN screener as an identifier, analyzed the out-of-pocket expenses of families with CSHCN (Newacheck & Kim, 2005). This analysis found that, overall, families of children with a CSHCN spend $6.20 a year per $1,000 of family income in out-of-pocket expenses, twice the amount ($3.06) spent by families who do not have a CSHCN. They also showed that out-of-pocket expenses in excess of 5% of family income occurred in 2.62% of families who had a CSHCN compared with 1.59% of families who did not. When analyzed by income status, 5.9% of families whose income was below 200% of the federal poverty level (FPL) have out-of-pocket expenditures in excess of 5% of family income, compared with 0.72% of families with incomes between 200% and 399% FPL and 0.86% of families with income levels above 400% FPL. This analysis included the entire CSHCN population, 15.6% of all children, without distinguishing children with minor problems from those with more severe conditions.

There are two conclusions to draw from this analysis: 1) Families with a child with special health care needs pay a considerable amount of their income for out-of-pocket expenses, and this amount increases depending on the severity of their child's special health care needs and mental health status; and 2) The ability of a family to keep insurance coverage is highly dependent on employment status. In addition, important questions remain unanswered: What should be the safety net for families who have diminishing health insurance coverage and increasing out-of-pocket expenses? Must these families impoverish themselves more to meet publicly supported insurance eligibility standards? Where does public responsibility begin and private responsibility begin and end?

COST OF PRESCRIPTION MEDICATIONS

Health care costs in general are increasing at double-digit rates of inflation (National Coalition on Health Care, 2004). The causes of this inflation include the increased age of the population, the increased use of health care services, and increased pharmaceutical costs. There is very little information on the costs of prescription drugs for the childhood population and even less for children with chronic conditions.

Percentage of Overall Costs

Ireys and colleagues analyzed this issue using CRGs for a large sample of commercially insured children whose insurance package included prescription drug usage for 3 years, from 1999 though 2001. In this analysis of more than 200,000 children, the authors found that prescription drugs represent 13.5% of the PMPM cost of all services for children with chronic conditions, and that these percentages vary by condition status and age. This percentage was higher in the older age group—17.9% to 20.9% in the 6–19-year age group compared with 4.5% in the 0–5-year group—and tended to increase in parallel with the severity of the health condition (Ireys, Humensky, Wickstrom, & Rheault, 2004).

Increasing Costs of Prescription Medications

Ireys and colleagues' 3-year analysis showed that, while the use of pharmaceuticals increased by 8.1%, their cost increased by 56.3%, indicating that in children, it is the cost of prescription medicines rather than the amount used that is contributing to inflation. The overall cost of prescription drugs increased from $28.40 PMPM in 1999 to $44.40 PMPM in 2001, and was exceeded only by the cost of inpatient care, which was $91.00 PMPM. Ireys and colleagues also found that prescriptions for central nervous system (CNS)/psychiatric medications were the most frequently prescribed pharmaceuticals and accounted for 32.2% of the entire prescription drug cost for children with chronic conditions. Finally, the number of medications used was high for children with chronic conditions. Each child with a chronic condition averaged 10 unique prescriptions in 2001 (Ireys et al., 2004).

The implications of this study are considerable, and many issues warrant further evaluation, including the increasing dependence of CSHCN on CNS/psychiatric medications and the ability or willingness of insurers to sustain this inflationary trend. Is the use of these medications appropriate? Can and should the use, and especially the cost, of individual prescription medications be controlled? Might improved access to and the quality of mental health services for children help reduce medication use?

COSTS TO PROVIDERS

The availability, provision, and continuity of comprehensive care management services for children with chronic conditions are considered essential to achieving better health, improved outcomes, and lower overall costs. Practitioners and other health care providers must receive appropriate reimbursement for the coordination of care they provide to CSHCN. Otherwise, this coordination will not occur or will need to be subsidized by another source. The entire medical home concept, addressed in Chapter 6 of this book, is based on the principle that children, especially those with special health care needs, require coordinated and comprehensive care to reduce the impact of these conditions on the child's health and the family's associated costs. Starfield and Shi, in a comprehensive review of the literature, concluded that a medical home with four essential features (accessibility for first contact care; long-term, person-focused care; comprehensive care; family orientation) correlates with better health outcomes on both an individual and population levels, as well as with lower overall costs and less disparity of care (Starfield & Shi, 2004). Gaps in insurance coverage, as well as in overall insurance status, are directly related to access and continuity of primary care (Kogan et al., 1995; Newacheck, Stoddard, Hughes, & Pearl, 1998). Starfield and Shi also concluded that insurance alone does not guarantee an appropriate medical home (Starfield & Shi, 2004).

Costs Related to Care Coordination

Care coordination, however, requires time and effort that is not generally reimbursed to practices through most private and public health insurance packages. Because there is a wide variety in costs and needs of CSHCN by condition and severity status, practitioners who provide comprehensive care management services for families of children with severe and complex conditions are at a distinct disadvantage financially compared with practitioners who either provide no comprehensive coordinated care and/or who have in their practices a small number of families who have children with more complex chronic conditions. This disadvantage will be accentuated as parents seek out practitioners who provide the most comprehensive care management. Without a method to identify and reimburse the extra costs accompanying care management services for these children, very few providers will be able to deliver needed care and still survive without some type of financial subsidization.

Richard Antonelli has been one of the few pediatricians to carefully document the estimated cost of unreimbursed time spent providing care and coordinated services for CSHCN in a community-based, general pediatric practice (Antonelli & Antonelli, 2004). During a 95-day study period, he documented 774 encounters for 444 separate patients who would benefit from care-coordination activities. The 11% of patients with the most complex conditions accounted for 25% of these encounters, which required four times more time per patient than encounters with children who had less complex conditions. Fifty-one percent of the encounters were for problems not typically thought of as medical (e.g., coordinating activities at school, providing oversight for psychosocial issues). The estimated unreimbursed care for the pediatric office for this coordination ranged from $22,809 to $33,048 a year.

Methods of Reimbursement

Although many insurance companies are aware of this issue, unfortunately, there are few, if any, methods to provide a consistent and acceptable system for reimbursement. This includes a uniform method to identify CSHCN according to severity level as well as agreement between providers and insurance companies on appropriate reimbursement and the most effective methods of care coordination. Finally, there should be agreement on acceptable outcome measures to assess the effectiveness of care coordination. Development of methods to evaluate long-term health and functional outcomes of the child, cost reductions over time, and emotional and economic viability of families is crucial.

The provision of coordinated comprehensive care takes professional time. The studies above demonstrate that if professional time is not reimbursed appropriately, coordination of care for CSHCN and their families may not occur within our health care delivery systems. Two questions must be answered: How do we identify and measure these activities and who will pay for them?

SOURCES OF FUNDING FOR HEALTH CARE

Health care funding for CSHCN is complex and uneven. It often is far from adequate, and, even when it is adequate, it may be discontinued due to changes in the insurance status of a child's parents, or, in the case of state or federal insurance, changes in the statutes that support state or federal insurance. The two general sources of health insurance for children are private employer-based insurance and government insurance programs. Unfortunately, neither has as its basic or even secondary goal the support of children with chronic conditions. While there are many sources of private insurance that can be purchased individually or are provided by an employer, government insurance is available primarily through Medicaid, State Children's Health Insurance Program (SCHIP), Supplemental Security Income (SSI), and, to a limited degree, MCHB Title V funds. (See Chapter 2 for more on these programs.)

To fund the care of a child with special health care needs, a family member has to work for an employer who provides insurance for dependent children, and this insurance must include a benefits package that meets the requirements of the child's specific condition. If this is not available, families are dependent on their own resources to purchase private insurance or to seek public support that generally has income eligibility standards or strict disability standards that must be met. Medicaid is funded generally, but with some variability, by formulas that provide approximately 50% from the federal government and 50% from the state. States establish rules for eligibility, reimbursement policies, and medical care coverage within existing federal guidelines. Originally, Medicaid was designed to support poor families and had very strict income requirements, often below and not exceeding 100% FPL. The SCHIP program was initiated in the late 1990s to provide insurance coverage for children who had no insurance but who were living in families with incomes above Medicaid income limits. SSI was designed to provide support for the people with disabilities and requires strict disability standards for eligibility. Title V funds also have disability standards for eligibility and are set individually by state. Title V funds, however, are not available for reimbursable patient care in states selecting to use these funds for non-direct patient care services (health information and assessment).

Another important issue is that the expenses of Medicaid, SSI, and SCHIP, the major public support programs for children, are shared to a significant degree by states. On the one hand, these health care expenditures represent a high proportion of state budgets. On the other hand, the expenses of Medicare and the health program of the Veteran's Administration system (VA)—the programs that provide the major medical support systems for the elderly and veterans—are supported entirely by the federal government and not by states. Eligibility for Medicare and VA support also do not require individuals to meet income eligibility standards, while all of the programs that support children do.

Patterns and degrees of dependency on public support vary according to ethnic status and whether or not a family has a CSHCN. Overall, in 2003, 61% of all children were covered by employer-based insurance, 27% by public insurance, and 12% were uninsured (Kaiser Family Foundation, 2004). When these rates were analyzed according to health and economic status, the results showed distinct differences be-

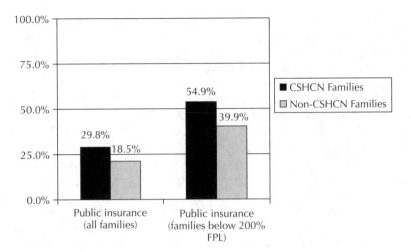

Figure 3.5. Likelihood of obtaining public insurance for CSHCN and non-CSHCN families. *Source:* Davidoff, 2004.

tween families with and without a CSHCN (Davidoff, 2004). CSHCN families were more likely to have public insurance than non-CSHCN families, 29.8% vs. 18.5%. For those below 200% FPL, 54.9% of CSHCN families were covered by public insurance compared with 39.9% of non-CSHCN families (see Figure 3.5).

Another analysis of the National Survey of CSHCN in 2001 (Honberg, McPherson, Strickland, Gage, & Newacheck, 2005) reported on the adequacy of insurance coverage for CSHCN using three essential components: 1) insurance had to be present at the time of interview, 2) coverage had to be continuous for the preceding 12 months, and 3) insurance had to be adequate from the family's perspective. In this analysis, only 59.6% of families of CSHCN reported meeting all three components. According to ethnic status, 45.2% of Hispanic, 57.6% of non-Hispanic Black, and 62.5% of White families of CSHCN met all three components of adequate insurance coverage. These ethnic differences were probably driven in part by the differences in the availability of health care services for these population groups.

Insurance Programs

The following is an outline, including strengths and weaknesses, of the various insurance programs that are available to CSHCN.

Employer-Based Insurance

Even though employers can be sympathetic to the need to provide coverage for CSHCN, the financial realities they face may prevent them from providing this support (Kaiser Family Foundation, 2004). Private industry must compete nationally and internationally, and costs must be carefully controlled. For small businesses, the margin of success may be so narrow that any added health insurance costs may make the difference between success and failure. Consequently, companies often find that they have to restrict coverage by

- Eliminating coverage for dependents entirely

- Increasing copays and deductibles

- Eliminating or decreasing the availability of certain specialty services

- Limiting or eliminating coverage for prescription drugs

- Decreasing or eliminating mental health and dental support

- Decreasing lifetime benefits (Kaiser Family Foundation, 2004; McManus, Fox, Perry, Stark, & Kennel, 1999)

In addition, there are a growing number of partially employed individuals who may not have any insurance at all because they do not meet employment standards (Collins, Davis, Doty, & Ho, 2004).

The strengths of employer-based insurance are realized if an adult family member has full insurance coverage for a child through work and also has a sympathetic employer. In such a case, there are no income eligibility requirements, and employment may provide some form of stability for the family. Weaknesses stem from the fact that because of current market pressures, the trend is for employers to decrease coverage: Dependents may not be covered, families may have to pay more out-of-pocket expenses, and continuity of coverage will depend upon continuity of employment.

Public Insurance

When employer-based insurance is unavailable or inadequate to meet the needs of CSHCN families, the only other resource is public insurance: Medicaid, Supplemental Security Income (SSI), State Children's Health Insurance Program (SCHIP), and the Title V program.

Medicaid

Medicaid is the principal public insurance source for children with chronic conditions and includes a wide range of benefits to cover the needs of these children. Medicaid originally was designed to provide a safety net for the poor, and consequently it has very strict income eligibility standards that vary from state to state. In time, in addition to supporting the poor, the program has in fact become the major safety net for people with disabilities and for the elderly requiring long-term care. The latter two groups, which do not include children, account for approximately 75% of Medicaid expenditures.

While Medicare is designed to cover the health care for people over 65, once a person needs long-term nursing care, families must provide this support from personal resources, additional long-term care insurance, or, as a last resort, Medicaid. This has put a significant burden on the Medicaid funds available for children. While children make up approximately 50% of Medicaid enrollees, they account for less than 25% of Medicaid expenditures. In 1996, more than one third of Medicaid's expenditures were for long-term care, 47% of the nation's $72 billion long-term nursing care bill (Feder, Lambrew, & Huckaby, 1997). This amount has increased over the past decade as the population has aged and is living longer.

Most states require a balanced budget, and Medicaid represents a major and growing part of states' budgets. When the pressures to cut Medicaid mount, children with and without special health care needs are competing for funds with adults in poverty, perinatal care, people with disabilities, and the elderly (Kuttner, 2005). In a broader sense, Medicaid funding is in competition with other state imperatives such as education, transportation, corrections, public health, and social services. States are responding in a variety of ways to this funding pressure, including but not limited to decreasing enrollments, increasing copayments, decreasing SCHIP programs, freezing reimbursement rates for physicians, and decreasing or excluding benefits such as nutritional supplements; ancillary therapies; and dental, vision, and mental health services (Ku, Nathanson, Park, Cox, & Broaddus, 2003). All of these measures affect families of CSHCN and leave them with no other source for these services except their own limited resources. The changes expose families with CSHCN to very unstable systems of support and undermine the long-term viability of Medicaid's safety net role (Berman, 2003; Huang, Kogan, Yu, & Strickland, 2005; Kogan et al., 1995; Newacheck, Pearl, Hughes, & Halfon, 1998; Weller, Minkovitz, & Anderson, 2003).

Supplemental Security Income

The Supplemental Security Income (SSI) program, established in 1972, is a means-tested, income-assistance program authorized by Title XVI of the Social Security Act and administered by the Social Security Administration (SSA; Social Security Act Amendments of 1972). SSI provides federal monthly cash payments for populations of the elderly, the blind, and people with disabilities following national standards of financial and health needs assessment. The Social Security Act intended that these populations would no longer have to subsist on below poverty-level incomes. Although national criteria were established, there was considerable local interpretation of who qualified as having disabilities. Once enrolled in SSI, Medicaid was a source of health care, while the federal government provided supplemental income.

By the early 1980s, approximately 200,000 children in the United States were covered by SSI. From 1990 to 1995, because of improved eligibility and broad interpretation of standards, childhood caseloads increased by 197%, from approximately 300,000 children in 1990 to more than 950,000 in 1995 (Schmidt, 2004). By 1997, a little more than one million children, 1.35% of all children in the United States, were on SSI (Loprest, 1997). This support was provided disproportionately to children with complex physical needs and high health care expenditures (Kuhlthau, Perrin, Ettner, McLaughlin, & Gortmaker, 1998; Neff et al., 2001; Perrin, Kuhlthau, McLaughlin, Ettner, & Gortmaker, 1999). In 1996, as part of the Personal Responsibility and Work Opportunity Reconciliation Act, and in response to the increasing enrollment of children in SSI, eligibility standards changed, placing greater emphasis on diagnostic or physical rather than functional criteria (Personal Responsibility and Work Opportunity Reconciliation Act, 1996).

The effect of this legislation was to decrease the enrollment of children in SSI by 135,000 and then effectively freeze the number enrolled at 1997 levels. In 2003, the level of enrollment of SSI children had just reached the 1996 level of about 1,000,000 children (Schmidt, 2004). It is likely that the restriction created by new eligibility standards, and the emphasis on physical rather than functional criteria, resulted in more children on SSI with medically expensive physical conditions such as cerebral palsy, quadriplegia, and multiple birth defects, in contrast with children who had less medically expensive disorders such as learning and mental impairments. The cash payments to children from the federal government may have stayed the same as part of welfare reform because enrollment has not increased, but in all probability, the average per child SSI health care expense has increased because of the increase in medical complexity of the children enrolled. This certainly has contributed in part to the SSI component of Medicaid inflation.

SSI, therefore, is not a safety net that can be expected to cover an increasing number of CSHCN. In a survey of children with disabilities under Medicaid in New York City in 1999 and 2000, 85% live in families with incomes of less than $20,000 a year (Long & Coughlin, 2005). If national patterns continue, more children with disabilities will be enrolled in Medicaid, not SSI, thus increasing the level of complexity of the Medicaid children and the per person expenditure. These families also will not have the benefit of cash assistance. The SSI program may not ensure that the nation's children with disabilities will live above the poverty level.

State Children's Health Insurance Program

In 1998, the U.S. government initiated a State Children's Health Insurance Program (SCHIP), which was designed to increase the number of insured children to include those at and above 200% of the poverty level. Incentives were provided in the form of an increase in general matching federal funds, and considerable latitude was provided for states to establish guidelines for enrollments, eligibility, benefits, and general cost sharing (Davidoff, Kenney, & Dubay, 2005; Fox, Levtov, & McManus, 2003). There has been broad and nearly universal statewide participation in this program, with states operating separate SCHIP programs either exclusively or in combination with Medicaid SCHIP programs. Most states have designed their programs to provide generous coverage with comprehensive benefit packages, but some states have limited their coverage to exclude ancillary therapies, home health care, durable equipment, and dental and mental health services. Most states also have imposed some form of cost sharing in the form of premiums or copayments for those with income levels above 150% FPL (Fox et al., 2003).

While SCHIP did result in a significant increase in the number of children with health insurance, the effect on CSHCN has been limited. In many states, funding from this program has been separate from Medicaid funding, and the benefits for CSHCN have not been as comprehensive as Medicaid benefits and have required cost sharing by families. Because of budgetary constraints, states are restricting SCHIP coverage even further. This can result in CSHCN facing more gaps in accessing needed services (Davidoff et al., 2005).

Title V Funds

Enacted as part of the Social Security Act of 1935, Title V is one of the nation's oldest health programs. Over the years, Title V has been implemented by states to improve all aspects of maternal and child care, including direct support for "children with crippling conditions." In 1981, Title V was incorporated into Maternal and Child Health Service Block Grants, and the term *crippled children* was changed to *children with special health care needs*. Over time, the use of Title V funds has expanded, allowing states the flexibility to support a wide variety of programs (Marcus, Rosenbaum, & Cyprien, 2004; see Chapter 7). A consequence of this expansion is that funding for direct support of medical care of CSHCN has diminished. In fact, some states no longer use these funds for direct medical services at all because they are considered to be duplicative of Medicaid support. Title V funds are available in some states for care of specific chronic conditions, but they are no longer the safety net that was once conceived, and they do not necessarily fill in the health care delivery gaps that CSHCN face (Marcus, Rosenbaum, & Cyprien).

Of all publicly and privately funded health insurance programs, Medicaid remains the most critical and reliable source of financial support for families with children with special health care needs. Any decrease in benefits from that source generally leaves families of CSHCN with no publicly or privately funded avenue of support. If Medicaid is inadequate what will be available for these families? If the intention of the federal government in the 1970s was to ensure that no families of children with disabilities live below the poverty line, what is the intention now?

MANAGED CARE INITIATIVES

In the early 1990s, as a result of a national effort to reform Medicaid and control costs, many states developed initiatives to contract directly with health care plans to provide managed care services and to distribute costs fairly according to risk.

Managed Care Contracts

Instead of following past practices of contracting directly with individual physicians for care of Medicaid patients, states developed managed care contracts with health care plans that would then be responsible for managing the care of these patients. States offered broad and variable quality assurance measures to be sure that appropriate care would be provided. For the first time, many Medicaid children were assigned a primary care provider. It was the expectation of the states and the federal government that these arrangements would reduce the existing double-digit inflation rate within the Medicaid program.

While in some ways these changes were welcome and beneficial, leading, for example, to more children with a designated primary care provider, they did not take into account the great variation in expenses that occurs as a result of the presence of chronic conditions, as well as the potential financial disadvantage to plans or programs that attract children with these conditions (e.g., plans associated with academic centers, hospitals that traditionally have taken care of the poor and disabled). In addition, quality assurance measures were inadequate to provide uniform and comprehensive protection for these children

(American Academy of Pediatrics, 1998; Neff & Anderson, 1995). If a plan, excluding administrative reimbursement, provided an annual payment for direct patient care in the range of $1,000 a year per child, and nearly 88% of children fall below that expenditure, then the providers for these basically healthy children will benefit considerably, while the providers for the remaining 12% of children who have special health care needs may lose significant revenue (Shenkman et al., 2001).

There are several potential solutions to this problem. One is to be sure that CSHCN are distributed evenly throughout all plans so that no one plan is disadvantaged. Other possible solutions include the development of risk adjustors that adjust projected payments according to the past analysis of costs, reinsurance programs that provide extra insurance for the very expensive patients, and exclusions (carve-outs) of certain population groups that can be expected to have high long-term costs. While in theory these solutions should help develop appropriate payment systems, in fact, all have major limitations (Shenkman et al., 2001).

Risk-Adjustment Method

Risk-adjustment payments are not highly predictive of expenditures and have been developed primarily for the adult Medicare population. There are two studies—one by Hwang, Ireys, and Anderson (2001) and the other by Madden, Mackay, and Skillman (2001)—that have evaluated several risk adjustment capitation payment systems in childhood populations. While the risk adjustment methods are somewhat comparable and significantly better than methods that use only age and sex, they are still not highly predictive of childhood expenditures year to year.

Reinsurance and Carve-Outs

Reinsurance is another method used to provide insurance payments to plans for children with very high expenditures. These insurance payments provide separate payments for the small number of patients with expenditures at the high end—greater than $50,000 per child per year. Carve-outs are arrangements that exempt (carve out) from managed care groups of children who can be expected to incur unusually high costs. These exemptions have been used only for a select group of CSHCN (e.g., SSI enrollees, foster care children, Title V recipients, children with HIV/AIDs). These children represent a very small portion of CSHCN.

At present, the methods to project future payments that include reinsurance, coupled with health status risk-adjusted payments, provide a better method of matching payments with health expenditures than the more commonly used methods that are based only on demographic conditions (e.g., age and sex) (Shenkman et al., 2001). Even with these adjustments, there may not be sufficient financial protection for plans that enroll a disproportionately expensive population.

Payments to Providers

Even if Medicaid patients could be evenly distributed by severity status among plans with optimal risk adjustment, payments from the plan to individual providers may not reflect the cost spectrum of patients in that provider's practice. We simply do not know the best way to determine how to distribute resources to individual practitioners within plans so that revenue matches expenses incurred for caring for a large number of patients at the high end of the severity spectrum.

One of the major underlying problems in all reimbursement strategies is that at the time contracted managed care was initiated for the Medicaid population in the early 1990s, the fee-for-service reimbursement rates for primary physicians taking care of Medicaid patients were very low and generally below reimbursement levels from commercial plans and Medicare. All of the newly initiated managed care methods did not infuse new revenue into the system to correct this inequity but counted on savings to provide incentives. The initial goals of Medicaid-managed care were to direct Medicaid patients to primary care providers and to reduce the episodic use of emergency rooms and urgent care facilities, not necessarily to improve care management for those with chronic conditions. During the 1990s, managed-care strategies, even without adequate risk adjustment, seemed to work as planned, reducing unnecessary utilization of services. This was especially true for children with ambulatory care-sensitive conditions—conditions that should be cared for in a primary care setting, which could decrease the use of the emergency services or hospital visits. During the mid-1990s, states experienced reduced (single-digit) inflation in Medicaid, and those plans that contracted for Medicaid patients in capitated arrangements did fairly well. These financial gains did not continue and were not passed on to primary care physicians frequently enough to correct old, inequitable patterns of reimbursement.

Return of Health Care Inflation

By the end of the 1990s, health care inflation returned, and by the year 2000, Medicaid expenses were back to double-digit increases. Capitated managed care achieved financial gains via reduced hospital and emergency department utilization to a certain point, but further reductions in utilization, in order to experience an ongoing annual reduction in costs, could not be sustained. In addition, there had been insufficient efforts to control the real drivers of health care inflation—the costs of medication and new technology, the increasing aging and chronic illnesses in the population, and the use of long-term care nursing facilities—all of which were a continuing drain on Medicaid resources. Without increases in Medicaid contracts from the states, many private health plans could not afford to continue to care for Medicaid patients and thus ceased to contract for the state's Medicaid population (Fox, Limb, McManus, & Levtov, 2005).

The result has been that certain plans, primarily those associated with community health centers or university academic plans, have contracted for Medicaid patients, their historic patient base, while other health plans have restricted their coverage to contracts for patients with commercial health insurance. Consequently, as plans have changed focus and Medicaid programs have been forced to move patients from one plan to another, there have been growing gaps in access to care and in insurance coverage for children, especially those with chronic conditions.

Thus, after a decade of efforts to manage patient care costs, families of children with chronic conditions are now left with a safety net, Medicaid, that cannot actually ensure comprehensive and consistent access to the services they need. Two important questions remain: How can families of CSHCN be ensured access to adequate primary and specialty care services? How can contractual agreements with the private sector be created to assure individual providers adequate support for the care and coordination of care that are so essential for optimal health outcomes?

WHAT FAMILIES CAN DO

Unfortunately, coverage of health care for CSHCN is often both fragmented and inadequate. The existing systems of financial support are subjected to the changing fortunes of employer-based insurance and political differences over the extent and depth of public support. There is no national agenda beyond the MCHB to provide children who have special health care needs with coverage that is present for all, adequate, and continuous. This leaves both providers and families in positions of vulnerability and requires considerable personal effort and planning to obtain the best support possible. In view of this, families are advised to take the following six steps to the best of their ability:

1. Be knowledgeable about the insurance coverage for their child and its potential limitations.

2. Be knowledgeable about the extent of the family's out-of-pocket expenses in order to budget carefully.

3. Explore every possible avenue of support for both family and child.

4. Engage in long-term financial planning.

5. Find the best possible medical home for the child with access to well-coordinated medical care, and work with providers to obtain optimal coverage for the child.

6. As much as possible, join practitioners and child advocacy groups in their efforts to obtain continuous and adequate health care coverage with access to services for all children, especially CSHCN.

CONCLUSION

Children with special health care needs, approximately 10% to 16% of the childhood population, are considerably more expensive to care for than healthy children, and they consume a high percentage of the health resources devoted to children. Their medical care costs increase according to the type and severity of their conditions and to the presence of complicating mental health illnesses.

Families of children with special health care needs are stressed by increasing financial burdens because of vulnerability of employment, their dependence on employment based-insurance, their rising out-of-pocket expenses, decreasing benefits, and long-term insurance limits. Furthermore, the principal safety net, Medicaid, is not available unless families meet certain poverty level limits. It may be restricted to certain plans and even then will not necessarily ensure comprehensive access to care, especially for mental health conditions. The health care system has been characterized by the Institute of Medicine as a system in crisis (Institute of Medicine, 2001). In the current situation, the following trends seem to be intensifying:

- Health care costs are escalating at double-digit rates of inflation without clear short- or long-term solutions in either the public or private sector.

- Employers are reducing insurance costs to be competitive in global commercial markets. They are reducing coverage for children and reducing lifetime insurance limits and benefits.

- CSHCN are increasingly dependent on Medicaid—the insurance of last resort—as a safety net.

- State governments, faced with escalating Medicaid costs, are under great pressure to reduce expenditures and are being forced to choose among the elderly, the poor, chronically ill adults, healthy children, children with special health care needs and chronic conditions, and other essential state services.

- Families of CSHCN are under considerable financial stress to care for their children. Any addition to their financial burden decreases their socioeconomic status, productivity, and ability to care for their child.

- Practitioners who are not appropriately compensated for the care of CSHCN are not able to provide the comprehensive coordinated service these children require.

- The numbers of CSHCN who do not receive comprehensive coordinated care is increasing. This has resulted in an upsurge in the use of emergency and hospital services, which adds costs to the health care system.

- Children and families with escalating financial and health burdens will add to the Medicaid enrollment and its per-child complexity of illness and expenditures. This increase in the Medicaid burden will add to inflation, and, without added revenue, will lead to another round of cost and health care containment measures, reductions in services, and an increased and costly use of hospital and emergency services. Unless these trends are reversed, CSHCN and their families will not be ensured access to the three components necessary for the services they need: presence of insurance, continuity of coverage, and adequate coverage.

Providing comprehensive, coordinated services for families of children with special health care needs is essential and remains the responsibility of all of us. The ultimate outcome that we all should seek is to help these children meet their maximum potential as adults. Our society can only improve if we are able help them attain this goal. If, however, we allow these children to become adults without reaching their potential in large part because of an inadequate health care system, the burden of their care will increase accordingly for all of us and especially for the next generation. We will be judged by our accomplishments on behalf of these vulnerable children.

REFERENCES

American Academy of Pediatrics: Committee on Disabilities. (1998). Managed care and children with special health care needs: A subject review. *Pediatrics*, *102*(3), 657–660.

Antonelli, R.C., & Antonelli, D.M. (2004). Providing a medical home: The cost of care coordination services in a community-based, general pediatric practice. *Pediatrics, 113*(Suppl. 5), 1522–1528.

Berman, S. (2003). Is Medicaid, the largest insurer of children with special health care needs, in danger? *Pediatrics, 112*(3 Pt. 1), 668–669.

Bethell, C.D., Read, D., Stein, R.E., Blumberg, S.J., Wells, N., & Newacheck, P.W. (2002). Identifying children with special health care needs: Development and evaluation of a short screening instrument. *Ambulatory Pediatrics, 2*(1), 38–48.

Collins, S.R., Davis, K., Doty, M.M., & Ho, A. (2004). *Wages, health benefits, and workers' health.* New York: The Commonwealth Fund; http://www.cmwf.org/usr_doc/Collins_workers_IB_788.pdf

Davidoff, A.J. (2004). Insurance for children with special health care needs: Patterns of coverage and burden on families to provide adequate insurance. *Pediatrics, 114*(2), 394–403.

Davidoff, A.J., Kenney, G., & Dubay, L. (2005). Effects of the state children's health insurance program expansions on children with chronic health conditions. *Pediatrics, 116*(1), e34–42.

Feder, J., Lambrew, J., & Huckaby, M. (1997). Medicaid and long-term care for the elderly: Implications of restructuring. *The Milbank Quarterly, 75*(4), 425–459.

Fox, H.B., Levtov, R.G., & McManus, M.A. (2003). *Eligibility, benefits, and cost-sharing in separate SCHIP programs* (No. 6). Washington, DC: Maternal and Child Health Policy Research Center.

Fox, H.B., Limb, S.J., McManus, M.A., & Levtov, R.G. (2005). *An analysis of states' capitation methods and pediatric rates, 1997–2003.* Washington, DC: Maternal and Child Health Policy Research Center; http://www.mchpolicy.org/publications/documents/MCHPolicyResearchCenterReport.PDF

Heck, K.E., & Makuc, D.M. (2000). Parental employment and health insurance coverage among school-aged children with special health care needs. *Am J Public Health, 90*(12), 1856–1860.

Honberg, L., McPherson, M., Strickland, B., Gage, J.C., & Newacheck, P.W. (2005). Assuring adequate health insurance: Results of the National Survey of Children with Special Health Care Needs. *Pediatrics, 115*(5), 1233–1239.

Huang, Z.J., Kogan, M.D., Yu, S.M., & Strickland, B. (2005). Delayed or forgone care among children with special health care needs: An analysis of the 2001 National Survey of Children with Special Health Care Needs. *Ambulatory Pediatrics, 5*(1), 60–67.

Hughes, J.S., Averill, R.F., Eisenhandler, J., Goldfield, N.I., Muldoon, J., Neff, J.M., et al. (2004). Clinical Risk Groups (CRGs): A classification system for risk-adjusted capitation-based payment and health care management. *Medical Care, 42*(1), 81–90.

Humensky, J., Ireys, H.T., Wickstrom, S., & Rheault, P. (2004). *Mental health services for children with special health care needs in commercial managed care, 1999–2001.* Washington, DC: Mathematica Policy Research; http://www.mathematica-mpr.com/publications/PDFs/menhlthchil.pdf

Hwang, W., Ireys, H.T., & Anderson, G.F. (2001). Comparison of risk adjusters for Medicaid enrolled children with and without chronic health conditions. *Ambulatory Pediatrics 1*(4), 217–224.

Institute of Medicine (2001). *Crossing the quality chasm: A new health system for the 21st century.* Washington, DC: National Academies Press.

Ireys, H.T., Humensky, J., Wickstrom, S., & Rheault, P. (2004). *Prescription drugs for children with special health care needs in commercial managed care: Patterns of use and cost, 1999–2001.* Washington, DC: Mathematic Policy Research. http://www.mathematica-mpr.com/PDFs/prescription.pdf

Ireys, H.T., Humensky, J., Peterson, E., Wickstrom, S., Manda, B., & Rheault, P. (2002). *Children with special health care needs in commercial managed care: patterns of service use and cost;* http://www.mathematica-mpr.com/publications/PDFs/childrenspecial.pdf

Kaiser Family Foundation. (2004). *Health coverage for low-income children.* Washington, DC: Author; http://www.kff.org/uninsured/upload/Health-Coverage-for-Low-Income-Children-September-2004-UPDATE.pdf

Kogan, M.D., Alexander, G.R., Teitelbaum, M.A., Jack, B.W., Kotelchuck, M., & Pappas, G. (1995). The effect of gaps in health insurance on continuity of a regular source of care among preschool-aged children in the United States. *Journal of the American Medical Association, 274*(18), 1429–1435.

Ku, L., Nathanson, M., Park, E., Cox, L., & Broaddus, M. (2003). *Proposed state Medicaid cuts would jeopardize health insurance coverage for one million people.* Washington, DC: Center on Budget and Policy Priorities; http://www.cbpp.org/12-23-02health.pdf

Kuhlthau, K., Hill, K.S., Yucel, R., & Perrin, J.M. (2005). Financial burden for families of children with special health care needs. *Maternal and Child Health Journal, 9*(2), 207–218.

Kuhlthau, K., Perrin, J.M., Ettner, S.L., McLaughlin, T.J., & Gortmaker, S.L. (1998). High-expenditure children with Supplemental Security Income. *Pediatrics, 102*(3 Pt. 1), 610–615.

Kuttner, R. (2005, February 16). Taming the Medicaid monster. *Boston Globe,* p. 1.

Long, S.K., & Coughlin, T.A. (2005). Access to care for disabled children under Medicaid. *Health Care Finance Review, 26*(2), 89–103.

Loprest, P.J. (1997). *Supplemental security income for children with disabilities: Part of the federal safety net* (No. A-10). Washington, DC: Urban Institute; http://www.urban.org/url.cfm?ID=307041

Madden, C.W., Mackay, B.P., Skillman, S.M. (2001) *Measuring health status for risk adjusting capitation payments.* Hamilton, NJ: Center for Health Care Strategies; http://www.chcs.org/publications3960/publications_show.htm?doc_id=211914

Marcus, A., Rosenbaum, S., & Cyprien, S. (2004). *SCHIP-enrolled children with special health care needs: An assessment of coordination efforts between state SCHIP and Title V programs* (No. 7035). Menlo Park, CA: The Henry J. Kaiser Family Foundation; http://www.kff.org/medicaid/upload/SCHIP-Enrolled-Children-with-Special-Health-Care-Needs.pdf

McManus, M.A., Fox, H.B., Perry, M., Stark, E., & Kennel, S. (1999). *Private health insurance coverage for children: A survey of 450 employers.* Washington, DC: Maternal Child Health Policy Research Center; http://www.mchpolicy.org/publications/pdfs/report1.pdf

McPherson, M., Arango, P., Fox, H., Lauver, C., McManus, M., Newacheck, P.W., et al. (1998). A new definition of children with special health care needs. *Pediatrics, 102*(1 Pt. 1), 137–140.

Medical Expenditure Panel Survey (MEPS). (2000). *MEPS HC-050 documentation. 2000 full year consolidated data file.* Retrieved June 29, 2006, from http://www.meps.ahcpr.gov

National Coalition on Health Care (2004). *Health insurance cost.* Retrieved June 29, 2006; http://www.nchc.org/facts/cost.shtml

Neff, J. M. (Fall 2002). Chronic conditions in children: A decade of change. *Children's Hospitals Today, 10,* 14–17. Retrieved July 13, 2006, from http://www.childrenshospitals.net/AM/Template.cfm?Section = Search&template = /CM/HTMLDisplay.cfm&ContentID = 10926

Neff, J.M., & Anderson, G. (1995). Protecting children with chronic illness in a competitive marketplace. *Journal of the American Medical Association, 274*(23), 1866–1869.

Neff, J.M., Muldoon, J.H., Gay, J.C., & Anderson, G.F. (2001). Profile of the SSI population enrolled in Washington State's Medicaid program with a diagnosis-based classification system: Managed care implications. *Journal of the Cost Quality and Quality Association, 7,* 1–15.

Neff, J.M., Sharp, V.L., Muldoon, J., Graham, J., & Myers, K. (2004). Profile of medical charges for children by health status group and severity level in a Washington State health plan. *Health Services Research, 39*(1), 73–89.

Neff, J.M., Sharp, V.L., Muldoon, J., Graham, J., Popalisky, J., & Gay, J.C. (2002). Identifying and classifying children with chronic conditions using administrative data with the clinical risk group classification system. *Ambulatory Pediatrics, 2*(1), 71–79.

Neff, J.M., Valentine, J., Park, A., Hicks-Thomson, J., Christakis, D.A., Muldoon, J., et al. (2002). Trends in pediatric hospitalizations of children in Washington State by insurance and chronic condition status, 1991–1998. *Archives of Pediatrics and Adolescent Medicine, 156*(7), 703–709.

Newacheck, P.W., & Kim, S.E. (2005). A national profile of health care utilization and expenditures for children with special health care needs. *Archives of Pediatric and Adolescent Medicine, 159*(1), 10–17; corrections: *Archives of Pediatric and Adolescent Medicine, 159*(4), 318.

Newacheck, P.W., Pearl, M., Hughes, D.C., & Halfon, N. (1998). The role of Medicaid in ensuring children's access to care. *Journal of the American Medical Association, 280*(20), 1789–1793.

Newacheck, P.W., Stoddard, J.J., Hughes, D.C., & Pearl, M. (1998). Health insurance and access to primary care for children. *New England Journal of Medicine, 338*(8), 513–519.

Nyman, R.M., Ireys, H.T., Wickstrom, S., & Rheault, P. (2004). *Family cost-sharing in employer-based managed care plans 1999–2001.* Washington, DC: Mathematica Policy Research; http://www.mathematica-mpr.com/publications/PDFs/familycost.pdf

Perrin, J.M., Kuhlthau, K., McLaughlin, T.J., Ettner, S.L., & Gortmaker, S.L. (1999). Changing patterns of conditions among children receiving Supplemental Security Income disability benefits. *Archives of Pediatric and Adolescent Medicine, 153*(1), 80–84.

Personal Responsibility and Work Opportunity Reconciliation Act (PRWORA) of 1996, PL 104-193, 42 U.S.C §§ 1305 *et seq.*

Schmidt, L. (2004). *Effects of welfare reform on Supplemental Security Income (SSI) program.* Ann Arbor: Gerald R. Ford School of Public Policy, University of Michigan; http://www.npc.umich.edu/publications/policy_briefs/brief4/brief4.pdf

Shenkman, E., Aydede, S., Dick, A. W., Sappington, D., Vogel, B., Youngblade, L., et al. (2004). *The development of financing and reimbursement strategies for children with special health care needs: A series overview.* Institute for Child

Health Policy, Gainesville, University of Florida; http://www.ichp.ufl.edu/documents/Overview%20reimbursement%20strategies.pdf

Shenkman, E., Vogel, B., Aydede, S., Wegener, D.S., Szilagyi, P.G., Dick, A., et al. (2001). *State strategies for financing CSHCN needs: How well do they work?* (No. 2). Gainesville: University of Florida; http://www.ichp.ufl.edu/documents/State%20Strategies.pdf

Social Security Act of 1935, PL 74-271, 42 U.S.C. §§ 301 *et seq.*

Social Security Act Amendments of 1972, PL 96–603, 42 U.S.C. §§ 1381–1383.

Spady, D.W., Schopflocher, D.P., Svenson, L.W., & Thompson, A.H. (2001). Prevalence of mental disorders in children living in Alberta, Canada, as determined from physician billing data. *Archives of Pediatric and Adolescent Medicine, 155*(10), 1153–1159.

Spady, D.W., Schopflocher, D.P., Svenson, L.W., & Thompson, A.H. (2005). Medical and psychiatric comorbidity and health care use among children 6 to 17 years old. *Archives of Pediatric and Adolescent Medicine, 159*(3), 231–237.

Starfield, B., & Shi, L. (2004). The medical home, access to care, and insurance: A review of evidence. *Pediatrics, 113*(Suppl. 5), 1493–1498.

Stewart, S.M., Rao, U., Emslie, G.J., Klein, D., & White, P. C. (2005). Depressive symptoms predict hospitalization for adolescents with type 1 diabetes mellitus. *Pediatrics, 115*(5), 1315–1319.

U.S. Department of Health and Human Services (USDHHS; 1999). *Mental health: A report of the surgeon general—Chapter 3 children and mental health.* Rockville, MD: USDHHS, Substance Abuse and Mental Health Services Administration, Center for Mental Health Services, National Institutes of Health, National Institute of Mental Health. http://www.surgeongeneral.gov/library/mentalhealth/chapter3/sec1.html

U.S. Department of Health and Human Services (USDHHS; 2004). *The National Survey of Children with Special Health Care Needs: Chapter 4 health care needs and access to care.* Health Resources and Service Administration, Maternal Child Health Bureau. Retrieved June 28, 2006, from http://mchb.hrsa.gov/chscn/pages/needs.htm#services

van Dyck, P.C., Kogan, M.D., McPherson, M.G., Weissman, G.R., & Newacheck, P.W. (2004). Prevalence and characteristics of children with special health care needs. *Archives of Pediatric and Adolescent Medicine, 158*(9), 884–890.

Weller, W.E., Minkovitz, C.S., & Anderson, G.F. (2003). Utilization of medical and health-related services among school-age children and adolescents with special health care needs (1994 National Health Interview Survey on Disability [NHIS-D] Baseline Data). *Pediatrics, 112*(3 Pt. 1), 593–603.

II

THE PARENT EXPERIENCE

Many of the problems that children with special health care needs (CSHCN) and their families experience stem from a lack of, or uneven access to, adequate primary care, preventive care, and specialist services. These problems often manifest themselves as systemic failures in communication and comprehensive care coordination. Many CSHCN have multiple medical complications, making management by a single physician, whether a primary care pediatrician or specialist, particularly difficult (Perrin, Kuhlthau, Gortmaker, Beal, & Ferris, 2002). Compounding the problem is the high degree of variability and complexity among programs and services utilized by CSHCN and their families and the extensive, intensive, and continuous interactions with the health care system that CSHCN and their families face.

Family caregivers may spend a great deal of time in various medical offices and clinics completing paperwork. They may have to actively search for physicians who are experienced with and knowledgeable about their child's complex needs, and they often have to battle with managed care organizations reluctant to provide the support needed for adequate care (Bryan & Burstein, 2002). The multitude of official entities and myriad funding requirements mean that families with CSHCN often have difficulty accessing services and may require assistance in obtaining them (American Academy of Pediatrics, Committee on Children With Disabilities, 1999). When the families are poor, of color, or culturally unfamiliar and uncomfortable with the biomedical model of illness and healing, barriers to quality care are magnified (Sobo, Seid, & Gelhard, 2006). In sum, parents of CSHCN must do many things other parents do not have to do—for example, fulfilling expanded roles as caregiver and knowledgeable advocate in partnership with health care professionals, in addition to satisfying the demands of managing households and families in a challenging sociocultural context.

Section II begins with a chapter by anthropologist Gail Landsman and nursing researcher Marcia Van Riper that addresses the way normal stresses of household life are compounded by the unique stresses that a CSHCN can add. Much current research focuses on the resiliency of families and their ability to recover from stressful life situations. Some of the issues highlighted in Chapter 4 include sources of stress such as increased time demands, changes in roles, additional caretaking responsibilities, and the mixed messages parents receive as they interact with adherents of a curative, biomedical model in the health care and early intervention systems.

Chapter 5 includes valuable first-hand information of the sort not generally shared in published papers. Parent advocate Nora Wells explains how parents of CSHCN learn to cope with the fragmentation and opaqueness of the health care system to access quality health care and help each child reach his or her maximum potential. After reviewing these processes, the chapter presents parent-derived strategies for advocacy within the health care system, and offers guidelines for support that can help parents adapt to the challenges of their roles. The chapter also suggests how providers can meet the information needs of the families they serve and discusses ways to build and support trusting partnerships between families and physicians.

REFERENCES

American Academy of Pediatrics, Committee on Children with Disabilities. (1999). Care coordination: Integrating health and related systems of care for children with special health care needs. *Pediatrics, 104*(4 Pt. 1), 978–981.

Bryan, T., & Burstein, K. (2002). *Parents as partners in the medical home helping children with special healthcare needs* (Exceptional Parent web site). Retrieved August 26, 2003, from http/:www.eparent.com/healthcare/medicalHome_hcsn.htm

Perrin, J.M., Kuhlthau, K.A., Gortmaker, S.L., Beal, A.C., & Ferris, T.G. (2002). Generalist and subspecialist care for children with chronic conditions. *Ambul Pediatr, 2*(6), 462–469.

Sobo, E.J., Seid, M., & Gelhard, L.R. (2006). Parent-identified barriers to pediatric health care: A process-oriented model and method. *Health Services Research, 41*(1),148–172.

4

Incorporating Children with Disabilities into Family Life

Gail Landsman and Marcia Van Riper

When a child is born with or develops impairments, the normal stresses of household life are compounded. This chapter outlines the main challenges associated with raising a young child with disabilities and provides an overview of our current knowledge concerning the impact on parents, siblings, and household systems. Cross-cultural variability in the meanings given to physical and cognitive differences and in how children with those differences are treated and incorporated into family life are considered, as are strategies for dealing with the variation of disabled children. Both positive and negative consequences of raising a child with disabilities will be discussed.

NOTE ON TERMINOLOGY

It should be noted from the outset that the terminology available to discuss these issues is laden with ambiguity and controversy. (See Chapter 1's discussion on terminology.)

Medical versus Social Focus of Terms

Special health care needs, impairment, disabling conditions, developmental delay, disability, and other current terms all carry particular connotations in particular contexts. For example, the term *children with special health care needs* (CSHCN) in general usage refers to children who have a chronic condition and who require health services of a type or amount beyond that required by typical children. The range of problems covered by this term is potentially quite broad. Does it include a child with vision problems that can be corrected with eyeglasses, or a child receiving orthodontia treatment over an extended period of time? In addition to its imprecision, the term (which does have a rather specific governmental definition; see Chapter 1) is rooted in a medical model or view that portrays a functional disability or a physical difference as an illness—i.e., as a medical problem within the child. This perspective implies that the child's difference is pathological, and that the appropriate response is to seek expert assistance from medical professionals to alleviate or eliminate an internal *defect*. It therefore focuses the parents' efforts on changing their child.

Many parents worry, however, that the problems faced by their child with physical, developmental, and/or cognitive differences have less to do with the child's medically defined health status than with society's negative response to those differences (see Landsman, 2005). Although they don't deny the existence of different health care needs associated with particular conditions, disability rights activists and scholars in the growing field of disability studies have argued that disability is primarily a consequence of societal barriers and discrimination rather than of health itself (Oliver, 1990; Read, 1998). Furthermore, the medical focus of the term *children with special health care needs* may appear to suggest the need or desire to provide not just health care appropriate to children with a particular chronic condition such as Down syndrome or cerebral palsy but also *cures* for those conditions. Although many parents do indeed seek cures, some parents and disability rights advocates interpret such cure-seeking behavior as attempts to eliminate diversity and as disrespectful to disabled people. For these reasons, in this chapter we do not regularly use the term *children with special health care needs*.

Alternative Terms

This is not to say that other available terms are without problems or controversy. The term *children with developmental delay* has the advantage of reflecting the inherent uncertainty of predictions about the eventual extent and/or permanence of a very young child's deviation from a measurable developmental norm, and many American parents prefer to use this term. In a society that values individual achievement and progress, its use may eliminate the stigma of labels implying that a child has reached a developmental plateau. However, physicians also report that the term *developmental delay* misleads, and many parents believe that it denies a child's individuality by measuring children against a standardized developmental sequence and rate (Landsman, 2003).

In response to such critiques, Russell Shuttleworth and Devva Kasnitz (2004, 2006) suggested the term *impairment-disability*. In their definition, *impairment* represents a "negatively construed, cultural perception of a bodily, cognitive, or behavioral anomaly in terms of function or some other ethnopsychological or ethnophysiological status," whereas *disability* is "a negative social response to a perceived impairment" (Shuttleworth & Kasnite, 2004, p. 141). The hyphenated term *impairment-disability* is a way to highlight both "their relationship and the need for their analytical separation" (2004, p. 141). Analytical separation is useful as a means to distinguish between problems deriving from a child's health status, for which the child is the appropriate site of intervention, and problems primarily due to discriminatory attitudes and/or public policies, which need to be addressed at other levels.

For Shuttleworth and Kasnitz, the term *children with disabilities*, preferred by many for its quality as so-called people first language, is also rejected in favor of the term *disabled children* as a way to reflect that "disability is not part of the impaired person but is a social process that disables" (2004, p. 141). In this chapter, which includes a discussion of just how *social process* can disable, we use the two terms interchangeably.

THE IMPACT OF DISABLED CHILDREN ON FAMILIES

Social scientists make a fine distinction between the concepts of *family* and *household*, both of which are culturally constructed organizing principles for social and economic life. Both are expressed as particular kinds of social systems, with particular kinds of ramifications for peoples' health and well-being. Although *family* refers, technically speaking, to kinship relations, *household* refers to the social unit occupying a shared dwelling space and cooperating in economic activities. Families can extend over many households, and households can include people who do not belong to the same family (Sobo, 2003).

In the United States, however, there is great conceptual overlap between family and household. Despite demographic evidence showing a different reality (*Economist*, 2001), the idealized household consists of a single-family dwelling shared by a nuclear family consisting of a married heterosexual couple and their biological offspring. Due in part to this belief, *family* and *household* often are used interchangeably. Following common parlance, then, in this chapter, we use one term to encompass both concepts. Except where the practical functioning of the socioeconomic household system is directly referenced, whether it consists of biological parents and siblings or some other social grouping such as a grandmother and cousins, we will refer to the household in which the disabled child lives (or would live, if possible) as a *family*.

Mainstream Studies of Familial Response to Disability

At the practical level of providing family support and early intervention services, "a family's response to their child's disability is important because if affects the kinds of support and services that can be offered" (Wayman, Lynch, & Hanson, 1990, p. 68). Much of the research on parental response that has been incorporated into health services delivery has been carried out by scholars in the field of psychology (social and health psychology, specifically), although research in the counseling field also has received some attention. Studies have proposed stages of grief and of mourning the loss of the idealized child in situations in which a child is identified as being different from the parents' expectations. They have largely ignored fathers, focusing instead on factors leading to or inhibiting eventual maternal adjustment to a child's disability.

A Brief History of Theoretical Perspectives

As Philip Ferguson argued, professional explorations of family reactions are, like families themselves, embedded in particular times and places and reflect not only research, but also cultural expectations and assumptions (2002, p. 124). From about 1820 to 1920, for instance, moral blame theories attributed childhood disability to parents—"especially those with the bad judgment to be both poor and female" (Ferguson, 2002, p. 124). Whether in the guise of reform schools, asylums, or residential schools for specific disabilities such as blindness, deafness, epilepsy, and insanity, there was a common concern throughout this period to develop institutionalized social programs to remove disabled children from their parents (Ferguson, 2001, p. 378).

Later, reversing the underlying assumption that parents damaged their children, most of the professional research from 1920 to 1980, perhaps influenced by the clinical orientation of serving families experiencing difficulties, instead emphasized the ways in which children with disabilities inevitably damaged their families. For example, Ferguson (2002) argued that, whether they used attitudinal categories (e.g., denial, guilt, displaced anger, grief) or behavioral categories (e.g., role disruption, marital cohesiveness, social withdrawal), the majority of scholars assumed that childhood disability was intrinsically harmful to family life. Analyses of parental adaptation during this period presented parents alternatively as being driven to neurotic or dysfunctional behavior, or as experiencing perpetual sorrow and suffering. "The challenge for research was to catalogue and sequence the evidence of parental damage and to argue for the efficacy of this or that therapeutic intervention" (Ferguson, 2002, p. 125).

Influence of Social Context on Family Adaptation

Underlying more recent research, however, is the recognition that social context, including available financial and emotional resources and social supports, influence family adaptation to disability. Emerging within the literature are depictions of families as adaptive, evolving, and active, with general agreement that family responses to disability are variable. Further, although having a disabled child may be stressful, a significant number of studies have shown that parents attribute positive outcomes to the experience of disability in the family (e.g., Cunningham, 1996; Flaherty & Glidden, 2000; Van Riper, 2004).

Among the benefits most commonly cited in an interview study of 60 mostly White mothers of disabled children was obtaining knowledge of the true meaning of unconditional love. This study was conducted across a broad range of socioeconomic and educational levels in rural, urban, and suburban neighborhoods in upstate New York (Landsman, 1999). The mothers described this knowledge not as inherent or natural but rather as acquired either through observing a disabled child model unconditional love through his or her behavior, or through the experience of raising a child who does not meet the normal developmental milestones, thus providing the mother an opportunity to reassess her priorities and values. As one mother in Landsman's study explained,

> "I had to shift my focus off the academic, which the world really throws in, you know, oh, your children have to succeed and they have to do this and they have to do that, and to come back to what we really feel is just simple unconditional love, just loving people for who they are and not putting all the conditions on how they perform. . . . When they're older, you think, sure, you have to deal with loving them unconditionally when they're really trying you as a teenager, and you're thinking way down the line, but it was a lesson that we were starting to learn already that we weren't anticipating."

In interpreting her disabled child as giving the gift of knowledge of unconditional love, a mother does not dismiss sorrow or the fear she feels as she anticipates a future of social discrimination for her child. She may feel that the benefits she has received from the experience of unconditional love also are at the cost of her child. A mother whose son was diagnosed with pervasive developmental disorder said, "Look at all the things he's taught me, patience, unconditional love. . . . I just hope that he doesn't have to suffer the rest of his life to teach me lessons." A mother who feels herself to be enriched by the experience of parenting a disabled child can and often does simultaneously regret the financial hardships, added care burdens, and perceived lost opportunities for herself, her family, and her disabled child. Mothers' stories of unconditional love do not deny but rather unify experiences that on the surface appear contradictory such as of hope and fear or joy and sorrow (Landsman,1998; Larson, 1998).

Current Psychological Research on Family Adaptation

As the field of research concerning families of disabled children grows, the health psychology literature is becoming more wide-ranging in focus, more international in scope, more methodologically diverse, and more theoretically and methodologically sophisticated. There has been a dramatic increase in the number of researchers exploring strengths and resilience in families that include a disabled child (e.g., Flaherty & Glidden, 2000; Scorgie & Sobsey, 2000). Moreover, it is now much more common for researchers to assess both the positive and negative consequences associated with raising a disabled child. In addition, the assessment of how, or if, these consequences vary over the life course of the disabled child has received increased attention (Nachshen, Woodford, & Minnes, 2003; Todd & Jones, 2005). Finally, more and more researchers are focusing their attention on the identification and measurement of *modifiable* variables (e.g., family demands, family resources, social support), which may play a pivotal role in how individuals and families respond to the challenges associated with raising a disabled child (Saloviita, Italinna, & Lenonen, 2003; Van Riper, 2000).

Much of the existing literature on family adaptation to a childhood disability is based on data from White, well-educated, middle-income families of disabled children living in developed countries. However, many researchers have acknowledged that this is a major limitation, and they have emphasized the need for including families who are more diverse in terms of ethnicity, education, residency status, and income. Concurrently, there is growing interest in research about families of disabled children who live in developing countries where resources for disabled children and their families may be severely limited (Bridge, 2004; Harley, Ojwang, Baguwemu, Ddamulira, & Chavuta, 2005). Anthropological analyses of cross-cultural interpretations of disability offer important insights for understanding variation in family experiences of disability (Devlieger, 1995; Ingstad & Whyte, 1995; Shuttleworth & Kasnitz, 2006).

Models for Coping with Stress

Although a variety of theoretical frameworks have been used to guide the recent research on family adaptation to childhood disability, the ones most commonly used in the mainstream health psychology literature are those that have been derived from early models of stress and coping or models of family life-course development. With the recent surge of interest in strengths and resilience in families of disabled children, many researchers have chosen to use models based on Hill's ABCX model (1949, 1958), which is designed to help explain why some families adapt and become stronger in the face of stressful circumstances, some remain vulnerable, and some deteriorate. In the ABCX model, family crisis (X) is defined as an interactive outcome of three factors: an initial stressor event (A), the family's resources for dealing with the stressful event (B), and the family's definition of the stressor event (C). Later versions of the ABCX model recognize that responses to stressor events are often cyclical and cumulative within the same family (Ferguson, 2002). That is, how a family responds to one stressor event may influence how it responds to subsequent stressor events in a domino-like fashion.

One of the most comprehensive outgrowths of Hill's ABCX model is the Resiliency Model of Family Adjustment and Adaptation (McCubbin & McCubbin, 1993; McCubbin, Thompson, & McCubbin, 1996). In this model, resiliency is defined as "the positive behavioral patterns and functional competence individuals and families demonstrate under stressful or adverse circumstances, which determines the family's ability to recover by maintaining integrity as a unit while ensuring, and where necessary restoring, the well-being of family members and the family unit as a whole" (McCubbin, Thompson, & McCubbin, 1996, p. 5). Family resources—the strengths and capabilities of individual family members, the household unit, and the community, including financial, social, and emotional resources—are taken into account. Successful adaptation (*bonadaptation*) occurs when the family is able to achieve a balance between the needs of the disabled child, the needs of other family members, and the needs of the family as a whole (Van Riper, 2000).

In research carried out by Saloviita and colleagues in Finland testing the model, the single-most important predictor of stress for the parents was the way they appraised or defined the situation. Parents who had a negative definition of their situation reported experiencing more stress. But the family resources variable accounted for 42% of the stress for mothers and 33% for fathers. In mothers, the most important resource was informal support, but in fathers it was spousal support. Overall, findings from this study suggest that the way in which parents define their situation and the various resources available to them is more important in the predication of parental stress than are characteristics of the child (Saloviita et al., 2003).

Time Demands and Caregiving Stresses

In addition to the demands faced by families with typically developing children, members of the families of disabled children are subject to changes in roles and increased caregiving difficulties and time demands. Some of the new roles include advocate, teacher, writer, parent-group leader, conference speaker, and member of advisory councils for schools, hospitals, and agencies representing individuals with disabilities (Scorgie & Sobsey, 2000). In one study of mothers of children with Down syndrome (Van Riper, in press), many mothers with very high scores on the family-demands measure noted that family members were constantly trying to juggle multiple demands. Many of the mothers also commented about time demands and the lack of time for social and recreational activities. There was a significant negative association between family demands and family adaptation. Mothers who reported higher levels of family demands, life-style changes, and unresolved strains rated their family adaptation lower.

Elsewhere (see Chapter 3 regarding financial costs), mothers of children with Down syndrome reported reducing time in paid work by about 7 hours per week and increasing their child care time by about 9 hours per week because of increased time demands (Barnett & Boyce, 1995). For some mothers of disabled children, not being employed outside the home may result in feelings of isolation, a lack of fulfillment, and low self-esteem (Shearn & Todd, 2000). Increased time demands also may result in parents of children with disabilities having less time to participate in valued social and recreational activities than do parents of children without disabilities (Barnett & Boyce, 1995; Scorgie & Sobsey, 2000). When the number of demands on or within the family unit is high, meeting the needs of the disabled child may take precedence over meeting the needs of other family members. This may ultimately result in family dysfunction.

Problem Solving and Coping Strategies

Family adaptation in stressful situations depends, in part, on the range and depth of the family's repertoire of problem-solving and coping strategies (McCubbin & McCubbin, 1993). Families of children with disabilities demonstrate considerable resilience in their everyday coping, as demonstrated by the number and range of coping strategies that they put into action. In a study of mothers of children with Down syndrome, the five most commonly reported items on the measure of family coping were 1) having faith in God, 2) knowing that we have the power to solve major problems, 3) facing problems head-on and trying to solve them right away, 4) sharing concerns with close friends, and 5) knowing that we have the strength within our family to solve our problems (Van Riper, in press).

Problem-solving and cognitive coping strategies appear to be more useful than stress reduction techniques (Grant & Whittell, 2000). The most frequently used and helpful strategies tend to build on personal experience and expertise, provide a regular routine or structure for coping, entail talking things over with a trusted person, involve setting priorities, and include a repertoire of coping processes that can be used when appropriate. In cognitive strategies, the focus is on reframing or changing the meaning of the situation by realizing that there is always someone worse off, seeing the funny side of the situation, and looking for—and finding—the silver lining. The use of cognitive coping strategies has been positively associated with maternal perceptions of the child with a disability as a source of happiness and fulfillment as well as strength and family closeness (Hastings, Allen, McDermott, & Still, 2002). In a study by Seltzer, Greenberg, Floyd, and Hong (2004), mid-life parents of children with mental health problems or developmental disabilities had lower levels of depression and higher levels of environmental mastery and self-acceptance if they used accommodative coping, which involves flexibly adjusting goals in response to a persistent problem.

Some coping strategies have been shown to be detrimental in the long run. Use of wishful thinking, a passive coping strategy, was negatively associated with measures of individual and family well-being (Cunningham, 1996). Avoidance coping strategies have been significantly correlated with both depression and anxiety in a study of parents of children with Down syndrome (Spangenberg & Theron, 2001). Another factor that may influence family adaptation to stressful situations is the type of communication that families use to problem solve. For example, families with an affirming style of problem-solving communication (conveys support and caring and exerts a calming influence) have been found to adapt more successfully to stressful situations than families with an incendiary style of problem-solving communication (inflames and exacerbates a stressful situation; McCubbin et al., 1996).

BROADENING OUR PERSPECTIVE: SOCIAL, HISTORICAL, AND CULTURAL CONTEXTS

Although family function in and of itself is a valid site for study, and quantitative measures of stress, resources, and adaptation can be informative, the data described above cannot be fully understood in isolation. A broader perspective, including analysis of the impact of social policies, gender roles, and cultural meanings of disability, among other variables, is important for understanding *why* the research shows the findings discussed above, as well as how disability is actually experienced in different families. Such analyses add to the health psychology

literature information that is critical for developing strategies to improve families' experiences.

The Role of Early Intervention

Although evaluations of the efficacy of intervention programs for infants, toddlers, and preschoolers have indicated both short- and long-
term benefits for children, researchers have paid less attention to assessing outcomes of early intervention (EI) programs for families (Bailey &
Bruder, 2005, p.1). This has occurred despite the fact that the EI programs that provide therapeutic services to young children in the United
States were established in the late 1980s with a mandate to be family-
centered (Leiter, 2004).

Family-Centeredness and Its Pressures

Family-centeredness refers to a particular set of principles and practices
that include "individualized, flexible, and responsive practices; infor-
mation-sharing so that families can make informed decisions; family
choice regarding . . . program practices and intervention options; parent–professional collaboration . . . and the . . . resources and supports
necessary for families to care for and rear their children in ways that
produce optimal child, parent, and family outcomes" (Dunst, 2002, p.
139). Although this is in part the outgrowth of parental activism, it is
important to note that the very legislation that enables and encourages
parents to become more involved in their child's early development
may ironically also place greater pressure on them (Cantor & Cantor,
1995, p. 108). For instance, although parents nominally have the power
to choose from whom to receive early intervention services, they do
not necessarily have the knowledge they need to feel comfortable doing
so. Some mothers have said that although they may appreciate having
options, they have little or no idea how to pick the best therapists
or educational programs for their children; after all, most had never
imagined needing such services. "Told to choose among their options
and in accordance with their family's own priorities, a mother may feel
as a burden the responsibility for making what may turn out to be the
wrong decision at a critical time in her child's development" (Landsman,
1998, p. 90).

Isolation can compound this sense of burden. The IDEA amendments of 1997 require states to ensure that to the maximum extent
appropriate to a child's needs, early intervention services are provided
in "natural environments." The natural environment for infants has
been widely interpreted in recent years to be the home or a typical
child care center as opposed to a facility designed specifically for disabled

children. As a consequence, parents who themselves grew up in environments in which they were isolated from people with disabilities are now the primary caretakers of such individuals. Although legislation has in many ways empowered parents of disabled children, keeping their children at home or in centers with nondisabled peers has had the unintended consequence of isolating members of this first generation of parents in early intervention programs from one another (Landsman, 1998, p. 89). They therefore have less access to parent support networks that can emerge from participation in center-based programs.

Parents as Therapists

Parents also may experience stress from exposure to what Valerie Leiter refers to as the "therapeutic imperative" inherent in family-centered early intervention (EI) programs (Leiter, 2004). Leiter's study of parents and professionals in EI programs in Massachusetts revealed that professionals expect mothers to carry over knowledge and skills gained during home visits by applying specific techniques and activities with their children in between such visits (2004, p. 840). As a result, Leiter found that mothers made a greater commitment of time to doing EI therapies with their child than did professionals, and that professionals tended to discuss parents' adherence to therapeutic norms in terms of compliance. Mothers often felt overwhelmed by these professional expectations and expressed concern that they lacked sufficient knowledge and/or time to provide therapeutic care such as physical therapy or occupational therapy tasks (2004, p. 844). Ironically, although mothers believed that therapy provided by professionals was the more effective intervention, professionals believed parents to be the more important means for influencing a child's development (Leiter, 2004, p. 845).

Leiter noted that some mothers refuse the therapy role; some do so because they feel overwhelmed by a difficult diagnosis or because of family responsibilities, including paid employment and care for other children. Yet parents also may refuse the therapy role because they wish to retain both the routines of typical family life and a relationship with their child, for example, as "just a mother" rather than as therapist or teacher (Landsman, 2005; Leiter, 2004). One mother in Landsman's interview study describes how the therapy role intrudes upon tasks as mundane as shopping. "When I'm searching in the store for toys . . . I'm thinking, what kind of skills does he need now? At this point, you know, how can I get these things so that it can help him pull and, you know, get good grasping skills. . . . So there are periods of time where you think, wow, this is all consuming!" (Landsman, 2005). Parents also may resist the therapy role because their child dislikes, is scared of, or seems to experience pain during therapy.

Challenges for Minority and Low-Income Families

The process of developing and carrying out an individualized education plan for a child in EI assumes parental involvement and advocacy that, as we have seen, may present difficulties for many parents. The challenges to effective participation in an early intervention program may be even greater for minority and low-income families (Harry, 2002). Among the reasons cited for this are the social stigma that has long been attached to the ethnicity or social status of minority and low-income families, with the result that the parents are treated with disrespect by professionals, and the barriers to effective parent–professional communication caused by culturally based differences in interaction styles (Harry, 2002).

The Variable of Gender

Although families make a variety of individual arrangements, research suggests that overall men and women tend to experience the challenges and rewards of a disabled child in the family differently. This is in part because men and women often play different roles in a household; as a consequence, although they are exposed to the same stressful life events, men and women may actually have to cope with different problems (Gray, 2003). Also affecting differences in how men and women experience a child's disability are broadly held cultural attitudes about causes of childhood disability.

Gender Roles in Caring for Children with Disabilities

David Gray's study of Australian parents of children with high functioning autism or Asperger's syndrome showed that fathers tended to describe the effect as indirect and less severe, primarily due to the role that work played in their lives. Raising a child with Asperger's tended to have a much more significant effect on the careers of mothers (2003). Women in the study, only half of whom were employed outside the home (mostly in part-time jobs or a family business), were far more likely to describe having to miss work or perform below their normal level. In short, Gray revealed the societal progress women have made toward more egalitarian workplaces as tenuous, with the presence of childhood disability in the family as potentially restricting or reverting women to traditional gender roles.

Reviewing the literature on allocation of responsibility for household work, Alice Home (2002) found that the replacement of institutional responsibility for disabled individuals by family care in the community has not been matched by effective changes in resources; this had led to increased caring burdens for mothers of disabled children. Analyzing data from three studies in Canada, McKeever and Miller (2004) similarly found that the shift of the site of care away from institutions is associated with an increasingly disproportionate share of the responsibility for disabled children's care, much of it technologically sophisticated, being borne informally by women as part of their role as mothers. Accordingly, although early intervention programs are designed to be family-centered, fathers participate relatively little (Turbiville, Turnbull, & Turnbull, 1995). This may reflect family choice or be a reaction to failures of service providers to engage with fathers. Traustadottir found that all of the mothers in her study of U.S. families with disabled children had the main responsibility for providing the care necessary to keep the child within the family (1991, p. 218). "Caring is seen as women's responsibility, and the division of labor assigns far more responsibility for caring to women than to men" (Traustadottir, 1991, p. 216). Such care includes traditional caring work (e.g., feeding, bathing, toileting) and the work involved in searching for and coordinating services a child might receive. Additional caring work may involve seeking alternative therapies (Prussing, Sobo, Walker, & Kurtin, 2005), advocating for their own child and for disabled children more generally (Landsman, 2004; Prussing et al., 2005), and facilitating friendships for a child with disabilities (Turnbull, Pereira, & Blue-Banning, 1999). Mothers in families living in poverty experience even greater burdens, have fewer options available to help them cope, and are more likely to experience mental health problems (Park, Turnbull, & Turnbull III, 2002).

Gender and Attribution of Blame for Disability

Women in the United States not only take on the greater share of responsibility for the care of disabled children, but also are ascribed a greater share of responsibility for the very existence of the child's impairment. Although this may appear to be merely a continuation of a longstanding tradition of blaming mothers for their children's behaviors and conditions, its strength is related to the successful and widespread dissemination of public health information about the relationship between women's behaviors and fetal health. Signs in bars and on wine and liquor bottles publicly proclaim drinking alcohol by pregnant women as detrimental to the fetus, anti-smoking ads target pregnant women (Oaks, 2001), pregnant drug users—particularly African Americans—are subject to arrest (Roberts, 1991), and popular pregnancy advice books discuss the importance of nutrition and raise issues of the presumed dangers of caffeine and over-the-counter medications.

American pregnant women and new mothers are keenly aware of

biomedical advice about appropriate nutrition (Markens, Browner, & Press, 1997), and when first encountering a diagnosis of a child's impairment, few women may fail to consider what they had personally done wrong to bring about their child's condition. Among the causes considered by women in Landsman's previously cited study (1998), having an alcoholic drink before they were aware they were pregnant, taking an over-the-counter pain medication such as Tylenol or ibuprofen, and eating fast food loomed particularly large. Even when mothers were themselves convinced they had behaved in compliance with expert advice, they worried that others blamed them for the child's impairment. "I've had people really openly ask me if I did drugs while I was pregnant," complained a mother of a child with mental retardation, "and that to me is like a knife in the chest."

In mainstream U.S. society, a woman's purported control of the uterine environment through diet and the culling out of fetuses with genetic abnormalities through pregnancy termination is largely understood to result in the birth of a perfect child (Landsman, 1999). The women's health movement, the fundamental premise of which is "that women must wrest back control of their bodies from physicians, especially during pregnancy and birth, reinforces the notion that positive birth outcomes are something women can control" (Layne, 2003, p. 243). In addition, the development of ultrasound technology, in which the fetus is portrayed as a person separate from the mother, has assisted in developing the concept of maternal–fetal conflict in which a woman, through "inappropriate choices," is a potential danger to the health of her fetus (Petchesky, 1987; Taylor, 1998). Media accounts publicizing so-called fetal abuse "reinforce and intensify the moral imperative that underlies health advice: To be a good mother, a woman must follow today's pregnancy rules" (Oaks, 2001). Thus, many historically and culturally specific factors, as well as women's own embodied experience of pregnancy, converge to place societal blame for a child's negatively construed impairment on the mother rather than on the father or on conditions beyond the mother's control. This is so despite documented existence of such conditions—for example, impact of paternal smoking and/or paternal exposure to toxic substances, some of which have been linked to specific occupations (see Daniels, 1999).

Mothers themselves describe gender variation in parental responses to a child's physical difference. A 32-year-old college-educated mother of a boy born with a radial club hand commented to Landsman on the difference between her husband's reaction to the impairment and her own. "He [husband] has always been like, 'He's going to be fine, it's just an arm, it's just a hand. . . .' " But, as the woman explained to her husband, "I suppose you didn't grow him." Another mother in

Landsman's study (1998) said that her husband reacts to such questioning by saying, "This is ridiculous, we don't know why it happened, who cares why it happened, that's not the issue," to which she responds, "You're absolutely right, but you don't understand; you've never carried a baby." Although the reactions of U.S. fathers to disability remain understudied, these comments reveal the mothers' sense of their own possible failure to control pregnancy outcome.

Cultural Context

Only relatively recently, with the mandate of family-centered practice in early intervention, has the cultural context of families of disabled children been addressed seriously by researchers. Harry attributed the former lack of concern with cultural context both to "a powerful ethnocentrism that made it difficult for mainstream practitioners or researchers to recognize and give credence to non-mainstream family patterns or practices" (2002, p. 131). She also attributed it to the fact that the disability advocacy movement had framed disabled people as a minority group and disability as a master status, strategically minimizing other aspects of identity such as racial and socioeconomic status so as not to diffuse the disability rights lobby (2002, p.132). More recent research recognizes that American families with disabled children may simultaneously participate in 1) a shared mainstream culture, 2) one or more minority cultures depending on their ethnic origin, and 3) the unique context of their own particular family life. This section will consider broad American cultural beliefs related to disability, and the range of intra-cultural variation within the United States.

The American Myth of Exceptional Parents

If one message of U.S. culture is that mothers of children with impairments are morally inferior and to be blamed for their role in bringing about childhood disability, another is that they are morally superior and to be admired for their extraordinary abilities (Landsman, 1999). The latter view is reflected in the adage that God gives special children to special mothers, and although in the image of the exceptional parent this perspective would appear to flatter parents, it carries a number of implications that may insult and provide an additional source of stress for mothers of disabled children. Some feel it candy-coats the adversity, belittling the hardships parents face in caring for a child with impairments. In the words of a mother of a child with a chromosomal impairment who participated in Landsman's previously described study (1998), "it undermines what you've been through." Others feel that it diminishes the value of the child, presenting him or her as exclusively a burden or tragedy beyond the capacity of most parents to love or nurture. Above all, it presents parents of disabled children as themselves inherently different from presumably typical parents. A mother of prematurely born twins, one of whom has cerebral palsy, told Landsman that she found the adage about being *special* annoying. Speaking about the experience of raising a disabled child, she explained, "I think it certainly *makes* you different, you know. . . . We're not special parents, we're average, normal people who had this crazy thing happen to us. And we're doing the best we can" (Landsman, 1999, pp. 144–145). In the view of such mothers, a woman's exceptionality does not precede the birth of a disabled child; if it exists, it is a product of parenting.

Moreover, the myth that parents of children with disabilities are exceptional may not serve families well. The danger in accepting the myth, Hebert (2000) pointed out, is that the real issues of caring for disabled children, which she likens to being the wizard in *The Wizard of Oz* frantically manipulating the switches behind the curtain, are hidden from view as supposedly *exceptional parents* try to maintain their public image. It is time, she argues, "that we parents of kids with disabilities pull back the curtain and expose ourselves as the mere mortals that we are" (Hebert).

Cultural Variation in Interpretation of Disability

Blaming mothers for bringing about a disability, and depicting parents of disabled children as exceptional people more capable than others of raising *special* children are culturally and historically specific portrayals. Rooted in the assumption that childhood disability is a tragedy to be avoided by typical families, they represent explanations for childhood impairment that are by no means universal. Women's conduct during pregnancy is not always interpreted as the cause of a child's impairment. In Israel, for example, many view the destiny of an infant as defined by its initial body composition rather than by its exposure to substances during a woman's pregnancy (Ivry, 2003). Among Puerto Rican families, a child's impairment may be attributed to the *evil eye*, a curse placed on him or her by an enemy (Rogers-Adkinson, Ochoa, & Delgado, 2003). In Pakistan, the most plausible explanation for mental retardation is that a child has been taken over by a *djinn*, a spirit, or that the child is a changeling (Miles, 1992).

Nora Groce notes the presence in many cultures of the belief that a disability can be caught, citing the example of some North American Indian tribes who discourage children from touching wheelchairs and other assistive devices for fear that contact will lead to an acquired disability. In those cultures in which there is a strong belief in reincarnation, the disabled child's status is understood to have been earned, and attempts to intervene may lessen the amount of suffering for the child and therefore compromise the possibility of future rebirth at a higher level of existence (2005, p. 7).

Nor is there universal agreement even on what constitutes an impairment or disability, as the anthropological literature attests (see Ingstad & Whyte, 1995). In the Micronesian Caroline Islands atoll societies, social isolation is the critical criterion. Individuals who are physically impaired from birth defects, accidents, or diseases affecting mobility, agility, or appearance usually continue to participate in everyday social relations and therefore do not fall into a category of *disabled* "unless the impairment is coupled with an inability to speak and/or hear—that is, with an inability to manipulate culture and to participate in the social life of the community" (Marshall, 1996, p. 254). Similarly, among the Cuna Indians of Panama in the early 20th century, albinism was not considered a disability but rather "one of the many characteristics of an individual" (Scheer, 1994, p. 249).

Among the Navajo, a child with an impairment-disability is understood to be different but in a good way; indeed, he or she may not receive specialized interventions because such interventions might interfere with the special gifts and lessons the child is believed to impart to the tribe (Rogers-Adkinson et al., 2003). Physically different Jewish and Arab children in Israel, on the other hand, have a high rate of abandonment at birth, and those appearance-impaired children who are brought home experience territorial isolation there (Weiss, 1997); metaphors of monsters, animals, and other stigmatizing terms are applied to such children, effectively denying their personhood (Weiss, 1998).

Cultural Competence

There is now widespread agreement that differences arising from culture affect the health, beliefs, and behaviors of patients, their families, and providers in the United States. Culture is associated with disparities in health and with barriers to health care (Betancourt, Green, Carrillo, & Ananeh-Firempong II, 2003). A family's core values, deeply influenced by cultural background, have been shown to affect what types of planning and interventions are appropriate or possible (Bui & Turnbull, 2003).

Accordingly, there have been calls from various medical and rehabilitation fields in the United States for what is popularly termed *cultural competence*. Cultural competency in rehabilitation services in particular refers to the "ability to adequately understand and respond to the needs and concerns of individuals with disability and their families from ethnic and minority communities, with responses based on an accurate understanding of their specific cultural practices" (Groce, 2005, p. 5).

Teaching Cultural Competence

One of the most popular texts used in teaching cultural competence is journalist Anne Fadiman's *The Spirit Catches You and You Fall Down: A Hmong Child, Her American Doctors, and the Collision of Two Cultures,* first published in 1997. Fadiman skillfully tells the story of Lia Lee, a child of Hmong immigrants from Laos, who settled in Merced, California. Lia began suffering seizures as an infant. Her devoted and hardworking doctors diagnosed her with epilepsy, and her parents diagnosed her with "soul loss." Eventually, Lia suffered irreversible brain damage, leaving her comatose, all the while lovingly cared for by her family. The Merced doctors saw Lia's parents as noncompliant with physician advice, and for a time Lia was removed from her home. The parents had used traditional healers in conjunction with Western medicine, and they blamed the doctors' prescribed medicines for Lia's brain damage. The lesson Fadiman draws for medical practitioners is that Lia's life "was ruined not by septic shock or noncompliant parents but by cross-cultural misunderstanding" (Fadiman, 1997, p. 262). The explanations of illness used by the Hmong family and American doctors were each rooted in their respective cultures. The participants' experience is portrayed then as a "tragedy of distinct 'cultures' because it was the difference between their respective cultures that sent Lia's parents and her doctors hurtling headlong toward each other" (Taylor, 2003, p. 165). Many educators, Landsman included, use this book in teaching to illustrate the powerful impact of culture on both family and medical decision making, and the life and death relevance of cross-cultural communication in daily life. Fadiman herself documents the growth of interest in cross-cultural training in medical school curricula and the use of her book in cultural competence training (Fadiman, pp. 270–272). Yet, as Janelle Taylor (2003) explained, the story Fadiman tells is emotionally engaging as tragedy precisely because it proceeds from an understanding of culture that is in fact out of step with current anthropological knowledge.

Recent Conceptualizations of Culture

Today, the notion that culture comprises internally consistent and bounded sets of beliefs and customs to which all members subscribe uniformly has been replaced by a vision of culture as subservient to social process. That is, members of a given culture are constantly engaged in making and negotiating meanings and social relations. Rather than being monolithic, culture involves competing sets of values and practices. Individuals are positioned differently within culture(s) based on a range of factors including gender, education, social status, stage in the life cycle, religion, dialect, geographic region, unique personal experiences, and location in a rural or urban environment. Therefore, the beliefs, values, behaviors, and expectations of one member of a culture do not necessarily match those of another member of that culture. Moreover, available cultural models and practices do not stand still; all cultures undergo change over time, as demonstrated in U.S. culture by changing gender roles, policies regarding racial segregation, and new styles of communication as a result of technological innovations such as e-mail and cell phones.

Culture is not biologically inherited from one's ancestors, it is learned and shared. Since the process of learning begins at birth, cultural beliefs are social constructions that may nevertheless appear to their adherents as inherently natural, as a *given* of what is and ought to be. Because the cultural beliefs are widely shared with others, their acceptance as real or appropriate tends to be reinforced daily. Yet, because culture is learned, concepts derived from new and different life experiences as well as from other cultures can be reworked and/or incorporated into an individual's worldview and values. Just as there is no *one* way to be a human being, there is also no *one* way to be a typical Chinese, Native American, Hmong, African American, Mexican, Korean, American, or Haitian family. Thus, there is no one set of rules to learn and apply in providing services to all families of any particular culture. Familiarity with the culture of populations being served is exceedingly valuable in optimizing care for children with impairment-disability, but current anthropological perspectives on culture suggest skepticism toward the more simplistic, cookbook interpretations of cultural competence.

Assisting in developing cultural competence, therefore, may be an awareness of the domains in which community members will respond in culturally defined ways rather than a list of what those ways *will* be. We have already considered cultural variation in explanations of causes for impairment-disability; other domains of importance are discussed below. The personal attributes that members of a cultural community value also will have a profound effect on how a child with disabilities will be treated, the extent to which resources will be expended for that child (Groce, 2005), and the goals a family may have for that child. This is particularly so when it comes to gender. If girls are in general valued less than boys in a particular culture, families will be less willing to spend scarce resources on disabled girls. In societies in which independence is valued, such as in the United States, efforts to ensure future employability and self-sufficiency may be encouraged. However, cross-culturally, in 94% of the world's societies, extended rather than nuclear families are the norm. In many instances, community members may regard sending a disabled family member into the workforce as a sign of abuse or neglect rather than of success (Groce, 2005; Ingstad, 1990), or may value chores performed at home as much as work that is economically productive (Harry, 2002). For another example, personal attributes or activities such as motherly sacrifice and devotion shaped in part by interpretations of Catholicism affect both the meaning of childhood disability and of parenting for Latinos. Contrary to the stories told by predominantly White U.S. mothers of disabled children, which *reject* the mainstream society's notion that God gives special children to special mothers, many Latina mothers tell stories in which they actively embrace that perspective. The culturally specific religious ideology validates a mother's sacrifice (Skinner, Bailey, Correa, & Rodriguez, 1999).

Culture can be expected to have an effect on the types of treatment families seek, including herbal remedies (Jezewski & Sotnik, 2005) and assistance from traditional healers, and on the role played by prayer and other forms of spiritual intervention for disability (Barnes, Plotnikoff, Fox, & Pendelton, 2000). Relationships with service providers also will vary based in large part on cultural differences. In some hierarchically structured societies, for instance, professionals have high status and their suggestions will always be met with polite affirmation, regardless of parents' true feelings. Similarly, attitudes toward the validity of the batteries of tests and evaluations professionals employ are not consistent across cultures (Groce, 2005). For instance, Harry noted that studies show that working class Puerto Rican and African American parents of children with mild retardation hold broader parameters of normalcy than allowed by school-based evaluations, with the result that a child defined by professionals as mentally retarded and in need of services may not be considered as such by family members (2002, p.134).

Many other beliefs and practices are influenced by culture of origin and by immigrant or ethnic experience. These include styles of verbal and nonverbal communication (e.g., eye contact, gestures, amount of personal space, use of silence), perception of time and punctuality, family decision-making patterns, level of directness in relaying a difficult diagnosis, intensity and types of emotion considered appropriate to express, methods of feeding and carrying children, infants' sleeping arrangements and scheduling, levels of personal modesty and privacy within the household, and concerns over surveillance by authorities. This is the case both for families of children with impairment-disability and for the professionals who provide services to them. Practitioners are encouraged to examine the role their own culture plays in their expectations (Kagawa-Singer & Kassim-Lakha, 2003) and to utilize parents' narratives (stories) as tools for understanding how the parental understandings of disability are informed by deeper levels of meaning that may account for families not responding or following through in ways health professionals might expect or wish (Landsman, 2003, 2005; Larson, 1998; Prussing et al., 2005).

Biomedicine as a Foreign Culture

Training programs have predominantly focused on cultural competence in terms of ethnoracial differences. Although awareness of and sensitivity to such cultural differences are helpful if practitioners are to work effectively with families from diverse backgrounds, it is important as well to understand that biomedicine itself constitutes its own foreign culture for most U.S. families (Sobo & Seid, 2003). Even when health care practitioners and parents of disabled children speak the same language (e.g., English) or are members of similar ethnic groups, medical miscommunication too often occurs. The more important issue is therefore for clinicians to develop communicative competence, and to provide education and assistance to families that will help them better navigate the health care system (Sobo & Seid, 2003, p. 99).

Mixed Messages: The Medical Model and Disability Rights

Regardless of the understanding of disability that families bring from their cultures of origin, parents of young children with developmental delays and impairments in the United States also are exposed to additional, sometimes competing, models for making sense of their experiences. Upon a child's evaluation or diagnosis, for example, parents are exposed to and often encouraged to use the medical, or rehabilitation, model of disability to communicate with the professionals who are assisting them. Yet, U.S. society also is the scene of an active and vocal disability rights movement, which provides access to an alternative perspective. Parents are not necessarily bound to any one model or view, but may interact with or draw upon competing disability models, blending them in complex ways as they experience impairment-disability in relation to their own child (Landsman, 2005).

Medical Model of Disability

The medical model of disability used in medical or rehabilitation settings portrays disability as a problem residing within the body of an individual. It is widespread in public culture and characteristic of most clinical professions. Parents may first encounter this model directly when a physician labels their child as outside the range of typical development; that is, the child has failed to meet developmental milestones or has a particular chromosomal anomaly (e.g., the extra portion of the number 21 chromosome associated with Down syndrome). In cases in which a problem is described by a physician as a chronic or permanent condition, parents may feel that their child has been dismissed or insulted because of the implication that he or she will not outgrow or overcome a disability in time (Landsman, 2003, 2005; Prussing et al., 2005). In behavior that health services professionals often label *denial*, parents may reject the placement of their child in the *disabled* category. Instead, they may point to contradictory prognoses offered by different biomedical (or other) professionals, to how the child's behavior is different at home than in the clinic, or to earlier instances in which the child has proven that a doctor's dire predictions were wrong. Often, parents do not reject the medical category of *disability*—only the accuracy of a particular professional's judgment in placing a particular child in a particular category (Landsman, 2005). In other words, some parents may indeed accept the professional's greater knowledge about specific disabilities, but they will claim for themselves a greater knowledge about their *particular* child.

In interactions with early intervention programs and various therapists, parents encounter the medical model in its rehabilitation variant. In these settings, the goal is to work toward approximating the norm in behavior and function. As an alternative to either resigning oneself to or rejecting the attribution of the label *permanently disabled* to a child, a parent may adopt for a child a cultural identity of what disability rights advocates refer to as the *supercrip*. In this model, a defect or deficiency can and should be overcome or compensated for through a child's strong will and a parent's love and commitment in efforts culturally defined as inspirational. Narratives collected from mothers in Landsman's (1998) study, as well as from parents of children with Down syndrome (Prussing et al., 2005), expressed a great deal of parental faith in therapeutic interventions, often framed in opposition to physicians' dismal predictions. As the mother of a boy with a chromosomal impairment explained to Landsman, "Had I been a parent who really believes in doctors and really thought that was it for Billy, I don't know if I would have gotten him the therapy and the services that he needed." Refusing to accept a clinician's dismal prognosis may be a strategy whereby parents retain hope and thereby their commitment to early intervention therapies that can benefit their child (Landsman 2003). Ironically, to receive the services necessary to assist in the efforts to move a child onto the culturally approved track of linear progress and out of the *disabled* category, parents must accept a medical expert's authoritative judgment that their child's development falls outside the norm. Eligibility for early intervention services is determined on the basis of a medical diagnosis or the degree of delay in meeting developmental milestones measured against a norm; this in turn becomes the basis for the written individualized family service plan (IFSP) that authorizes therapies. A mother quite literally, and often painfully, signs onto her child's labeled deficit when signing the IFSP. Whether understood as a permanent or temporary impairment, the medical model treats the disability as intrinsic to the child and assumes a binary opposition of the categories of typical and disabled (Landsman, 2005). By virtue of giving birth to a child with impairments in an American hospital or by seeking early intervention services, a parent in the United States is compelled to engage with this model.

Disability Rights Perspective

The medical model, however, coexists in American culture with competing perspectives, especially those emerging from the disability rights movement. These offer a distinction between impairment, defined as a bodily dysfunction, and disability, which refers to the social processes of oppression applied to impaired individuals. In the United States the disability rights movement has cast disabled people as a minority group in which *disability* is defined as a matter of policy not health. This represents a shift from an agenda of rehabilitation and cure to one of political change in which activists argue that "A disability comes not from the existence of an impairment, but from the reality of building codes, educational practices, stereotypes, prejudicial public officials . . . ignorance and oppression" (Pfeiffer, 1999, p. 106).

Although there is variation in specific arguments put forward, what became known as *the social model* in Britain and *the minority group model* in the United States denaturalized the disadvantaged position of disabled people in society. Disability was not a problem located in anatomy but a process rooted in social relations. The model put forward in the public arena by disability rights advocates underlies legislation such as the Americans with Disabilities Act and the Individuals with Disabilities Education Act and provided a vocabulary through which parents understand and give meaning to a child's disability (Landsman, 2005).

Activists have portrayed parents' cure-seeking efforts as misguided and as distractions from the more important goal of obtaining rights and of eliminating barriers to full participation in social life (Hershey, 1993; Oliver, 1990). Although U.S. parents of children with an impairment-disability may not be aware of the critique disability rights activists offer, in research, mothers themselves often express their own belief that the real disability a child faces is not the bodily impairment but the discrimination and social isolation experienced by people who are deemed to be different. That is, they make the distinction between the impairment and the disablement process. For example, when Landsman asked mothers their greatest concern for their disabled child, answers consistently referred to fears that their child would suffer from prejudice and social isolation. Mothers described concerns that their child would be teased or picked on in school, would be taken advantage of, would have nobody willing to hold the child's deformed hand in preschool, would not get a date to the prom, and would never marry or have friends. In short, the mothers worried that their children would not be recognized and included as a full person with value. "I mean, what does the future hold for her?" reflected the mother of a girl with Down syndrome. "Do they get to have a family life or do they live singly by themselves, so that's sad? That part bothers me, I think, more than anything else. What happens when I die and she's left here by herself? Is she going to be by herself the rest of her life? Is she ever going to have a partner?"

The real problem, as some parents have defined it, was not located within the child, rather it was located within society. Yet, in contrast to their general commitment to therapeutic interventions as offering hope for change in their son or daughter, mothers in Landsman's (1998) study expressed little faith that society could be changed in time to benefit their own child. Parental efforts to render their child *typical* through interventions, or to portray their child as nondisabled, may therefore not necessarily reflect parental acceptance of the medical model or a denial of the reality of their child's impairment. Rather, it may represent attempts to shield a loved and valued child from a future of discrimination culturally understood to follow from impairment.

For parents seeking the best lives for their children with disabilities, neither the medical model nor the minority group model is adequate in itself, and together they send American parents of disabled children mixed messages about how to proceed. The medical model as used by physicians all too often fails to acknowledge the positive qualities that parents attribute to their disabled children and to their experience of raising them. As applied in the rehabilitation fields, the medical model may engage parents, particularly mothers, in an exhausting, all-consuming, and sometimes demoralizing or family-damaging effort to change a child. A minority group or social model utilizing the vocabulary of rights speaks to many of the very real concerns parents feel about discrimination and prejudice, but offers little guidance about how to bring about the immediate changes parents feel are necessary to ensure a happy life for their own child and therefore for their family (Landsman, 2005).

IMPLICATIONS FOR PRACTITIONERS

Daily activities and the narrative accounts of them are sites for constructing the meaning of disability in family life and are opportunities for researchers and service providers to do the important work of listening to and understanding families' own expectations and norms (Ferguson, 2001). Concurrently, those working with families with disabled children can leverage the process whereby families give meaning to their experience, helping parents to reshape or refine the sociocultural resources they bring to bear on their situation and to adopt patterns shown to be more beneficial to the family. For instance, the dependency of disabled children may be cast as an opportunity to know unconditional love (Landsman, 1999; Larson, 1998), to reassess the values of a consumer culture (Landsman, 2004), to redefine the concept of "normalcy" (Landsman, 1998, 2005; Read, 2000), and to give a voice to the essential human rights of children (Landsman, 2004; Prussing et al., 2005; Read, 2000).

Described as a "thread that connects love with loss, desire with despair, hope with humiliation" (Hebert, 2000), raising children with disabilities involves the embrace of paradox and contradiction. Families of children with disabilities often are in the position of simultaneously engaging in efforts to change their child and defending the value of the child as she or he is. Practitioners can assist families to retain the hope necessary to sustain a commitment to intervention therapies, to seek solutions to specific problems, and to find joy in their child's unique accomplishments and characteristics. Strategies may include keeping prognoses relatively open and honest, and behaving in a way that indicates one's recognition of the disabled child as a valued person. By referring to the child by name rather than by diagnosis, commenting on a child's specific personality traits (e.g., strong will, determination, sense of humor, attentiveness, curiosity, friendliness), and communicating directly with the child about matters other than his or her medical condition, health practitioners model an understanding of a child as first and foremost a child.

Families with disabled children in which parents have the information, confidence, and support to problem solve show resilience. Families may benefit from having strong support systems involving family members, institutions, and/or other parents and from developing communication competence to successfully interact with the biomedical system. Problem-solving strategies may be directed in many ways, however.

Although parents seek treatments for and ask health professionals questions regarding their child's impairment, of equal or greater concern to them may be their child's future as a valued member of a community. Practitioners can contribute to successful incorporation of a child into family and community life by providing assistance and encouragement to parents as they seek resources—financial, informational, and emotional—and devise strategies to include their children in family, school, and community activities. Parents, engaged in the often-demanding responsibilities of daily care for children with disabilities, are well served by support in their efforts not only to provide care within the family, but also to increase the rights and opportunities of children in a more inclusive society.

CONCLUSION

Research suggests overall that families with disabled children fare no better or worse than families with typical children (Ferguson, 2001, p. 386). This is not to say that their lives are the same. At the same time that they experience greater stress, exhaustion, sorrow, and fear, many parents of disabled children also acquire profound and positive new understandings about society, about their own strengths, and about what constitutes true value in a person. Interpretations of disability may vary, certainly across cultures but also over time for any particular family member, as disruptions of the expected life course and new relationships become opportunities for reflection and creativity.

The experience of having a disabled child in the family always takes place within a specific cultural and historical context. This context constrains both what seems possible and what is desirable. Nevertheless, there is room for creativity and variation within this context. Individuals and families are not passive, but rather exert agency and give meaning to their experience. The current U.S. context provides models and resources from which parents may draw as they serve as intermediaries between children with impaired bodies and a society that simultaneously discriminates against them and articulates new policies of rights and inclusion. Seeking to improve their children's opportunities, parents may at times comply with the mainstream medical model. They also may at the same or another time draw on a social model's rejection of this problem-based definition of disability as inherently caused by impairment. Above all, families may use their own particular strengths to cope with disability, and, with adequate social and cultural support, gain resilience and strength from the intimate, caring relationship that they build with their disabled children.

REFERENCES

Americans with Disabilities Act (ADA) of 1990, PL 101-336, 42 U.S.C. §§ 12101 *et seq.*

Bailey, D., & Bruder, M.B. (2005). *Family outcomes of early intervention and early childhood special education: Issues and considerations.* (third version). Menlo Park, CA: Early Childhood Outcomes Center.

Barnes, L, Plotnikoff, G., Fox, K., & Pendleton, S. (2000). Spirituality, religion, and pediatrics: Intersecting worlds of healing. *Pediatrics, 106* (Suppl.), 899–908.

Barnett, W.S., & Boyce, G.C. (1995). Effects of children with Down syndrome on parents' activities. *American Journal of Mental Retardation, 100,* 115–127.

Betancourt, J.K, Green, A., Carrillo, E., & Ananeh-Firempong, O., II (2003). Defining cultural competence: A practical framework for addressing racial/ ethnic disparities and health and health care. *Public Health Reports, 118,* 293–302.

Bridge, G. (2004). Disabled children and their families in Ukraine: Health and mental health issues for families caring for their disabled children at home. *Social Work and Health Care, 39,* 89–105.

Bui, Y., & Turnbull, A. (2003, March). East meets west: Analysis of person-centered planning in the context of Asian American values. *Education and Training in Developmental Disabilities, 38*(1),18–31.

Cantor, R., & Cantor, J. (1995). *Parent's guide to special needs schooling: Early intervention years.* Westport, CT: Auburn House.

Cunningham, C. (1996). Families of children with Down syndrome. *Down Syndrome Research and Practice, 4,* 87–95.

Daniels, C. (1999). Rethinking gender differences. In L. Morgan & M. Michaels (Eds.), *Fetal subjects, feminist positions* (pp. 83–98*).* Philadelphia: University of Pennsylvania Press.

Devlieger, P. (1995). Why disabled? The cultural understandings of physical disability in an African society. In B. Ingstad & S. Whyte (Eds.), *Disability and culture* (pp. 94–106). Berkeley: University of California Press.

Dunst, C. (2002). Family-centered practices: Birth through high school. *The Journal of Special Education, 36*(3), 139–147.

Economist (2001, July 28–30). At last, good news on the family (probably). *Economist, 360*(8232), 29–30.

Fadiman, A. (1997). *The spirit catches you and you fall down: A Hmong child, her American doctors, and the collision of two cultures.* New York: Farrar, Straus and Giroux.

Ferguson, P. (2001). Mapping the family: Disability studies and the exploration of parental response to disability. In G. Albrecht, K. Seelman, & M. Bury (Eds.), *Handbook of disability studies* (pp. 373–395). Thousand Oaks, CA: Sage Publications.

Ferguson, P. (2002). A place in the family: An historical interpretation of research on parental reactions to having a child with a disability. *The Journal of Special Education, 36*(3), 124–130, 147.

Flaherty, E.M., & Glidden, L.M. (2000). Positive adjustment in parents rearing children with Down syndrome. *Early Education and Development, II,* 407–422.

Grant, G., & Whittell, B. (2000). Differentiated coping strategies in families of children or adults with intellectual disabilities: The relevance of gender, family composition, and the life span. *Journal of Applied Research in Intellectual Disabilities, 13,* 256–275.

Gray, D. (2003). Gender and coping: The parents of children with high functioning autism. *Social Science & Medicine, 56*(3), 631–642.

Groce, N. (2005). Immigrants, disability, and rehabilitation. In J.H. Stone (Ed.), *Culture and disability: Providing culturally competent services* (pp. 1–14). Thousand Oaks, CA: Sage Publications.

Harley, S., Ojwang, P., Baguwemu, A., Ddamulira, M., & Chavuta, A. (2005). How do carers of disabled children cope? The Ugandan perspective. *Child: Care, Health and Development, 31,* 167–180.

Harry, B. (2002). Trends and issues in serving culturally diverse families of children with disabilities. *The Journal of Special Education, 6*(3), 131–138.

Hastings, R., Allen, R., McDermott, K., & Still, D. (2002). Factors related to positive perceptions in mothers of children with intellectual disabilities. *Journal of Applied Research in Intellectual Disabilities, 15,* 269–275.

Hebert, M.J. (2000, September). *The unexceptional parent.* Paper presented at the 63rd annual conference of the American Association on Mental Retardation (AAMR) Region X, Saratoga, New York.

Hill, R. (1949). *Families under stress.* New York: Harper & Row.

Hill, R. (1958). Generic features of families under stress. *Social Casework, 49,* 139–150.

Home, A. (2002). Challenging hidden oppression: Mothers caring for children with disabilities. *Critical Social Work, 2*(2), 88–103.

Hughes, B., & Paterson, K. (1997). The social model of disability and the disappearing body: Towards a sociology of impairment. *Disability and Society, 12,* 325–340.

Individuals with Disabilities Education Act (IDEA) of 1990, PL 101-476, 20 U.S.C. §§ 1400 *et seq.*

Ingstad, B. (1990). The disabled person in the community: Social and cultural aspects. *International Journal of Rehabilitation Research, 13,* 187–194.

Ingstad, B., & Whyte, S.B. (Eds.). (1995). *Disability and culture.* Berkeley: University of California Press.

Ivry, T. (2003). *The Ultrasonic horror picture show: Obstetrical ultrasound in Israeli public spheres.* Paper presented at the Annual Meeting of the American Anthropological Association, Chicago, Illinois.

Jezewski, M.A., & Sotnik, P. (2005). Disability service providers as culture brokers. In J. Stone (Ed.), *Culture and disability: Providing culturally competent services* (pp. 31–64). Thousand Oaks, CA: Sage Publications.

Kagawa-Singer, M., & Kassim-Lakha, S. (2003). A strategy to reduce cross-cultural miscommunication and increase the likelihood of improving health outcomes. *Academic Medicine, 78,*(6), 577–587.

Landsman, G. (1998). Reconstructing motherhood in the age of "perfect" babies: Mothers of infants and toddlers with disabilities. *Signs: Journal of Women in Culture and Society, 24,* 69–99.

Landsman, G. (1999). Does God give special kids to special parents?: Personhood and the child with disabilities as gift and as giver. In L. Layne (Ed.), *Transformative motherhood* (pp. 133–166). New York: NYU Press.

Landsman, G. (2003). Emplotting children's lives: Developmental delay vs. disability. *Social Science & Medicine, 56,* 1947–1960.

Landsman, G. (2004). "Too bad you got a lemon": Peter Singer, mothers of children with disabilities, and the critique of consumer culture. In J. Taylor, L. Layne, & D. Wozniak (Eds.), *Consuming motherhood* (pp. 100–121). New Brunswick, NJ: Rutgers University Press.

Landsman, G. (2005). Mothers and models of disability. *Journal of Medical Humanities, 26, (2/3)* 121–139.

Larson, E. (1998). Reframing the meaning of disability to families: The embrace of paradox. *Social Science & Medicine, 47,* 865–875.

Layne, L. (2003). *Motherhood lost: A feminist account of pregnancy loss in America.* New York: Routledge.

Leiter, V. (2004). Dilemmas in sharing care: Maternal provision of professionally driven therapy for children with disabilities. *Social Science & Medicine, 58,* 837–849.

Markens, S., Browner, C.H., & Press, N. (1997). Feeding the fetus: On interrogating the notion of maternal–fetal conflict. *Feminist Studies, 23*(2), 351–372.

Marshall, M. (1996). Problematizing impairment: Cultural competence in the Carolines. *Ethnology, 35*(4), 249–263.

McCubbin, H.I., Thompson, A., & McCubbin, M.A. (1996). *Family assessment: Resiliency, coping and adaptation.* Madison: University of Wisconsin–Madison.

McCubbin, M.A., & McCubbin, H.I. (1993). Families coping with illness: The resiliency model of family stress, adjustment, and adaptation. In C. Danielson, B. Hamell-Bissell, & P. Winstead-Fry (Eds.), *Families, health and illness: Perspectives on coping and intervention* (pp. 21–63). St. Louis: Mosby.

McKeever, P., & Miller, K. (2004). Mothering children who have disabilities: A Bourdieusian interpretation of maternal practices. *Social Science & Medicine, 59*(6), 1177–1191.

Miles, M. (1992). Concepts of mental retardation in Pakistan: Toward cross-cultural and historical perspectives. *Disability, Handicap & Society, 7*(3), 235–255.

Nachshen, J.S., Woodford, L., & Minnes, P. (2003). The Family Stress and Coping Interview for families of individuals with developmental disabilities: A lifespan perspective on family adjustment. *Journal of Intellectual Disability Research, 47,* 285–290.

Oaks, L. (2001). *Smoking and pregnancy: The politics of fetal protection.* New Brunswick, NJ: Rutgers University Press.

Oliver, M. (1990). *The politics of disablement.* London: Macmillan.

Park, J., Turnbull, A., & Turnbull, H.R., III. (2002). Impacts of poverty on quality of life in families of children with disabilities. *Exceptional Children, 68*(2), 151–170.

Petchesky, R. (1987). Fetal images: The power of visual culture and the politics of reproduction. *Feminist Studies, 13*(2), 263–292.

Pfeiffer, D. (1999). Clinical commentary: The categorization and control of people with disabilities. *Disability and Rehabilitation, 21*(3), 106–107.

Prussing, E., Sobo, E., Walker, E., & Kurtin, P. (2005). Between "desperation" and disability rights: A narrative analysis of complementary/alternative medicine use by parents for children with Down syndrome. *Social Science & Medicine, 60,* 587–598.

Read, J. (1998). Conductive education and the politics of disablement. *Disability and Society, 13*(2), 279–293.

Read, J. (2000). *Disability, the family and society: Listening to mothers.* Buckingham, England: Open University Press.

Roberts, D. (1991). Punishing drug addicts who have babies: Women of color, equality, and the right of privacy. *Harvard Law Review, 104,* 124–155.

Rogers-Adkinson, D., Ochoa, T., & Delgado, B. (2003). Developing cross-cultural competence: Serving families of children with significant developmental needs. *Focus on Autism and Other Developmental Disabilities, 18*(1), 4–8.

Saloviita, T., Italinna, M., & Leinonen, E. (2003). Explaining the parental stress of fathers and mothers caring for a child with intellectual disability: A Double ABCX Model. *Journal of Intellectual Disability Research, 47,* 300–312.

Scheer, J. (1994). Culture and disability: An anthropological point of view. In E. Trickett, R. Watts, & D. Birman (Eds.), *Human Diversity* (pp. 244–260). San Francisco: Jossey-Bass.

Scorgie, K., & Sobsey, D. (2000). Transformational outcomes associated with parenting children who have disabilities. *Mental Retardation, 38,* 195–206.

Seideman, R., & Kleine, P. (1995). A theory of transformed parenting: Parenting a child with developmental delay/mental retardation. *Nursing Research, 44,* 38–44.

Seltzer, M.M., Greenberg, J.S., Floyd, F.J., & Hong, J. (2004). Accommodative coping and well-being of midlife parents of children with mental health problems or developmental disabilities. *American Journal of Orthopsychiatry, 74,* 187–195.

Shearn, J., & Todd, S. (2000). Maternal employment and family responsibilities: The perspectives of mothers of children with intellectual disabilities. *Journal of Applied Research in Intellectual Disabilities, 13,* 109–131.

Shuttleworth, R., & Kasnitz, D. (2004). Stigma, community, and ethnography: Joan Ablon's contribution to the anthropology of impairment-disability. *Medical Anthropology Quarterly, 18*(2), 139–161.

Shuttleworth, R., & Kasnitz, D. (2006). Cultural context of disability. In G. Albrecht (Ed.), *Encyclopedia of disability* (pp. 330–337). Thousand Oaks, CA: Sage Publications.

Skinner, D., Bailey, D., Correa, V., & Rodriguez, P. (1999). Narrating self and disability: Latino mothers' constructions of identities vis-à-vis their child with special needs. *Exceptional Children, 65*(4), 481–495.

Sobo, E.J. (2003). Prevention and healing in the household: The Importance of socio-cultural context. In E.J. Sobo & P.S. Kurtin (Eds.), *Child health services research: Applications, innovations, and insights* (pp. 67–119). San Francisco: Jossey-Bass.

Sobo, E.J., & Seid, M. (2003). Cultural issues in health services delivery: What kind of "competence" is needed? *Annals of Behavioral Science and Medical Education, 9*(2), 97–100.

Spangenberg, J., & Theron, J. (2000). Stress and coping in parents of children with Down syndrome. *Studia-Psychologica, 43,* 41–48.

Taylor, J. (1998). Image of contradiction: Obstetrical ultrasound in American culture. In H. Ragone & S. Franklin (Eds.), *Reproducing reproduction* (pp. 15–45). Philadelphia: University of Pennsylvania Press.

Taylor, J. (2003). The story catches you and you fall down: Tragedy, ethnography, and "cultural competence." *Medical Anthropology Quarterly, 17*(2), 159–181.

Todd, S., & Jones, S. (2005). Looking at the future and seeing the past: The challenge of the middle years of parenting a child with intellectual disabilities. *Journal of Intellectual Disabilities Research, 49,* 389–404.

Traustadottir, R. (1991). Mothers who care: Gender, disability and family life. *Journal of Family Life, 12*(2), 211–228.

Turbiville, V.P., Turnbull, A.P., & Turnbull, H.R., III. (1995). Fathers and family-centered early intervention. *Infants and Young Children, 7*(4), 12–19.

Turnbull, A., Pereira, L., & Blue-Banning, M. (1999). Parents' facilitation of friendships between their children with a disability and friends without a disability. *Research and Practice for Persons with Severe Disabilities, 24*(2), 85–99.

Van Riper, M. (2000). Family variables associated with sibling well-being in families of children with Down syndrome. *Journal of Family Nursing, 6,* 267–286.

Van Riper, M. (2004). What families need to thrive. *Down Syndrome News, 27,* 18–22.

Van Riper, M. (in press). Families of children with Down syndrome: Responding to a "change of plans" with resilience. *Journal of Pediatric Nursing.*

Wayman, K., Lynch, E., & Hanson, M. (1990). Home-based early childhood services: Cultural sensitivity in a family systems approach. *Topics in Early Childhood Special Education, 10*(4), 56–75.

Weiss, M. (1998). Ethical reflections: Taking a walk on the wild side. In N. Scheper-Hughes & C. Sargent (Eds.), *Small wars: The cultural politics of childhood* (pp. 149–162). Berkeley: University of California Press.

5

LEARNING TO CARE AND ADVOCATE FOR CHILDREN WITH SPECIAL HEALTH CARE NEEDS:

A FAMILY PERSPECTIVE

Nora Wells

Aaccording to the National Survey of Children with Special Health Care Needs, 2001, one in five families in the United States has a child who is born with, or acquires, a special health care need (Child and Adolescent Health Measurement Initiative, 2004). Each of these families must learn about the challenges this special health need will mean for their child and about how they can help him or her best meet those challenges. This chapter explains how parents of a child with special health care needs (CSHCN) can best cope with a fragmented and opaque health care system so that they can access quality health care and help their child reach his or her maximum potential. Without central sources of information regarding services, parents with a CSHCN often turn to other CSHCN parents—individually, through groups, or on the web—to learn about various services available as well as how to navigate the system. As they learn, many parents express the desire to pass along their hard-won knowledge to help other parents who face similar experiences.

After reviewing these processes, this chapter presents parent-derived strategies for adapting to the challenges of their roles. The strategies take into account findings from a national survey conducted by Family Voices and Brandeis University of more than 3,000 families regarding their experiences in finding health care for their children (Wells, Doksum, Martin, & Cooper, 2000; Wells, Kraus, et al., 2000), and reflect this author's own experiences over the past 30 years as a parent of, and an advocate for other parents of children with special health care needs. The chapter also suggests ways that providers can proactively support the information needs of the families they serve and discusses ways to build and support trusting partnerships between families and physicians and other providers.

FAMILY EXPERTISE

In the context of this chapter, references to *parents* represent those who are most responsible for the care of the child. Generally, this is the biological mother, but it also may be the biological father, an adoptive or foster parent, a grandparent, or another family member or guardian. For this reason, and because people who live together are intertwined in many ways, we sometimes use the term *family* to refer to the context of those in this caregiving role. Further, as children may live with one or multiple parents, and as child care can be a singular as well as a joint or team task, the terms *parent* and *parents* are used interchangeably.

In contemporary U.S. society, parents are the most important people in a child's life and their most consistent caregivers. Although providers and staff of service systems fluctuate, parents and other family members are in most cases the constant in a child's life. Because of this caregiving experience, parents know their children in ways that no one else does. Indeed, no one has a more vested interest in being sure that the health care provided meets the needs of a child than his or her parents. They are often the ones most aware of when things are not going well for the child. Parents know when their children are happy or sad, comfortable or afraid. They also know when something is different or not right with their child's health. Parents are essential sources of information in identifying when something is wrong with their child and providing critical clues as to what the problem may be. They are crucial partners with health care providers in ensuring that their child receives the highest-quality medical care.

However, when a child is first diagnosed with a special health care need, parents may not realize how valuable their instincts and knowledge will be to ensuring effective quality health care for the child. This may be the case even though parents are responsible for making informed medical decisions on behalf of their child and for carrying out a great deal of his or her medical care.

Encouragement from health care professionals as well as support from other parents helps families learn to trust their instincts and to develop the confidence in their family expertise that allows them to assume the important roles of caregiver and advocate for their child. The expert medical training of the professional and the unique knowledge and commitment to the child of the family are each critical elements in a child's medical care. Respecting the expertise that each member brings to a partnership between parent and professional is essential to providing quality care. Often, however, it is only through other parents that parents of a newly diagnosed child learn the value of their active participation and advocacy.

Connecting with Other Families

Family Voices is a national grassroots organization of families and friends, speaking on behalf of children with special health care needs, that helps link CSHCN families with similar families, other resources, and support. The national Family Voices web site (www.familyvoices.org) provides information on many family friendly resources and links to Family to Family Health Information Centers in every state that assist families in finding the specific help they need. Family Voices has learned that helping families connect with other families as soon as possible after they learn or suspect that their child has a special need opens up whole new worlds of information and support. First, and most important, families realize that they are not alone in their experience, and second, they learn that there are many sources of practical information that will guide them in navigating the health care system. For example, in response to the Family Voices/Brandeis national survey about how she found information, one parent said, "No one has ever told me about what is available, really. Other parents telling parents is where I get 99.9% of information. My child would not have Early and Periodic Screening, Diagnosis, and Treatment (EPSDT), nursing care, a handicap placard, and diapers paid for if not for parents telling me" (Wells, Krauss et al., 2000, p. 7).

When a family first receives a diagnosis of a child's special need, however, parents are unlikely to be aware of the many options for and the value of connecting with families who share similar experiences. A provider who offers to help a family connect with a parent organization is providing an invaluable referral. In every state, there is a Family Voices contact as well as a parent-to-parent mechanism for connecting parents who have children with similar special health care needs so that they can provide emotional support for and exchange information with one another. Supporting parents receive training in how to supply information and encouragement, and most programs recruit supporting parents across many different disabilities, social economic groups, family structures, and cultural and ethnic backgrounds. Parent to Parent USA, an alliance of state parent-to-parent programs following established best practice standards, has a web site with background information about parent-to-parent support as well as links to state-specific parent-to-parent matching programs (www.p2pusa.org). Information about state-specific parent-matching programs also can be found at www.familyvillage.wisc.edu/cof_p2p. Another source of information about parent-to-parent matches for families whose child has a rare disorder is www.netnet.net/mums/. Families may also find one another through informal places such as hospitals or doctor's offices, or through structured environments such as support groups in hospitals and care settings, schools, and special programs. When a special need is identified in a child under the age of 3, a parent should be referred to an early intervention program. This often provides a first opportunity for parents to meet other parents in similar situations. When a special need is identified in an older child, it might take longer to find other families with whom to connect, but many parents find success through their health care providers, schools or churches, friends or neighbors, and the Internet.

Parent organizations specific to many diagnoses can be located by searching the Internet or the phone book. Disability-specific parent organizations provide a wide variety of resources—from referrals to medical research and journal articles to opportunities to participate in Internet chat rooms. The National Dissemination Center for Children with Disabilities (www.nichcy.org) is a helpful link to disability groups as well as to information about specific disabilities and special education.

Sharing Information with Other Parents

Once parents make a connection with other parents, they frequently report how valuable they find the opportunities to gather and share information about all kinds of issues related to caring for their child. Parents may share with other parents emotional and peer support; concrete information about programs, services, and resources; experiences with health care providers and care and treatment protocols; and practical solutions to specific problems. Parent organizations share family friendly information broadly through newsletters and web sites; offer advice, support, and referrals to individual parents seeking help in navigating systems and finding needed resources; and provide avenues for equipment exchange or the sharing of books and other resources. Parent organizations also provide parents with opportunities to learn and develop important advocacy and communication skills through materials, conferences, workshops, and trainings.

Families of children with special health care needs connect with other families in many ways and on many levels. Ideally, a community offers a variety of parent-provided support and information opportunities so that an individual parent can find the kind of support that best meets his or her needs. Such opportunities might include parents connecting individually with each other in person, by phone, or through the Internet, or a group of parents meeting for discussions of issues of mutual interest. These parent connections help parents not only to ensure quality care for their child with special health care needs, but also to participate in activities that will affect health care policy and programs at the local, state, and national levels.

BUILDING PARTNERSHIPS WITH PROVIDERS

Although it may take time for parents to connect with other parents, the partnership between a child's parents and health care providers begins at diagnosis and is thus a critical piece in helping parents to become effective advocates for their child. The most fruitful parent–provider partnerships are built on mutual trust and honesty. From the beginning, providers have a responsibility to model an open exchange of information and to show respect for the unique perspective of each family. They must be considerate of the strengths and individuality of each family and of that family's specific methods of coping. On the family side, parents have the responsibility to share fully their concerns about their child and their expectations of the partnership. To build effective partnerships, both families and professionals need time to learn each other's styles and expectations.

Although some providers enter the lives of a child and his or her family in response to a medical crisis, others are purposefully brought in. Parents usually have some leeway, however constrained by insurance status and regulations, in choosing their child's providers. To choose effectively, they need to consider carefully what qualities are most important to them in a provider. Often, health coverage plans require that a child have a primary care provider who is responsible for referring the child to all specialists and other providers and services and for coordinating the child's care. Having a good relationship with a primary care provider who serves in this referral role is especially important for a child with special needs who may have to rely on a number of specialty providers.

Often parents turn to other parents of children with special needs for advice on finding a provider who will meet their needs. Parents ask one another for information regarding their experiences with various providers and make suggestions about the best questions to ask to evaluate a provider or treatment option and to gain more complete information to help them make informed decisions.

Parents need to be comfortable with a provider's training and experience and with the hospitals and specialists to whom the provider refers them. Parents want to know how much experience a provider has with their child's special need, and, if they do not have experience, how willing they are to become knowledgeable about it. They want to feel comfortable with the personality and style of the provider and to understand his or her approach to sharing information. Families want to know if the provider will allow parents to be with their children during treatments and procedures. They want to know if the provider will help the family find community services and payment for needed services.

Other factors parents consider in choosing a provider include whether the provider's location and office hours are convenient for them, how easy it is to get an appointment, whether there are special considerations given for extra time, if it is needed, during medical appointments or special waiting room procedures for a child who might need them, as well as how the provider handles emergencies. Frequently, parents advise other parents to get to know all the providers within a group practice, and to ask questions about how the group practice handles coverage in complicated cases of children with special needs.

Families advise one another to learn about the provider's approach to sharing decisions about the child's care. It is critical that a family is comfortable with the provider's approach to communicating with them and their child. Parents advise one another to ask: How will the provider help us gather the information we need to take part in decision making, and how will the provider help us think these decisions through? Further, parents encourage one another to include the child as a partner in his or her own care as early as possible. Parents want the providers they choose to respect their child, to communicate effectively and directly with him or her, and to help the child learn about his or her own health care.

Parents must fully understand medical instructions they are given and feel comfortable asking questions to clear up uncertainties they might have. The best intended medical care will not succeed if parents do not understand or follow instructions for the care they are responsible for carrying out. Providers cannot make appropriate adjustments to care plans if they do not understand a parent's concerns or hear a parent's perceptions of how a child is reacting to treatment. Parents urge one another to speak up with regard to any confusion they have about a treatment regimen or observations about a child's response to treatment. Parents advise other parents to learn as much as they can about care and treatment and to take as much responsibility for their child's care as they feel comfortable doing.

Family members and professionals share responsibility for being honest with one another about their relationship. If a parent is not comfortable with a provider's approach or treatment, it is important to talk with the provider about his or her concerns and ask for clarification or support for the provider's treatment plan. If they wish, parents should ask for time to seek out other opinions or to think thoroughly about a suggested treatment before making a decision to go ahead with it. Providers should welcome and honor a request for a second opinion, and parents should be concerned about providers who refuse or limit additional opinions. In many cases, parents and professionals can work out difficulties in a relationship over time. Not all families and providers work effectively together, however. If parents feel that they are not able to build a beneficial partnership with a provider, they should not hesitate to make a change. If they do, parents should explain to the current provider why they feel such a change is necessary, and they should give feedback to the provider about their impressions of the partnership. If such an exchange takes place, providers should listen: Parents talk to other parents and reputations may precede providers in ways that are not productive for those who are unresponsive.

Obtaining Information from Providers

One thing that families most frequently say they need is access to sources of information that will help them learn as much as they can about their child's special needs and the services available to help them. Although parents are helpful to one another in this regard, finding information about the specific medical care begins with the child's initial health care providers. When parents first suspect that there might be something wrong with their child's health, they naturally have many questions. They will likely think of additional questions as they learn more about the diagnosis and suggested treatments and as they have an opportunity to gather information from a variety of sources. Families also express the hope that providers will keep them updated with information on medical research that might help their child.

Providers who are receptive to parent inquiries can be an enormous help to parents. When professionals share clear and complete information about what they know and don't know about a diagnosis and direct parents to where to get additional information, they model an expectation that the parent will be an informed, active participant in their child's care. When providers explicitly reassure parents that their questions and opinions are valid and important, they are encouraging parents to become confident advocates for their child. When parents are connected to other parents and have an opportunity to discuss their experiences around diagnosis, treatments, or decisions, they are encouraged and strengthened in their confidence to become active, informed partners in their child's care. Sharing experiences and hearing others' questions and reactions help parents build effective advocacy skills.

Families gain important perspectives by searching widely for as much information as possible about their child's diagnosis and suggested treatments. It is often reassuring for a family member to have an opportunity to talk with more than one provider about his or her questions, either by getting a second opinion from another physician or by speaking to a nurse or physician's assistant who works with the child. It also can be helpful for parents to hear their own or other providers give presentations about their child's diagnosis at conferences or meetings, when they can listen to a provider talk in a more general way about health care instead of a more emotionally charged discussion of their own child's situation. Families can gain further insight by asking questions of teachers, caregivers, neighbors, or friends who work with their child. All the information they learn about their child will help parents seek the best care and become the best partner in providing and participating in health care for their child.

Obtaining Information from Other Sources

Many families like to learn more about a diagnosis or treatment by reading and investigating on their own. As one parent said in the Family Voices/Brandeis survey, "I have done a lot of independent research regarding all of my children's needs. I have learned how to coordinate the teams who provide services to [both my children with special needs]. I have had to rely on my own so much I have become able to help others. . . . I have a high school education and am a stay-at-home mom. I've learned a lot on my own [about] the system" (Wells, Doksum et al., 2000, p. 7). Parents like this tell one another, for example, that many children's hospitals have family resource rooms with a variety of information and often have staff to help a family find answers to specific questions. Further, each state has a Maternal and Child Health Bureau Title V program for children with special needs, which is a source of information for families about health care and community resources within the state.

The Internet can be a rich source of information, and families often help other families by suggesting particularly good web sites, articles, books, or other sources of material that might lead them to information about a condition or treatment options. Family Village (www.familyvillage.wisc.edu) provides access to a wide range of family friendly information in an online library about disability and special needs topics. One tip from parents is about the importance of sharing information they've found with their child's provider and giving the provider feedback on the value of Internet or written resources, so that the provider can pass this information on to other families.

MEDICAL RECORDS AND INFORMED CONSENT

Although generic information about conditions or procedures is important, information specific to each child is critically important for families to become effective advocates for their children.

Reading the Medical Records

Families should ask to read their child's medical record, and providers should offer families the opportunity to do so. Reading the medical record helps the family to understand more fully the information their provider has given them about treatment and diagnosis. It can also help a family to recognize which questions they need to ask to fully understand their child's condition and treatments and to make informed decisions about options. By carefully reading medical records, parents can play an important role in ensuring that their child receives quality care. Parents may find omissions in the record, such as a missing report from a specialist; they may find an error such as an inaccurate measurement or medication dose that could be critical to accurate treatment; or they may want to add comments to the record. A parent also has the right to make copies of their child's medical records, reproduced at a reasonable cost.

The medical record contains not only important case history information but also legal forms regarding consent to treat. Once a treatment or procedure has been recommended, the parent is required to provide such consent, acknowledging that they understand the nature, extent, and consequences of the treatment or procedure to which they are consenting. Families must rely on providers to give them the appropriate medical information, in terms they can understand, to make these decisions. Support and information they have received from other parents regarding their rights and responsibilities to ask questions and require clear answers can be critical in such situations; parents might otherwise find themselves confused and anxious about signing an informed consent form. It is very important that parents feel comfortable asking questions about what they don't understand to make sure that their consent is based on a solid understanding of what they are signing.

Including a Child in the Consent Process

As soon as they are able, the child should be included in providing this consent. Parents and providers should encourage the child to be part of this process of assent. If a child does not have the physical dexterity to write his or her signature but is able to understand the treatment options, the child can participate in this important process if provided with a signature stamp. This is the kind of information that one parent might learn from another parent. It is a simple strategy that parents might provide on their own, especially when a hospital might not offer this approach.

SUPPORTING A CHILD THROUGH MEDICAL PROCEDURES

Medical exams, tests, and treatments may be a frequent and regular part of the lives of children with special health care needs. Learning to cope with these experiences not only can make the test or treatment more successful, but it also helps the child gain mastery over his or her environment and approach each future experience with increased confidence.

Preparing a Child for Medical Tests and Procedures

Parents share with other parents ideas about how to prepare their children for medical tests or procedures or other medical experiences. To prepare a child, parents must first know themselves what to expect. By seeking information in advance from other parents and providers, parents can gather information about a test, treatment, or procedure that they can share with their child. When possible, as the child becomes older, the parents can help the maturing son or daughter learn how to seek and gather this kind of background information him- or herself.

Preparing children includes helping them understand what the treatment or test is for, how it will be done, and what the child might experience. Families and children want to know why a given treatment is being proposed, how it might benefit the child, and what risks are involved. They want to know how long the treatment will take and how its efficacy will be judged. What can they expect to change as a result of the treatment, test, or procedure? How and when might they expect to get the results for a test? When medication is recommended, what possible effects will it have, how will it be administered, are there contraindications to its use?

Being with a Child During Tests or Procedures

Having a parent present during a child's medical exam, test, or procedure or while the child is in the hospital can be enormously reassuring to both the child and the parent. Parents who have consulted with other parents may have selected a primary care provider who supports their desire to remain with their child through medical experiences. Other parents will learn the hard way that they will need to ask questions in advance in every setting to be sure that a hospital or doctor will follow the parent's wish to be present. If the law requires a parent to give informed consent, a hospital cannot restrict the parents' right to visit their child in the hospital at any time unless it would interfere with the care of other patients. But parents often do not know this unless other parents tell them.

COORDINATING CARE AND CONNECTING PROVIDERS

Children with special health care needs often see several different providers. One of the keys to helping families learn to advocate effectively, whether in coordinating care from a variety of providers or ensuring their child's access to certain services, is to help them understand the various agencies and systems that actually provide or pay for their child's care, including what each agency/system does and does not provide, the connections (and disconnections) between the agencies/systems, and how to work within those that are central to the child in question. For example, for a child who will frequently be in a hospital, a family needs to learn who makes decisions within the hospital setting, how to ask questions and get answers, how to complain if something is not going well, and how to provide feedback. Learning how each agency/system operates and how to identify allies within each can help a family navigate them more effectively.

Maintaining Accurate Records

Families are likely to be the only ones who have a complete picture of all the doctors, therapists, treatments, medications, school programs, and community services that a child is receiving. For this reason, it is important for families to maintain a complete record of information important to their child's care. This kind of information should include information on diagnosis, history, immunization/shot records, providers, medications prescribed, treatments and procedures, and details of medical orders to be carried out at home. It should include dates and details of all phone and in-person contacts with health care providers and providers of related services. Documentation of health insurance coverage and any communication with the coverage plan is also an important part of a child's health care record. It helps to include school records and records from community programs and public or private agencies that have been contacted. There are a variety of hard copy and electronic models for keeping personal medical or health records. Such records maintained by families can provide essential additional information, along with hospital or provider records, about a child's medical care. These records are important because without them a provider may not have all the information needed to make a decision on a treatment or medication at the time of a visit. The concept of a *medical home* (see Chapter 6) emphasizes the importance of a central health care provider, usually a primary care provider, who coordinates all aspects of a child's medical care and assures that all appropriate care is provided. Unfortunately, many families do not report that their child's care includes all aspects of a medical home. In the National Survey of Children with Special Needs sponsored by the Maternal and Child Health Bureau in 2001, almost half (47%) of respondents reported that a medical home for their child had not been achieved (Child and Adolescent Health Measurement Initiative, 2004). Many of the surveyed parents commented that coordinating multiple providers and payment sources is frequently left to them. For example, a parent replying to the Family Voices/Brandeis national survey reported, "I feel the concept of 'care coordination' is a myth. All of my son's health care is fragmented and left to parents to 'coordinate' as best we can. . . . I make a lot of phone calls and coordinate most of it myself. It would be nice to have some qualified help" (Wells, Krauss et al., 2000, p. 6).

Communication Between Parents and Providers

An effective partnership between parents and provider can greatly improve how care is coordinated for a child with special health care needs. For example, the provider could ask the family how the coordination of their child's care is working, what further help they need, and how the provider can help to find the needed assistance in coordinating care for the child. Providers should be concerned about and ask questions regarding all aspects of the child's care and life. They could greatly enhance the coordination of care by promoting communication among the child's health care providers and by consistently supplying records to the primary care provider to ensure accurate documentation of care. When a child relies on care from a number of providers, it is helpful when key providers and family members meet at least once a year to discuss the child's health care and to develop a coordinated written plan for that care.

UNDERSTANDING HEALTH CARE COVERAGE

No matter how good a parent becomes at connecting the providers who care for his or her child, without learning to work with the child's health care insurance company, or public program paying for health care, parents will have a difficult time ensuring that their child gets all the necessary care. Here again, parents learn an enormous amount from other parents about how to work with health coverage companies and programs to ensure that their child gets that care. If the health coverage is provided through an employer, the employer's benefits representative may be able to help a child gain access to a needed service or provider. When the child's health coverage is through a public program such as Medicaid, the family will want to identify key program staff that can help them negotiate within the program.

Having Access to Providers

One of the most important features to understand about a health coverage plan is how to access providers. For children, access to providers trained in pediatric care is particularly important; however, all providers are not covered by all health plans. Many families find themselves having to switch health coverage plans because of a change in job or in a child's eligibility for a program. This can be particularly troublesome when such a change in plans means not only learning how a new plan works but also having to change a child's health care providers to ones who are part of the new health coverage plan.

To understand a health plan, it is helpful for a parent to request a copy of the actual contract or legal document that defines the relationship. It is critical that a family learn all they can about the specifics of the health insurance plan covering their child—for example, what is covered, how to accurately submit claims, and how to appeal if a claim is denied. Whenever possible, families should carefully check the medical bills for potential errors. To meet the requirements of a child with special health care needs, experienced parents have advised other parents to ask for special services or exceptions to policies in a friendly manner, carefully explaining the child's need in medical terms, personalizing the request, emphasizing cost savings, and being ready and willing to negotiate. Particularly for a child who needs a great deal of medical care, it can be critical to identify key allies within the insurance company or public program paying for services. If a claim is denied, the family can seek clarification of the denial and resubmit the claim providing additional information. It is extremely helpful to be persistent, to learn about and be willing to pursue the appeals process, and to be willing to seek legal assistance and/or file a complaint if the parents feel that the child's claim has been wrongfully denied.

Assuring funding for the medical care that providers recommend for a child with special health care needs can be a very complex process. Many families must seek more than one source of payment to fund the health care that their child needs, so it is helpful to learn about all of the programs and services that a child may be eligible for and how each program or provider works.

The family may need to seek a secondary health coverage plan, for example, through a public program such as a Medicaid Waiver in their state. To do so, they first need to know that the program exists, whether their child is eligible, how to apply, and what supporting information may be needed to document their need. Often families require help in understanding all the potential sources of health care coverage, how such sources might be blended to pay for medical services, and how these coverage options can meet their child's needs. A child with special health care needs may be eligible for special education services that can cover related services such as physical therapy, occupational therapy, speech therapy, behavior supports, or counseling. Other sources of funding can be found in community programs or private foundations. Parents need to know about care coordinators in physician's offices and public programs and case managers within insurance plans who may be able to help find sources of payment to cover services their child needs (Wells et al., 1999). Family Voices (kidshealth@familyvoices.org) can help families in every state understand how to navigate these complex funding sources (see also Chapters 2 and 3 regarding funding and related policies).

Becoming Advocates for Their Children

Through learning all about their child's special health care needs and the services and systems that can serve them, most parents become, over time and through necessity, strong and effective advocates for their children. The persistence and insight of families during the past 50 years have not only helped ensure quality care for their own children, but also have helped to shape extraordinary changes in the way health care is provided to all children. These families have revolutionized the expectations that parents, providers, and other health care professionals have for parental roles in medical care for children. Today, there is a great deal of knowledge about what helps families take on the critical role of advocate for their children. Many levels of our health care systems are now seeking and supporting this role for families. Through honest communication, clear expectations, and mutual support, parents and professionals together can build the partnerships that will improve the quality of care for each child with special health care needs, and in turn will enhance health care for all of our nation's children.

REFERENCES

Child and Adolescent Health Measurement Initiative (2004). *National survey of children with special health care needs.* Retrieved February 14, 2005, from

Data Resource Center on Child and Adolescent Health web site, http://www.cshcndata.org

Wells, N. (1995). *Parents as health care consumers*. In Marc S. Miller (Ed.), *Families USA guide to quality and cost: Health care choices for today's consumer* (pp. 119–136). Washington, DC: Living Planet Press.

Wells, N., Brown, L., Cole, M., Gionet, A., Gresek, C., Mitchell, M., et al. (1999). *Paying the bills: Tips for families on financing health care for children with special needs* (2nd ed.). Boston: New England SERVE. Retrieved March 25, 2005, from http://www.neserve.org/neserve/ptb.html

Wells, N., Doksum, T., Martin, L., & Cooper, J. (2000). *What do families say about health care for children with special health care needs in California? Your voice counts!! Family survey report to California participants* (May). Boston: Family Voices at the Federation for Children with Special Health Care Needs. Retrieved March 20, 2005, from http://www.familyvoices.org/YourVoiceCounts/CA%20Famrpt.pdf

Wells, N., Krauss, M.W., Anderson, B., Gulley, S., Leiter, V., O'Neil, M., et al. (2000). *What do families say about health care for children with special health care needs? Your voice counts!! The family partners project report to families* (April, 2nd ed.). Boston: Family Voices at the Federation for Children with Special Health Care Needs. Retrieved March 20, 2005, from http://www.familyvoices.org/YourVoiceCounts/National%20Famrpt.pdf

III

THE PROVIDER EXPERIENCE

T he provision of high-quality care for children with special health care needs (CSHCN) is constrained by time and financial limitations, by a lack of clarity regarding the proper advocacy role of the provider, and by a lack of clarity regarding care coordination or case management responsibilities and location of the medical home. Further, different specialists have different types of interactions with CSHCNs, their families, and their primary care physicians (PCPs). The proliferation of managed care programs raises even more concerns and obstacles, as many managed care plans "are not routinely designed to respond to the special needs of children who have disabilities and chronic illnesses" (American Academy of Pediatrics Committee on Children with Disabilities, 1997).

Each chapter in this section acknowledges the constraints of funding arrangements and addresses the tension between specialist and PCP care. Each chapter also acknowledges the need for good communication and team-based care and the important role that therapists and other allied health professionals play. All of the chapters in this section offer a synopsis of the system that the authors work within, ways in which they improved that system, and ways that the system could work even better for CSHCN. Each chapter discusses a particular issue (as identified in the title of the chapter) that is relevant to his or her specialization. Chapters in this section are experience-based and include information of the sort not generally shared in published papers or presentations—practical information that will be of great value to health care professionals working on the front lines and seeking to better serve CSHCN and their families. This information is also of value to families: It helps them better understand how providers can, in some instances, work effectively within the system while at other times the system constrains their ability to provide care in the manner they think is best for the child.

In Chapter 6, pediatricians Charles Homer and Carl Cooley address models of care. The delivery of excellent health care for children with a chronic illness has long been hampered by the absence of a conceptual model with enough specificity to provide practical guidance to frontline physicians seeking to improve care. Two parallel efforts—the medical home concept and the chronic care model—have arrived at similar conclusions about a system of care that works. The medical home refers to the main source of care and care coordination or case management; the Chronic Care Model (Wagner, Austin, & Von Korff, 1998) provides guidance on conceptualizing roles and relationships for and between the patient, family, care team, and community. In its focus on the medical home, this chapter describes each of these approaches, including their vast overlap and subtle differences. It proposes their formal integration and explains how this has worked in dozens of practices with whom Homer and Cooley have worked. It also reports on several successful programs in other practices that resulted in improved care.

In Chapter 7, pediatrician Thomas McInerny specifically addresses the poorly defined role of the PCP in caring for CSHCN. PCPs are torn by a triad of conflicting forces, including the desire to provide comprehensive, family-sensitive care; the rapid advancement of technology and therapeutic modalities; and the increasingly complex regulations of and demands for so-called cost-effectiveness from managed care organizations. These forces press many PCPs to leave the care of CSHCN to specialists in tertiary care centers. After describing these very real competing forces, the chapter demonstrates how a busy PCP can balance or even diffuse his or her pressures and partner with families and specialists to provide up-to-date, sensitive, and coordinated care for CSHCN. The chapter begins by describing a typical practice morning, following a typical PCP from room to room, and phone call to phone call, as she or he sees patients for well-child health assessments, acute illnesses, and, most important, care coordination activities for CSHCN. In the process, this chapter describes how the PCP can learn continuously in an efficient manner; communicate effectively with specialists; utilize allied health professionals (e.g., nurse practitioners, physician assistants) and other office personnel to assist in care coordination, data gathering, and communication; interact positively with third party payors to demonstrate the value of, and be appropriately rewarded for, services; and utilize systems changes and technology advances to streamline and organize multiple consultations, lab tests, treatments, and so forth so that they are readily accessible when needed. The chapter concludes with a discussion of the basic principles of providing comprehensive, family-sensitive care to CSHCN: partnering with families to help them navigate the health care system; explaining complex diagnoses and treatments in terms understandable to the family; and monitoring and assisting the family in maintaining its stability, which is essential to achieving the optimal outcomes for their special children. Although providing this comprehensive care is demanding, the reward—improved well-being of children with special health care needs and their families—is great.

In Chapter 8, pediatric rheumatologist Robert M. Sheets and nephrologist and quality improvement specialist Paul S. Kurtin explore the comprehensive case management role of physicians treating children with special health care needs. After defining *case management,* Sheets and Kurtin reflect on their own experiences both in case managing care for CSHCN and in delegating case management. They examine the assumptions that Sheets had about case management as a pediatric PCP and explore the implications that his experiences as a specialist have had for his approach to case management. By examining examples of both failures and successes, and showing how the assumptions of PCPs regarding specialist care in particular can be in error, the chapter illustrates the issues at stake. Patient variables such as morbidity, chronicity, and curability affect the case management decision, and the chapter discusses how and why this is so. In certain conditions (e.g., dermatomyositis, an acquired muscle disease entailing profound weakness), the pediatric rheumatologist must be the case manager and educator of the patient, family, and general pediatrician. With direct communication, the pediatric rheumatologist can enlist the support of the PCP in providing ongoing well-child care. Both should agree on respective roles and responsibilities, and the family should be part of this agreement. Care can be compromised if the PCP tries to manage rare or complex cases, or if the rheumatologist tries to case manage simple cases that really should be the purview of the PCP. The care also can be suboptimal if the family is uncomfortable with the distribution of case management duties.

Chapter 9 takes us back full circle to the family experience as viewed through the eyes of developmental specialists Laurel Leslie and Kristin Gist. When parents are first informed that their child may have special health or developmental needs, their dreams for their child's life may shatter. Their own lives may change immediately and drastically. It is during this period, which can occur at or before birth (e.g., when a child is born prematurely or with complications, when genetic tests reveal a potential chronic condition before the child is born) or many months later (e.g., following an episode of meningitis or the detection of early signs of autism), that parents have their most intensive contact with the health care system. This chapter addresses the educational, developmental, and support needs that face a child and his or her family as they revise their dreams and make new discoveries regarding abilities and potentials. The chapter emphasizes the need for early identification and intervention, and offers strategies for dealing with the complexity of the present system and establishing interdisciplinary, interagency partnerships. It explores how both parents and pediatricians must work within the health care, insurance, and educational systems to ensure that their children and patients receive the services they need.

Not all specialist care is medical; in fact, allied health professionals carry out much of the care for many children with special health care needs. The chapter explains what types of care therapists in developmental services offer and asks what the therapist's and primary care physician's roles are (and should be) in screening for and assessing problems, securing referrals, and advocating for families and children. The latter may include preparing parents to experience a dramatic learning curve and providing them with the information and authority to advocate for their children in an increasingly complex system. This chapter emphasizes the importance of effective relationships and communication among the parents, pediatricians, and various specialized service providers. It also discusses therapists empowering parents to educate their children's physicians and to navigate the system in ways that both respect system limitations and optimize child and family functioning and outcomes.

REFERENCES

American Academy of Pediatrics Committee on Children with Disabilities. (1997). General principles in the care of children and adolescents with genetic disorders and other chronic health conditions. *Pediatrics, 99*(4), 643–644.

Wagner, E.H., Austin, B.T., & Von Korff, M. (1996). Organizing care for patients with chronic illness. *Milbank Quarterly, 74*(4), 511–544.

6

CREATING A MEDICAL HOME FOR CHILDREN WITH SPECIAL HEALTH CARE NEEDS

Charles J. Homer and W. Carl Cooley

C hildren with special health care needs (CSHCN)[1] are a diverse
group. Some have complex, multisystem disorders and require
technology to fulfill the basic functions of life such as eating or
breathing, while others have conditions that affect a single organ system
or are only intermittent in their effects on the child. Some children
have conditions that are well described, with a known trajectory, while
others have conditions that are exceedingly rare or difficult to catego-
rize and predict. Some children's conditions are present at birth while
others are acquired sometime after.

The families in which CSHCN live are as diverse as are the children's conditions. Some families are poor and some are affluent. Some
live in major cities near abundant sources of specialized care, and others
live in remote locations. Some families have a single parent and others
have two (or more) parents. Some families have just one child and
others have many children.

Given the diversity of children with chronic conditions and their
family situations, how can we say which type of care (*care model*) best
meets the needs of this heterogeneous group? On some level, models
of care must be as diverse as the individual needs and circumstances
they have been developed to address.

Yet, survey data collected from families over the past several decades are remarkably consistent in identifying what families want for
their children, regardless of illness or disability type, cultural background, or household configuration (Hobbs, Ireys, & Perrin, 1991; Orr,
Weller, Satterwhite, & Pless, 1984; Perry & Ireys, 2001; Pless, Satter-

---

[1] Children with special health care needs (CSHCN) are a subset of the larger population referred to in many program and policy documents as CYSHCN (children and youth
with special health care needs). Although none of the contributors to this book would
ignore the challenges that accompany older children (youth), this book focuses on children ages 0–5. Therefore, we use the acronym CSHCN throughout the chapter. Please
note, however, that many of the surveys and data sets that we draw on are not limited
to that age range, and therefore findings must be interpreted with caution in relation to
younger children and their families.

white, & Van Vechten, 1976, 1978). Families want care that is timely and technically expert. They want care that provides the right diagnosis, the right treatment, the right procedures, and the right follow-up. They want up-to-date information related to their child's condition— treatments, outcomes, and the like. They want care that encompasses the full spectrum of their child's needs, including prevention and education, not just a single bodily system or condition. They want care that addresses the mental as well as the physical health needs of their child and family, and they want care that helps them prepare for the future. They want an approach to communication that respects their particular cultural and linguistic heritage, including their religious beliefs.

The same type of survey data also show that the care that CSHCN now receive falls far short of what is desired. For example, using the National Survey of Children with Special Health Care Needs (2001), we found that 23% of parents reported being unable to get key family support services, and 33% reported not receiving family-centered care (National Survey of Children with Special Health Care Needs, 2001).

THE MEDICAL HOME

Responding to this clear and consistent message, the Maternal and Child Health Bureau (MCHB), part of the Health Resources and Services Administration within the U.S. Department of Health and Human Services, and the American Academy of Pediatrics (AAP), the professional organization of pediatricians in the United States, formulated the concept of the *medical home* (AAP Medical Home Initiatives for Children with Special Needs Project Advisory Committee, 2004; American Academy of Pediatrics [AAP] Ad Hoc Task Force on Definition of the Medical Home,1992; see also, Sia, Tonniges, Osterhus, & Taba, 2004).

The *medical home* is the organizational setting that not only provides specific health care services, but also integrates preventive services and acute illness and chronic condition management. An effective medical home seeks to identify the broad spectrum of the needs of a CSHCN and his or her family at a given point in time (including preventive care and psychosocial items), as well as to anticipate and design care to address the child's future needs. The medical home coordinates among agencies and services in the child's community (*horizontal coordination*) and within the health care system (*vertical coordination*) to address current health needs. It also provides continuity over time to address future health care needs. Care in a medical home spans childhood through adolescence and facilitates a smooth transition to adult services. The medical home fosters competence in patients and families as its key strategy to achieve positive results. This conceptual framework addresses the commonality of needs of CSHCN and their families, and at the same time is flexible enough to provide for the diversity of needs outlined above.

This definition of the medical home overlaps substantially with the most widely accepted definition of primary care: ". . . the provision of integrated, accessible health care services by clinicians who are accountable for addressing a large majority of personal health care needs, developing a sustained partnership with patients, and practicing in the context of family and community" (Donaldson, Yordy, Lohr, & Vanselow, 1996, p. 1). The medical home definition does not prescribe what type of clinician (e.g., generalist versus *specialist*[2]) or what type of setting can constitute a medical home, but it does make clear that the entity that assumes responsibility for the medical home function must assume responsibility for all of the components, not just some of them.

Although rooted in the clear articulation of patient needs and wishes, the medical home is not seen as immediately useful by all involved. Many parents are reluctant to entrust the care of their child with a chronic condition to a primary care clinician out of fear that such providers won't be up-to-date on the latest treatments. In addition, if families are already seeing a specialist, they may resent having to make additional visits to a different clinician.

Many primary care physicians (PCPs) are reluctant to care for CSHCN because they also fear that they are not up-to-date, particularly if a child has an uncommon condition. Moreover, primary care physicians often are concerned about the increased time required in providing care for children with chronic conditions, particularly complex ones, assuming that this time may not be well reimbursed.

At the same time, pediatric specialists are in short supply and great demand, and they have many priorities (research, teaching) that compete with their patient care responsibilities. Moreover, many specialists view providing preventive care, addressing family needs, and coordinating with community resources as outside the scope of their expertise. In addition, these aspects of comprehensive care are rarely better reimbursed in the specialty setting than they are in primary care, and reimbursement concerns may discourage them from providing such comprehensive care (Jewett, Anderson, & Gilchrist, 2005; Mayer, Skinner, & Slifkin, 2004).

As a result of the tension among the beliefs held by these three

---

[2] General pediatricians and family physicians view themselves as *specialists* in the care of children and families, respectively. Reflecting common usage, the term *specialist* is used throughout this book to refer to pediatricians with advanced training in a narrower clinical aspect of pediatrics such as nephrology or hematology.

stakeholder groups, the medical home concept has been slow to spread, with, at most, 54% of families with CSHCN reporting that they have a medical home (McPherson et al., 2004). Parents too often remain stuck in the middle—unhappy with care in both primary care and specialty settings.

The question we have wrestled with is how to implement care *on the ground* that better meets the expressed needs of children and their families, while at the same time addresses the constraints that confront both primary care and specialty physicians and the programs in which they work. We quickly realized that one barrier to widespread implementation of the medical home was the lack of specificity about which systems are required to support this approach to care. Our previous work had familiarized us with another model for the provision of care for people with chronic conditions: the Chronic Care Model developed by Edward Wagner and his colleagues Brian Austin and Michael Von Korff at the MacColl Institute of Group Health at Puget Sound (Wagner, Austin, & Von Korff, 1996a, 1996b). Their approach, while not specific to children and therefore missing some key factors related to the differences between care of children and care of adults (e.g., involvement of parents as partners in care), provides more operational guidance than the medical home concept as initially specified.

THE CHRONIC CARE MODEL

The Chronic Care Model[3] developed by Wagner and colleagues (1996b; see Figure 6.1) starts with the assumptions that care for people with a chronic illness is best delivered not by an individual provider alone but by a health care *team,* and that the team will best serve the patient if it can anticipate patient needs and act accordingly. The team can function most effectively when supportive clinical information, decision support, care delivery, and self-management support systems are in place within a practice or clinic, and when larger organizational systems also are aligned in support of the overall approach.

The Chronic Care Model further asserts that patients must participate in their own care as members of the care team. To do this, patients need sufficient knowledge, skills, and abilities to monitor and manage their conditions and their well-being. In caring for CSHCN, of course,

---

[3]The Chronic Care Model itself has continued to evolve and now incorporates more of these elements than it did when we adapted it for children's health care (see http:// www.improvingchroniccare.org). Also, because this model applies to the full spectrum of care—preventive and acute as well as chronic care—we have dropped the modifier *chronic* from the name.

Chronic Care Model

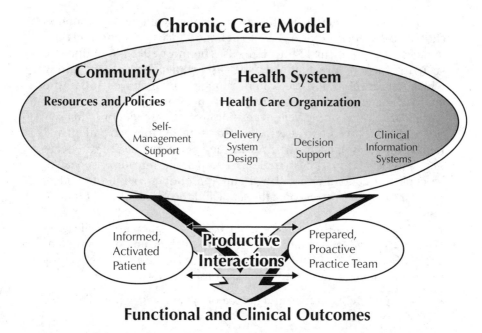

Figure 6.1. The Chronic Care Model. (From Wagner, E.H. [1998]. Chronic disease management: What will it take to improve care for chronic illness? *Effective Clinical Practice, 1,* 2–4; reprinted by permission.)

it is most often a parent who serves as the patient's voice and agent. The Chronic Care Model advises that health care practices and systems draw on community resources to help patients achieve better outcomes, and in one sense the child's parent is the most proximate member of his or her community circle.

Practices with appropriate *clinical information systems* are able to note which of their patients have specific clinical conditions (e.g., asthma), the severity or complexity of those conditions (e.g., severe persistent asthma), and whichever other information is relevant to the patient management question at hand (e.g., "Are all eligible children with asthma using the proper dosage of anti-inflammatory medication?"). Some practices have registries or clinical information databases devoted specifically to patients with particular ailments or conditions or to patients with chronic conditions more generally. Practices that not only have clinical information systems but that use them actively to assist in the management of individual patients to monitor performance overall and for specific subgroups of patients (e.g., patients with severe asthma who are African American) have greater potential to enhance patient outcomes (Bodenheimer, Wagner, & Grumbach, 2002a, 2002b).

Interactions among health care providers, patients, and families should be designed to address issues of importance to patients and their families and to anticipate future needs. The most effective settings for such interactions are planned visits—scheduled encounters during which matters of importance can be thoughtfully reviewed and future approaches developed (e.g., changes in medication management for particular seasons of the year, transition to a new school or living setting). In order for care to be effectively customized for each patient and family, the roles of each participating member of the health care team (e.g., physician, nurse, desk clerk, parent, patient, nutritionist) need to be explicitly defined and clarified and appropriate training provided. Written care plans can become the script and the record of such planned visits.

Chronic care itself needs to be based, Wagner and colleagues (1996b) asserted, on evidence where it is available and on expert guidance where evidence is not available or needs interpretation. Basing care on evidence requires a mechanism for practices

- To determine what type and degree of evidence is required to drive change

- To review and obtain evidence-based recommendations

- To share such information with patients and families so that there is common understanding

- To embed the evidence in clinical information or medical records systems so that faulty memory does not impede delivery of evidence-based care

- To maintain ready access to specialty expertise—either through referral, discussion and consultation, or specialty assumption of ongoing care if a need for this becomes clear (Feifer, Ornstein, Nietert, & Jenkins, 2001)

The most critical component of the Chronic Care Model is what Wagner and colleagues (1996b) termed *self-management support*—that is, the provision of care in a way that promotes patients' ability to provide and manage their own care. This framing acknowledges that professional health care providers are really facilitators, and the decisions, behaviors, and actions of patients are the final determinants of what happens. The core aspect of self-management support is the development of shared goals between patients and clinicians and the subsequent development of specific, mutually agreed-upon plans to achieve these goals.

The Chronic Care Model highlights two additional areas that are crucial to meeting the needs of persons with chronic conditions: 1) the alignment of provider activities with organizational aims and 2) community mobilization.

The activities of frontline providers and those who support them (e.g., clerks, lab staff) can only be sustained over time if the activities are aligned with organizational priorities and goals. Specifically, reimbursement systems and career advancement opportunities must reward the types of activities that the provision of excellent chronic care requires. In addition, effective strategies such as longitudinal training using practice data, role play, and the like should be undertaken to support behavior change (Davis et al., 1999).

Individuals with chronic conditions must be assisted in drawing on the resources of the larger community. This includes not only accessing formal supports and entitlements such as housing, employment-support, and special education services, but also informal and natural supports provided by community resources such as churches, libraries, family, and friends.

THE CARE MODEL FOR CHILD HEALTH IN A MEDICAL HOME

As noted above, the Chronic Care Model developed by Wagner and colleagues (1996b) was not designed specifically for children, although the overall framework is based in part on evidence of what works for both children and adults. The National Initiative for Children's Healthcare Quality and the Center for Medical Home Improvement, working together, adapted the Chronic Care Model in subtle ways to make it more suitable for the health care of children and more consistent with the terminology of the medical home (see Figure 6.2, Table 6.1). That model is called the Care Model for Child Health in a Medical Home.

Comparing the Care Model for Child Health and the Chronic Care Model

The Care Model for Child Health in a Medical Home places relatively greater emphasis on establishing close and effective linkages among the health care system, the family, and the community. Schools, child care, housing resources, community counseling programs, transportation systems, and the like must be responsive to the needs of CSHCN and their families. Formal and informal links need to be established between the medical home and these resources so that child and family needs

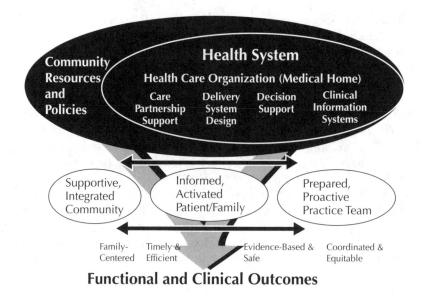

Figure 6.2. The Care Model for Child Health in a Medical Home.

are met consistently and expeditiously. We reflect this increased emphasis by specifying that a connected and responsive community is a key intermediate outcome of having the model in place.

Children with special health care needs by definition require greater services than other children (McPherson et al., 1998). These services are found in the community (horizontal) and the health care system (vertical). The complexity of these services and the typical fragmentation in their provision requires a greater emphasis on the function of care coordination. We place the locus of responsibility for performing care coordination on the effectively designed care team (delivery system design). Office-based care coordination may include the development of resource manuals, facilitation of referrals to community-based agencies, follow-through communication with local resources, and establishment of working relationships with key agencies such as schools and early intervention programs. Care coordination

Table 6.1. Areas of emphasis in the care model for child health in a medical home

- Increased emphasis on role of community
- Critical nature of care coordination
- Integration of self-management and family partnership
- Importance of cultural competency

also entails coordination of referrals and a seamless flow of information among primary care, specialty care (including mental health), and allied health providers. A designated office staff member may provide care coordination, or care coordination functions may be distributed in explicit ways among several individuals.

Also, because care for CSHCN includes supporting both the family's ability to provide care and the child's ability, in many cases, to assume self-care, we differentiate between *self-management support* and *family partnership*. For example, children with diabetes or asthma need to take increasing responsibility for monitoring their own condition and for adjusting their own medical regimen as they approach adolescence. The medical home needs to support the child's increasing competence in managing his or her own well-being and to counsel and support the family in monitoring the success of that effort while also maintaining the child's safety. We use the term *care partnership support* to encompass both self-management support and support of families as well as to provide an emphasis on the shared stake that families, patients, and professional have in the outcomes of care.

Finally, because children are ethnically and culturally diverse, we emphasize the critical role of delivering culturally effective care, weaving the concepts of cultural competency throughout each aspect of the care model. For example, we emphasize the importance of capturing information about ethnicity in patient registries so that practices can examine their care and outcomes by a patient subgroup. Similarly, we highlight the importance of using trained interpreters as a component of care partnership support to enable appropriate goal setting and care planning.[4] (For a more in-depth discussion of culture and care, see Chapter 4; see also Sobo 2003; Sobo & Seid, 2003.)

Implementing the Medical Home Model

As noted above, implementation of the medical home concept has been slow and inconsistent, in part because the concepts of the medical home have been difficult to measure and make operational. The Care Model for Child Health in the Medical Home addresses operationalization. Meanwhile, the Center for Medical Home Improvement developed and standardized a scoreable measure of *medical homeness* called the Medical

---

[4] One useful tool is the *Self-Assessment Checklist for Personnel Providing Services and Supports to Children and Youth with Special Health Needs and Their Families* at http://gucchd.georgetown.edu/nccc/nccc7.html (National Center for Cultural Competence, 2002). See also the National Initiative for Children's Healthcare Quality (NICHQ) 2005 publication: http://www.nichq.org/NICHQ/Programs/CollaborativeLearning/CulturalCompetency2005.htm

Home Index, which allows practices to assess their baseline and on-going implementation of the medical home concept and to target fruit-ful areas for further improvement (Cooley, McAllister, Sherrieb, & Clark, 2003).

In addition, efforts to spread implementation of the medical home did not take into account the complexity of making changes in what we have found to be a poorly operational and often demoralized health care system. Most previous efforts, in our view, focused on the name-able attributes of good care, which should be accessible, family-centered, continuous, comprehensive, coordinated, compassionate, and culturally competent. These efforts sought to inspire change by referring to how much families appreciated the medical home approach but ignored the pragmatic question: "How do I change my practice to get there?"

Based on our experiences, we believe that change in clinical prac-tice can be effectively accomplished by

1.   Directly involving families in the process of change

2.   Using an effective approach to improvement

3.   Participating in a structured learning or support process to maintain momentum and overcome barriers, such as the office-based im-provement model developed by the Center for Medical Home Im-provement (Cooley & McAllister, 2004) or the learning collabora-tive model developed by the Institute for Healthcare Improvement and applied to child health by the National Initiative for Children's Healthcare Quality

Engaging the family in this type of effort to change the delivery of care is critical. First, when families are involved, the focus of change efforts necessarily remains on meeting child and family needs (versus de-touring onto secondary issues such as reimbursement). Second, family engagement sustains attention over a long period of time, keeping prac-tices from falling victim to the fad of the month or year and the starting and stopping of programs based more upon the current trend and not on the ultimate health and well-being of children, youth, and families. Third, families provide a vast resource for talents and skills that are relevant to the improvement task, with many bringing expertise in a variety of disciplines that can be helpful to the improvement process such as education, business, communication, and, of course, parenting.

Engaging families is not a simple matter, however. Families need to be truly welcomed into the process and often must be trained in how to interact effectively as team members with health care pro-fessionals. For example, we have used the Center for Medical Home Improvement's manual for parent partners (www.medicalhomeim-provement.org) in quality improvement activities to explain to both practice staff and families how to negotiate this new relationship. Similarly, health care professionals often need coaching on how to effectively partner with families as fellow team members rather than as subordinates.

Once parents are engaged, an effective model to implement change and improvement is critical. One widely used and highly effective approach is the model for improvement developed by Associates in Process Improvement (Langley, Nolan, Nolan, Norman, & Provost, 1996). This model outlines a systematic approach to making productive changes in any organization. It starts by asking three questions: 1) What are we trying to accomplish? 2) How will we know if change is an improvement? 3) Which ideas are likely to lead to improvement? Once these questions are answered, the model emphasizes the critical importance of simple experimentation to test the new ideas, focusing participants on four types of activities:

1. Planning to make a change

2. Making the change on a very small scale

3. Studying the impact of the change

4. Reflecting on that impact to determine the next action, that is, if the change should be modified, expanded in scope, or sustained

We have found the combined use of the Care Model for Child Health in a Medical Home, the partnership with families, and the explicit improvement model effective in promoting implementation of the medical home. We have used this approach intensively in dozens of individual primary care practices in rural New England and other regions of the country and in two yearlong learning collaboratives involving almost 60 primary care practices in 20 states. Both the intensive, practice-based facilitation model and the learning collaborative model provide a disciplined approach to keep the efforts in a given practice moving forward and also provide access to external expertise and the shared experience of other practices that have undertaken the journey.

THE PRESENT: IMPLICATIONS FOR ACTION

Practitioners can commit to implementation of high-performing medical homes in their practices. Engaging parents, studying and adopting the Care Model for Child Health in a Medical Home, and then implementing that model through the use of the model for improvement is now feasible. Resources on both the medical home, the instruments for its assessment, and tools for implementation are available at a number of web sites (e.g., www.medicalhomeinfo.org, www.medicalhomeimprovement.org, www.nichq.org), as are resources on methods for improvement (e.g., www.ihi.org, www.improvingchroniccare.org, www. nichq.org). Training sessions on applying the model for improving children's health care are available (e.g., www.nichq.org), and, increasingly, state chapters of professional societies, state Title V programs, and other regional improvement programs are capable of supporting some form of collaborative learning and improvement (see www. med.uvm.edu/vchip/). Use of appropriate billing codes and effective negotiation with public and private payers often succeeds in securing sufficient reimbursement for undertaking this work.

Parents, too, can be both catalysts and enablers of change. Parents should maintain high expectations from their child's health care providers, and they also can connect with other parents both to address specific needs of their child and to learn how to negotiate more effectively with health care providers. The connections can take place through organizations such as Family Voices and the Institute for Family Centered Care, as well as condition-specific programs such as the Cystic Fibrosis Foundation, Epilepsy Foundation, and numerous others. Parents can become involved in improvement efforts in practices, and, once experienced, mentor other parents for similar roles.

Working together, parents and practitioners, supported by proven models and tools, can create medical homes that truly are responsive to the needs of children and their families.

THE FUTURE: POLICY CHANGES THAT COULD ACCELERATE IMPROVEMENT

Specification of an appropriate approach and the use of an effective change model have significantly accelerated improvement in provision of care for CSHCN through a medical home framework. Obstacles remain, but they are within our reach to address.

For instance, the reimbursement issues noted earlier are still a barrier for many physicians and systems—at both the primary care and specialty levels. Newer approaches that provide enhanced reimbursement for achieving improved outcomes (including patient experience of care and care coordination) or for having appropriate systems in place such as the Bridges to Excellence program[5] support provision of better care by rewarding providers financially for doing so.

---

[5] Bridges to Excellence is a program sponsored by employer groups, health plans, quality-related organizations, and provider groups whose purpose is to create programs that will realign everyone's incentives around higher quality. Their Physician Office Link program (http://www.bridgestoexcellence.org/bte/physician/officeassess.htm) enables physician office sites to qualify for bonuses based on their implementation of specific processes to reduce errors and increase quality (see http://www.bridgestoexcellence.org).

The use of electronic patient/family-controlled personal health care records—particularly with interfaces to their actual clinical electronic health care records—also holds promise for accelerating improvement. Such systems will enhance communication between primary care and specialty care and between health care and community resources. Health information can travel with the child (or his or her family), and therefore can be accessible in times of emergency, geographic moves, and developmental transitions.

REFERENCES

American Academy of Pediatrics Ad Hoc Task Force on Definition of the Medical Home. (1992). The medical home. *Pediatrics, 90*(5), 774.

American Academy of Pediatrics Medical Home Initiatives for Children with Special Needs Project Advisory Committee. (2004). Policy statement: Organizational principles to guide and define the child health care system and/or improve the health of all children. *Pediatrics, 113*(Suppl. 5); 1545–1547.

Bodenheimer, T., Wagner, E.H., & Grumbach, K. (2002a, October 9). Improving primary care for patients with chronic illness. *JAMA, 288*(14), 1775–1779.

Bodenheimer, T., Wagner, E.H., & Grumbach, K. (2002b, October 16). Improving primary care for patients with chronic illness: The chronic care model, Part 2. *JAMA, 288*(15), 1909–1914.

Cooley, W.C., McAllister, J., Sherrieb, K., & Clark, R. (2003). The Medical Home Index: Development and validation of a new practice-level measure of implementation of the Medical Home model. *Ambulatory Pediatrics, 3*(4), 173–180.

Cooley, W.C., & McAllister J. (2004). Building medical homes: Improvement strategies in primary care for CSHCN. *Pediatrics, 113*(5), 1499–1506.

Davis, D., O'Brien, M.A., Freemantle, N., Wolf, F.M., Mazmanian, P., & Taylor-Vaisey, A. (1999, September 1). Impact of formal continuing medical education: Do conferences, workshops, rounds, and other traditional continuing education activities change physician behavior or health care outcomes? *JAMA, 282*(9), 867–874.

Donaldson, M.S., Yordy, K.D., Lohr, K.N., & Vanselow, N.A. (Eds.). Committee on the Future of Primary Care, Institute of Medicine (1996). *Primary care: America's health in a new era.* Washington, DC: National Academies Press.

Feifer, C., Ornstein, S.M., Nietert, P.J., & Jenkins, R.G. (2001). System supports for chronic illness care and their relationship to clinical outcomes. *Topics in Health Information Management, 22*(2), 65–72.

Hobbs N., Ireys, H., & Perrin, J. (1991). *Chronically ill children and their families: Problems, prospects, and proposals from the Vanderbilt Study.* San Francisco: Jossey-Bass.

Jewett, E.A., Anderson, M.R., & Gilchrist, G.S. (2005, September 30). The pediatric specialty workforce: Public policy and forces for change. *Pediatrics, 116*(5), 1192–1202.

Langley, G.L., Nolan, K.M., Nolan, T.W., Norman, C.L., & Provost, L.P. (1996). *The improvement guide: A practical approach to enhancing organizational performance.* San Francisco: Jossey-Bass.

Mayer, M.L., Skinner, A.C., & Slifkin, R.T. (2004). Unmet need for routine and specialty care: Data from the National Survey of Children with Special Health Care Needs. *Pediatrics, 113*(2), 109–115.

McPherson, M., Arango, P., Fox, H., Lauver, C., McManus, M., Newacheck, P.W., et al., (1998). A new definition of children with special health care needs. *Pediatrics, 102* (1 Pt. 1), 137–140.

McPherson, M., Weissman, G., Strickland, B.B., van Dyck, P.C., Blumberg, S.J., & Newacheck, P.W. (2004). Implementing community-based systems of services for children and youths with special health care needs: How well are we doing? *Pediatrics, 113*(Suppl. 5), 1538–1544.

National Center for Cultural Competence. (2002). *Self-assessment checklist for personnel providing services and supports to children and youth with special health needs and their families.* Adapted from Tawara D. Goode, *Promoting cultural competence and cultural diversity in early intervention and early childhood settings.* Retrieved January 11, 2006, from http://gucchd.georgetown.edu/nccc/nccc7.html

National Initiative for Children's Healthcare Quality. (2005). *Improving cultural competency in children's health care: Expanding perspectives.* Boston: National Initiative for Children's Healthcare Quality; http://www.nichq.org/NICHQ/Programs/CollaborativeLearning/CulturalCompetency2005.htm

National Survey of Children with Special Health Care Needs. (2001). Retrieved December 26, 2005, from http://cshcndata.org

Orr, D.P., Weller, S.C., Satterwhite, B., & Pless, I.B. (1984). Psychosocial implications of chronic illness in adolescence. *Pediatrics, 104*(1), 152–157.

Perry, D.F., & Ireys, H.T. (2001). Maternal perceptions of pediatric providers for children with chronic illnesses. *Maternal and Child Health Journal, 5*(1), 15–20.

Pless, I.B., Satterwhite, B., & Van Vechten, D. (1976). Chronic illness in childhood: A regional survey of care. *Pediatrics, 58*(1), 37–46.

Pless, I.B., Satterwhite, B., & Van Vechten, D. (1978, January–February). Division, duplication and neglect: Patterns of care for children with chronic disorders. *Child Care Health Development, 4*(1), 9–19.

Sia, C., Tonniges, T.F., Osterhus, E., & Taba, S. (2004). History of the medical home concept. *Pediatrics, 113*(Suppl. 5), 1473–1478.

Sobo, E.J. (2003). Prevention and healing in the household: The importance of socio-cultural context. In E.J. Sobo & P.S. Kurtin (Eds.), *Child health services research: Applications, innovations, and insights (*pp. 67–119). San Francisco: Jossey-Bass.

Sobo, E.J., & Seid, M. (2003). Cultural issues in health services delivery: What kind of "competence" is needed? *Annals of Behavioral Science and Medical Education, 9*(2), 97–100.

Wagner, E.H. (1998). Chronic disease management: What will it take to improve care for chronic illness? *Effective Clinical Practice, 1* 2–4.

Wagner, E.H., Austin, B.T., & Von Korff, M. (1996a). Improving outcomes in chronic illness. *Managed Care Quarterly, 4*(2), 12–25.

Wagner, E.H., Austin, B.T., & Von Korff, M. (1996b). Organizing care for patients with chronic illness. *Milbank Quarterly, 74*(4), 511–544.

7

PRIMARY CARE PRACTICE AND CHILDREN WITH SPECIAL HEALTH CARE NEEDS:

ACTUAL AND IDEAL

Thomas K. McInerny

The role of a primary care pediatrician (PCP) in caring for children with special health care needs (CSHCN) is poorly defined. PCPs want to provide comprehensive family-centered care to all patients, but the need to keep up with the rapid advancement of technology and therapeutic modalities and the increasingly complex regulation of and demands for cost effectiveness from managed care organizations have led many PCPs to leave the care of CSHCN to specialists and tertiary care centers. Notwithstanding these pressures, authorities feel that the PCP should provide a medical home and act as a care coordinator for CSHCN (see Chapter 6). This chapter will augment that discussion by describing a typical PCP office setting and the morning schedule of patient visits, including a visit from a child with Down syndrome. In the form of a point-counterpoint discussion, the chapter contrasts this physician's ideal system of care with the actual patterns of care for CSHCN, especially with regard to care coordination, family involvement, and finance. It concludes with a discussion of seven principles of caring for CSHCN that address the concerns of PCPs noted above.

PRIMARY CARE PEDIATRICIAN SETTING

This section first will outline the characteristics of the practice and then discuss a hypothetical visit by a child with special health care needs.

Practice Location, Size, Operation

The primary care pediatrician in this example, a composite of many PCPs, belongs to a suburban pediatric practice located about 12 miles from a tertiary academic medical center with a large, comprehensive department of pediatrics (also a composite invention). There are eight pediatricians and four nurse practitioners in this office caring for about 16,000 patients, generating approximately 50,000 visits per year. Approximately 450 newborns visit the practice each year, with a similar

number of patients aging out annually. Each physician cares for a co-
hort of approximately 2,000 patients, alternating well-child visits with
the nurse practitioners. The pediatricians and nurse practitioners are
organized into three teams, each with its own receptionist and telephone number so that the members of each team are familiar with the
other team members' patients. In a typical 8-hour day, the pediatrician
will see 24–30 patients, approximately one-half of whom are visiting
for a health assessment and the other half for acute needs. Infant, child,
and preteen well-child visits are scheduled in 20-minute time slots and
well adolescents in 30-minute slots. Ten minutes are allotted for an
acute visit for an uncomplicated illness. Built into each pediatrician's
weekly schedule is a conference afternoon where two or three patients
with either complex medical or behavioral conditions are scheduled
over a period of $1\frac{1}{2}$ to 3 hours. Most telephone calls are handled by
the receptionist, a trained nurse, or the nurse practitioners so that the
pediatrician will usually need to return only four to five telephone calls
per day. Thus, a typical 4-hour session would be filled with approximately six well-child visits scheduled in advance and about 10 acute
illness visits usually scheduled that day.

Patient Visit

This discussion focuses on Down syndrome because patients with this
condition often have both somatic and cognitive challenges or problems, embodying a good portion of the range of issues PCPs serving
CSHCN may need to deal with. Given the relatively low incidence of
Down syndrome, each pediatrician has about two or three such patients. An illustrative example is the 18-month health assessment visit
of a child with Down syndrome and an atrioventricular septal defect.
Since this is a CSHCN, 30 minutes have been allotted for the visit.
During the interval between the 15-month visit and the current 18-
month visit, the patient has had two episodes of otitis media, which
responded promptly to high-dose amoxicillin. The pediatrician observes
in the history that the patient saw the cardiologist three months ago,
reviews the consult note from that visit, and reminds the parent to
keep the next appointment with the cardiologist in three months. The
patient also is followed by a developmental behavioral pediatrician in
the Diagnostic Clinic for Developmental Disorders at a nearby academic
medical center, and receives early intervention services in the form of
twice weekly visits by a speech therapist and an occupational therapist.
The child was last seen by the developmental behavioral pediatrician
two months ago; that note is reviewed by the pediatrician, and the
parent is reminded to be sure to attend the next scheduled visit.

The pediatrician then discusses feeding and development and behavioral issues with the parent, reviews progress, ascertains if there are concerns, and answers questions. One of the parental concerns is poor language development. The pediatrician plots the child's height, weight, and head circumference on the growth charts developed for children with Down syndrome and assures the parent that they are within normal limits. On physical exam, the heart rate is slightly elevated and the liver edge is palpable (slightly enlarged), but all else is normal for a child with Down syndrome. The pediatrician provides anticipatory guidance following the *Healthcare Guidelines for Individuals with Down Syndrome: 1999 Revision* (Cohen, 1999) and indicates to the parents that she will call the cardiologist regarding the slightly elevated heart rate and palpable liver edge and will consult the developmental behavioral pediatrician regarding the concern about language development.

During the remainder of the morning the pediatrician continues to see other patients, with two interruptions to speak with the cardiologist and the developmental behavioral pediatrician. At the end of the morning session, the pediatrician calls the patient's parent to discuss the cardiologist's and developmental pediatrician's recommendations.

In this scenario the pediatrician feels satisfied that she has met the needs of the patient within the constraints of a typical office setting using paper charts and the telephone as the main method of communication with specialists. Many experts considered this the standard of care for CSHCN in 2005, but with a more thorough understanding of how to coordinate care in a medical home setting and with the use of electronic medical records and e-mail for communication, this standard of care could be significantly improved. The next sections will contrast the current, actual practice with the ideal practice in four major areas: coordination of care, family involvement, financial considerations, and mental health care.

COORDINATION OF CARE

This section will illustrate the significant improvements in coordination of care for CSHCN that will occur when PCP's implement electronic medical records in their practices.

An Actual PCP Practice

In the vast majority of pediatrician offices, record keeping is on paper charts with handwritten or perhaps typewritten office notes, growth charts, correspondence from physicians and allied health professionals,

lab reports, X-ray reports, communications from early intervention programs, and schools—all on pieces of paper placed in the chart. In some
cases, there may be tabs separating the different categories of information, but in others the filing is more random. Clearly, this makes it
difficult, if not impossible, for the pediatrician to track myriad pieces
of information from multiple sources. It is not uncommon for charts
for young children to be two to three inches thick, and multiple volumes are required for older children.

In many cases, pediatricians will attempt to summarize the important aspects of caring for CSHCN by using a front sheet with a problem
list, current medications and doses, significant allergies, and so forth.
However, over time these front sheets can be almost as confusing as
the entire record itself because of numerous entries, changes in medications and dosages, and crossing out resolved conditions and discontinued treatments.

Another paper technique to follow the critical aspects of a patient's
illness (e.g., lab tests, consultations, clinical parameters) is to maintain
a flowchart tracking this data over time. This can be particularly helpful
for adjusting medications based on laboratory results. Again, however,
this can be quite laborious and time consuming to maintain. Given the
constraints imposed by paper charts, pediatricians often waste precious
office-visit minutes shuffling through the chart to find a recent lab test,
a note from a consultant, or which medications have been prescribed
over the past several months. Furthermore, in a large, busy practice,
the chart itself may be in one of a dozen locations ranging from the
desks of physicians, nurse practitioners, and correspondence-filing secretary to the billing office. Thus, locating the chart to assist in answering
a telephone call or preparing for an acute visit can involve a major
search of up to 30 minutes. Clearly, there must be a better method of
tracking and coordinating care.

An Ideal PCP Practice

The advance of electronic information technology has revolutionized
everything from accounting to zebra husbandry. However, medicine
has been far behind the information technology revolution, with only
a small percentage of primary care physicians' offices, hospitals, and
medical centers adopting electronic medical records. Fortunately, medical policy makers, large health care purchasers and payers, and the
federal government are proposing that EMR be instituted nationwide
within the next few years, offering to standardize electronic medical
language to facilitate communication among physicians and hospital
systems.

EMR will revolutionize how we provide care for patients, particularly those with chronic illnesses. The history and physical exam findings from office visits will be documented electronically as will lab test orders and results and prescriptions. Correspondence will be scanned and filed electronically in an orderly fashion so that rapid retrieval will be possible. Databases of physical findings such as height, weight, blood pressure, and lab tests will be automatically maintained and converted to graphs for easy viewing of changes over time. Most important, programs can be developed that will prompt physicians when certain tests or visits to specialists are due so that parents can be reminded of the appointments in a timely fashion. Pediatricians will need to adapt their practice styles to take advantage of these improvements by accurately entering information and paying close attention to the prompts. The PCP can be most helpful to the family and patient by assisting them in tracking and coordinating the many visits to the medical center for specialist consultations and evaluation and treatment by other professionals. Ideally the PCP will develop a master plan flowchart in the EMR indicating the appropriate intervals for follow-up appointments with the various specialists and therapists. This electronic flowchart would ideally provide a reminder/recall function to ensure that all appointments are kept in a timely fashion.

Furthermore, physicians, nurse practitioners, and others may access the patient's record from computer terminals throughout the office, thereby eliminating the chart search and unavailable record problems. In most instances, with proper conformity to health care privacy laws that require certain safeguards on software and limits to data sharing, physicians will be able to access the patient's EMR from a home computer by a secure encrypted Internet link. The improvement in providing after-hours telephone care in this scenario is a huge leap forward. In addition, it will be possible to electronically link the PCP's office record to the specialist in the medical center so that he or she will have access to the latest entries. Furthermore, within the academic medical center, a single electronic record will replace the multiple paper charts maintained by different specialists and will be accessible to all, including emergency room physicians and those caring for inpatients.

Finally, implementation of an EMR in the inpatient setting will vastly improve care and safety for patients. Computerized physician order entry has been shown to eliminate many drug errors and has led to shortened lengths of stay in the hospital (Potts, Barr, Gregory, Wright, & Patel, 2004). Patient discharge summaries can be prepared electronically and transmitted via the Internet to the primary care physician's office.

FAMILY INVOLVEMENT

As family-centered care becomes more commonly utilized in caring for CSHCN, there will be significant improvements in the outcomes of care for these children as the following two scenarios demonstrate.

Actual Family Involvement

Provider allowance for family involvement in the decision making and care of CSHCN is sporadic and inconsistent. Information sharing with families is often uncoordinated among various providers, and information that *is* shared with families can be quite confusing. As a result, families often lack the information they need to make truly informed decisions. The PCP can try to assist the family by pulling together and summarizing the multiple sources of information; however, this allows the PCP to interject his or her biases, thus influencing the family's decision in ways that go beyond the sharing of medical expertise. For example, a PCP may make value judgments regarding therapies based on his or her own personal biases rather than on scientific evidence. Furthermore, it is difficult for PCPs and families to keep up with the rapid advances in knowledge regarding care of patients with chronic illnesses. As a result, families have minimal understanding and input regarding the care of their CSHCN and are not true partners in the process of care.

Ideal Family Involvement

Some medical centers are pioneering family-centered and directed care, intimately involving the family in all decisions regarding the care of their child. This approach requires providing families with all the necessary information, including the pros and cons of the various treatment modalities they will need to make informed decisions. Family-centered care requires the parent to have access to the patient's medical record, hopefully in an electronic format, as well as to the latest evidence-based guidelines and/or expert consensus recommendations. Indeed, several software vendors have developed programs for families to document and track their medical care on their home computers. These personal health records will lead to significant improvements in a family's ability to participate actively in the care of their child.

True family-centered care is often a difficult process for physicians, as it requires that they give up control to families, which is contrary to their training and culture. Furthermore, providing families with full information may lead to their discovering that better outcomes and results are achieved at medical centers in other parts of the country. This process of sharing information, even when one's own practice or institution is not shown in the best light, is known as *transparency,* and it requires physicians to be honest with themselves about their need to improve their patterns of care. Another complicating factor is that not all families want the same amount of information or involvement, and it is notoriously hard to differentiate families on these dimensions or to meet exactly the information and involvement needs of each. Yet, as difficult as it may be to make the transition to family-centered care, early studies have shown improved outcomes for CSHCN when families are thoroughly involved in the decision making (McMenamy & Perrin, 2004).

FINANCIAL ASPECTS

One of the major problems faced by families with CSHCN is insufficient health insurance coverage. The following two sections will demonstrate how this problem can be resolved with a better design of the benefits package for these families.

Actual Financial Aspects

Health insurance coverage for the care of CSHCN is extremely complex, often inadequate, and sometimes frustrating for physicians and families (see Chapter 3). Insurance plans are not designed well enough to cover chronic illness care, which leads to gaps in coverage. Families often have great difficulty in dealing with insurance bureaucracies to obtain reimbursement for visits to specialists and therapists and for the purchase of drugs and durable medical equipment. Further, if pediatric specialists are out of network, families may endure a prolonged preauthorization process to obtain approval for referrals to these specialists, after which they will be required to pay an increased copay for the visit as an out-of-pocket expense.

Care coordination and case management activities by primary care physicians, specialists, nurse practitioners, and social workers often are not covered benefits, as these activities are usually done over the telephone and most insurers do not reimburse providers for these calls. Also, it is often the case that CSHCN have mental health issues requiring counseling by child and adolescent psychiatrists, child psychologists, and mental health social workers. Sometimes mental health benefits are *carved out* by the insurance company (covered under a separate policy arranged by the insurer, often with a mental health benefits management company) and managed by a mental health management company. This makes coordinating care more difficult. In many cases, insurance panels of providers contain an insufficient number of mental health professionals skilled in dealing with children with emotional problems, especially CSHCN, which can lead to major access-to-care difficulties. Also, in many cases, insurance companies reimburse families for only 50% of the cost of mental health care services, adding significantly to the out-of-pocket expense burden for such families.

The net result of these financial restrictions leads to incomplete care coordination and case management. Ultimately, it leads to a deterioration in the patient's health, resulting in excess emergency room visits and hospitalizations, offsetting initial cost savings for all involved.

Ideal Financial Aspects

Insurance companies should provide adequate reimbursement (e.g., case management fees) for physicians and allied health professionals to provide true case management and care coordination. For example, pediatricians in North Carolina have developed a care coordination program for CSHCN that provides a case management payment to pediatricians, which has led to markedly improved care and health outcomes (Piehl, Clemens, & Joines, 2000).

Patients should be provided access to pediatric specialists and mental health professionals without restrictions. Copays and deductibles for these services as well as for drugs and durable medical equipment should be minimal. Insurers should encourage health care that will prevent complications of chronic illnesses, thereby reducing costly hospitalizations and emergency room visits. Indeed, one study from Rochester, New York, has demonstrated that good preventive care for CSHCN can save insurers millions of dollars over time (Liptak, Burns, Davidson, & McAnarney, 1998). Insurers should use a combination of risk adjustment (e.g., clinical risk groups) and reinsurance to limit their costs of covering CSHCN (University of Florida Institute for Child Health Policy, 2004).

MENTAL HEALTH CARE

Improving mental health services for CSHCN is critically important to optimizing their care and outcomes. A change in the relationship between PCPs and mental health providers will allow such improvement to occur.

Actual Mental Health Care

It is well documented that 30% of children with special health care needs develop mental health problems at some point in their childhood years (Ganz & Tendulkar, 2006). The PCP, by virtue of his or her intimate knowledge of the patient and family, is in the best position to detect the development of emotional problems at an early stage when they are more easily treated. Therefore, it is important that the PCP assess the child at regular intervals to determine if he or she is developing mental health problems. The most common disorders are adjustment reaction, depression, learning disabilities, and attention-deficit/hyperactivity disorder. Less common disorders include oppositional defiant disorder in younger children and conduct disorder in adolescents.

In many cases, the PCP may be the appropriate individual to treat mild-to-moderate cases of the more common disorders, perhaps with the assistance of a mental health professional. In fact, due to the woefully inadequate supply of mental health professionals skilled in treating children, it is often the case that the PCP is the only one available to care for these patients. Many PCPs have developed the expertise necessary to care for these patients by taking continuing medical education (CME) courses on the diagnosis and treatment of mental health disorders in the primary care setting. Several texts and reference works are available to assist the PCP in this endeavor. Among them are the *Diagnostic Statistical Manual of Mental Disorders*—Primary Care Version—which lists the criteria necessary for the diagnosis of mental health disorders, and *Child and Adolescent Mental Health* (Kaye, Montgomery, & Munson, 2002). Learning how to diagnose and treat mild-to-moderate mental health problems allows the PCP to provide an extremely valuable service to his or her patients with chronic illness.

Ideal Mental Health Care

Rather than attempt to provide mental health care alone or with infrequent, irregular consultations with a mental health provider (MHP), the PCP should develop an ongoing collaborative arrangement with a child psychiatrist, child psychologist, mental health social worker skilled in caring for CSHCN, or psychiatric pediatric nurse practitioner. Ideally, the MHP would spend some time counseling the pediatrician's patients in his or her office, allowing for frequent, regular communication. Increasingly, pediatric practices are developing such relationships, leading to a significant reduction in barriers to receiving high-quality mental health care (Klinepeter, Williams, Shore, & Foy, 2005).

LESSONS LEARNED

The preceding point-counterpoint discussions indicate that there are important lessons to be learned that suggest several basic principles of care.

Basic Principles for Parents

Parents should decide whether their PCP or specialist should be the care coordinator for their CSHCN. This will vary according to their child's condition and how PCPs and specialists function in their community. For straightforward, single-system illnesses (e.g., asthma, diabetes), the specialist may assume the role of case manager, often with the assistance of associated allied health professionals. For more complex illnesses involving several systems (e.g., cerebral palsy, spina bifida) and requiring coordination of therapists in the patients' schools, the PCP may be best suited to coordinate the many aspects of care. In either case, the parents and physicians should reach a clear understanding of their roles in caring for a CSHCN, and parents should hold the physicians accountable for their roles. Responsibility for all aspects of care must be appropriately assigned and agreed on so that some aspects don't fall through the cracks.

Basic Principles for Excellent Primary Care

Emerging from the foregoing discussion regarding the roles and responsibilities of those caring for CSHCN is the lesson that there are eight basic principles that must be followed by the primary care pediatrician in caring for CSHCN (see Table 7.1).

Medical Home

First and foremost is the principle of the *medical home,* which is defined as providing accessible, family-centered, continuous, comprehensive, coordinated, compassionate, and culturally effective care. Because of the unique, continuous, and close relationship between the PCP and the family, some physicians skilled in caring for CSHCN believe that the medical home should be in the PCP office, but there are alternate viewpoints. (See Chapter 6 for more on this subject.)

Table 7.1. Principles of excellent primary care for children with special health care needs

Medical home concept honored

Noncategorical case management and care coordination practiced

Coordinated partnership across continuum of care enacted

Involvement with the educational system

Quality improvement practices in process

Longitudinal continuity of care attempted

Preparation for care transition anticipated

Family-centered care practiced

Noncategorical Care

The second principle is that care coordination for CSHCN should be *noncategorical;* that is, case management and care coordination are generic and should be applied to all CSHCN regardless of their specific diagnoses. This noncategorical approach is particularly necessary for children with complex medical conditions such as cerebral palsy and spina bifida. Although the specific conditions of chronic illnesses may vary, CSHCN share common issues of concern such as chronicity, need for frequent medical attention, interference with normal lifestyle, and family stress. Thus, the PCP caring for these children needs to be skilled in dealing with these generic issues to be of maximal help to CSHCN families.

Coordinated Partnership

Another important principle is the formation of a true *coordinated partnership* among the family, PCP, specialists, allied health providers, educators, social workers, and insurance companies, with open communication among all parties. Since advances in the treatment of chronic illnesses occur rapidly, it is impossible for the PCP to be aware of the latest recommendations for treatment of all of these patients. By partnering with the specialists who can provide the most up-to-date recommendations for care, the PCP can ensure that his or her patient is receiving optimal attention. This coordination and cooperation is the most difficult aspect of providing care for CSHCN, particularly those with multiple medical problems. Failure of coordination leads to suboptimal care and outcomes and extreme frustration for the families, patients, and caregivers. Several scholars have described the role of the primary care physician in coordinating the care of CSHCN as analogous to that of the orchestra conductor working with musicians. Without the conductor, even highly accomplished musical specialists playing independently will create a cacophony, but with the conductor's skillful leadership they will produce a beautiful symphony.

Involvement with the Educational System

One of the most important roles the PCP can play is as a link between the educational and medical systems. Clearly, the educational system faces significant issues and challenges in educating CSHCN in the *least restrictive environment* as prescribed by the federal government under the Individuals with Disabilities Education Act (IDEA) and the Americans with Disabilities Act (ADA). As the PCP's practice often is located in the region of school districts attended by his or her patients, he or she often is more familiar with the educators than the specialists and therapists who may be some distance removed. In many cases, the PCP may be the school physician for a particular school district or districts. This familiarity provides the PCP with an opportunity to demystify various aspects of the patient's chronic illness and to assist the teachers, nurses, guidance counselors, therapists, and administrators in adapting the school and classroom environment to meet the needs of CSHCN. In addition, the PCP can help translate recommendations made by specialists into understandable and straightforward actions by school personnel as part of his or her care-coordination efforts.

Quality Improvement

Another major principle is that of *quality improvement*. The PCP needs to be aware of evidence-based guidelines for care that reduce unnecessary variability and lead to improved health outcomes. However, simple awareness is not sufficient; the PCP also must strive to implement these guidelines into practice. This goal can best be accomplished by utilizing continuous quality improvement methods (e.g., the plan-do-study-act small cycles of improvement model) to change patterns of care in the desired direction. The Institute of Healthcare Improvement (www.IHI. org) and the National Initiative for Children's Healthcare Quality (NICHQ; www.NICHQ.org) are two excellent organizations promoting and guiding quality improvement in medicine in general and pediatrics specifically. Also, the American Academy of Pediatrics has developed an online resource meant to help pediatricians learn how to improve care for children with chronic illnesses through use of the principles developed by NICHQ called Education in Quality Improvement for Pediatric Practice (eQIPP; www.eqipp.org). Pediatricians should make quality improvement efforts a regular part of their practice processes. This is becoming a necessary skill to maintain certification by the American Board of Pediatrics.

Longitudinal Continuity of Care

One of the most important principles in providing care for CSHCN is that of the *longitudinal continuity of care*. Ideally, the family of a child with a chronic illness will have the same PCP from the onset of the illness until age 21 and care is transferred to an internist or family medicine physician. In this situation, the same PCP sees the child and family for all the health assessment and maintenance visits as well as most acute illness visits. When the PCP is not available for an acute illness visit, the substitute physician makes the PCP aware of the visit at the earliest opportunity, thus allowing the primary physician to follow up with the patient to ensure that all is proceeding appropriately. This longitudinal continuous care also allows the PCP to develop an ongoing long-term relationship with the specialists caring for these patients, thereby enhancing communication between them. In this situation, the family develops a strong sense of trust with their PCP, who, in turn, develops an in-depth understanding of the family composition, dynamics, and capabilities. This sense of trust and understanding leads to a bonding of the physician and family, invaluable as decisions regarding care are mutually discussed and agreed on, which in turn leads to true family-centered care. Similarly, as the patient with a chronic illness enters adolescence, the trust developed between the pediatrician and patient will be an important factor in the adolescent's ability to remain compliant with his or her treatment program.

Orderly Transfer of Care

One of the last principles to consider is the *orderly transfer of care* from the pediatrician to the internist. Fortunately, due to advances in the diagnosis and treatment of CSHCN, an increasing number of these children are *aging out,* that is, becoming young adults for whom care by a pediatrician is no longer appropriate. There are now well-developed guidelines (Blum, 2002) to assist the PCP in the transfer of care process. The basic principle is that care transfer planning should start early in adolescence, allowing several years for the family and adolescent to prepare mentally, emotionally, and physically for the transition.

In addition, it is critically important that the receiving physician understands the principles of case management and care coordination for chronically ill patients. Unfortunately, this is not always the case, and therefore the PCP should assist the family in selecting the appropriate internist. In many communities there are now a significant number of *med-peds,* physicians who are board certified in both pediatrics and internal medicine who often have the knowledge and interest necessary to provide excellent care for adults with special health care needs.

Family-Centered Care

The final principle is the importance of *family-centered care* in which the PCP supports the family as a whole as the parents care for their chronically ill child, siblings, and one another. It has been well documented that families with CSHCN have increased levels of stress, which manifests itself in several ways, including increased rates of separation and divorce (see Chapter 4). Siblings of CSHCN can often feel neglected and resentful of the increased parental attention being paid to the chronically ill child, as well as either guilt for feeling resentful or an imagined role in the causation of their sibling's illness. Since the PCP cares for the siblings of the CSHCN, she or he should counsel parents about the importance of relieving stress in appropriate ways and of paying attention to the needs of the chronically ill child's siblings. Furthermore, the PCP should monitor the family for early signs of emotional problems in parents or children, counseling and/or referring them to mental health providers as appropriate. In addition, assisting parents in obtaining respite services at regular intervals can be extremely helpful in maintaining family stability.

The PCP should counsel parents on the prevention of the development of the *vulnerable child syndrome,* which can be psychologically debilitating for CSHCN. Parents can be inclined toward overprotecting chronically ill children based on unrealistic fears of their vulnerability. Under these circumstances, CSHCN are not permitted to participate in the full range of activities essential for normal development, which can lead to developmental and emotional limitations. The PCP needs to inform parents regarding which activities may truly endanger their child and which should be allowed because they do not lead to a significant risk for adverse outcomes. Numerous examples exist of CSHCN who become, despite significant physical limitations, outstanding leaders, educators, artists, and athletes as a result of being encouraged by parents and others to test their limits and develop their special talents.

CONCLUSION

Clearly, provision of care for CSHCN by PCPs is a demanding and time-consuming process. However, most PCPs have only a handful of patients with complex chronic illnesses in their practice at any given time, so this commitment can be quite manageable. Furthermore, as electronic medical records utilization becomes more widespread, providing this comprehensive care will become easier.

As is usually the case, hard work often leads to significant rewards. Working closely with families of CSHCN provides the PCP the opportunity to optimize the physical, emotional, developmental, and social outcomes of these patients. Most physicians would agree that this is why many of us embarked on a career in medicine in the first place. Over time, the process of assisting families in the transition of their care to internists, after a decade or two of close involvement with these families, has led to favorable outcomes and provides the PCP with the opportunity to reflect on and rejoice in his or her sublimely humane practice of the art and science of medicine. After 33 years as a primary care pediatrician, this PCP can think of no greater satisfaction.

REFERENCES

Americans with Disabilities Act (ADA) of 1990, PL 101-336, 42 U.S.C. §§ 12101 *et seq.*

Blum, R.W. (Ed.). (2002). Improving transition for adolescents with special health care needs from pediatric to adult-centered health care. *Supplement to Pediatrics, 110,* 1301–1335.

Cohen, W.I. (Ed.). (1999). Health care guidelines for individuals with Down syndrome: 1999 revision, *Down Syndrome Quarterly, 4,* 1–15.

Individuals with Disabilities Education Act (IDEA) of 1990, PL 101-476, 20 U.S.C. §§ 1400 *et seq.*

Ganz, M.L., & Tendulkar, S.A. (2006). Mental health care services for children with special health care needs and their family members: Prevalence and correlates of unmet needs. *Pediatrics, 117*(6), 2138–2148.

Kaye, D.L., Montgomery, M.E., & Munson, S.W. (Eds.). (2002). *Child and adolescent mental health.* Philadelphia: Lippincott Williams & Wilkins.

Klinepeter, K., Williams, J., Shore, S., & Foy, J. (2005). Co-location of a mental health professional in a primary care setting. "Connecting for Children's Sake" [Abstract]. American Academy of Pediatrics—Pediatrics for the 21st Century. Elk Grove Village, IL: American Academy of Pediatrics; www. aap.org/peds-21

Liptak, G.S, Burns, C.M., Davidson, P.W., & McAnarney, E.R. (1998). Effects of providing comprehensive ambulatory services to children with chronic conditions. *Archives of Pediatric and Adolescent Medicine, 152,* 1003–1008.

McMenamy, J.M., & Perrin, E.C. (2004). Filling the gaps: Description and evaluation of a primary care intervention for children with chronic health conditions. *Ambulatory Pediatrics, 4,*(3), 249–256.

Piehl, M.D., Clemens, C.J., & Joines, J.D. (2000). Narrowing the gap: Decreasing emergency department use by children enrolled in the Medicaid program by improving access to primary care. *Archives Pediatric Adolescent Medicine, 154*(8), 791–795.

Potts, A.L., Barr, F.E., Gregory, D.F., Wright, L., & Patel, N.R. (2004). Computerized physician order entry and medication errors in a pediatric critical care unit. *Pediatrics, 113*(1), 59–63.

University of Florida Institute for Child Health Policy, National Center on Financing for CSHCN (2004). State strategies for financing care for CSHCN: How well do they work? *Focus on Child Health Policy, 2,* 1–7.

8

CASE MANAGEMENT OF CHILDREN WITH SPECIAL HEALTH CARE NEEDS:

THE PEDIATRICIAN PERSPECTIVE

Robert M. Sheets and Paul S. Kurtin

M anaged care systems *manage* patient care by establishing and enforcing guidelines for providing care and services often based on the best available science. Within such a system, whose job is it to provide case management for children with special health care needs (CSHCN), and whose job should it be? Who is most knowledgeable about and most capable of deciding the frequency of visits, which tests will be allowed, and which medications should be prescribed? Should it be the primary care physician/pediatrician (PCP), the pediatric specialist, or another physician or nurse reviewing the care plan for a medical group or insurance company? These three decision makers vary in expertise and usual role and sometimes in incentives to provide or deny specific care and services. Thus, the fundamental question we address in this chapter is: Who should be making which case-management decisions and when, with the health of the child always the first concern?

WHAT IS CASE MANAGEMENT?

Case management is the process of determining when and which visits, admissions, consultations, and other appropriate services a child will receive, and how those services can be best coordinated to optimize health outcomes and minimize the burden on the child, family, and providers. Case management has three components: clinical care of the child, coordination and management of the resources needed to provide appropriate care for the child, and patient and family education and self-management. Case management thus entails overseeing an individual patient's medical and sometimes social and financial needs, and assuring that all necessary services are obtained at the right time and in the right place.

It also entails the collaboration and cooperation of all involved in the care of the child. For example, specific decisions in any one of the three areas of case management may be made by the PCP, by the specialist, or even by an organization such as an insurance company or a medical group that has financial responsibility for the care provided. Each potential decision maker has an important, yet usually separate, role to play in directing what and how care is delivered. When all three decision makers work collaboratively, care and services proceed smoothly for the most part. However, if legitimate differences of opinion exist among the three, or if rules and regulations of the party financially responsible for the care interfere with this collaborative approach, care and services may be delayed or at least become laborious and time consuming to obtain.

For example, some treatments for rheumatic diseases were effective in adults, yet they also were expensive and consequently not tested for effectiveness in children. Because there was no evidence that the treatments could help children, some insurance companies balked at paying for them to treat children. Eventually, however, children were given the same treatment with success, and as the medical evidence of the effectiveness in children grew, and as pediatric rheumatologists around the country actively advocated for their patients with insurance companies, insurance companies agreed to pay for the treatments, which are now routinely available for children.

How Are Cases Managed?

Children have special health care needs for a variety of physical, mental, and behavioral conditions that vary greatly in duration, severity, availability, and cost of treatment. Although most children have only a single, long-term condition, some have several long-term, complex, often congenital conditions. Children in both categories require frequent outpatient visits; sometimes frequent hospital admissions; usually additional care in the home and/or school; and myriad tests, procedures, therapeutic processes, treatments, and devices.

In contrast, healthy children receive routine and acute care from their primary care physician, and no multidisciplinary case-management decisions are required. The PCP thus serves as a *medical home* (see Chapter 6) for the child and meets their preventive, routine, and acute health care needs in a manner mutually agreed on by the physician and family.

In contrast, the PCP who chooses to provide case management for a child with special health care needs (CSHCN) has many additional duties to perform. The first and most basic is to properly evaluate and diagnose the child. For many children with the first onset of a potentially chronic condition, the PCP will be fully able to make a diagnosis based on the child's history and the results of routine diagnostic tests.

The PCP often contacts a specialist after a diagnosis is made because the next step is to decide what therapy, if any, is needed for the specific condition.

The PCP and the specialist will discuss questions ranging from what, if any, therapeutic intervention or medication is required at this time to deciding if the child needs to be admitted to a hospital for further diagnostic testing or for therapy. The PCP and the specialist also will decide if the child needs to see the specialist at this or any other point in the child's evaluation or treatment. In this example, the PCP is serving as the case manager by deciding which tests, referrals, and/or treatments are needed to provide the best care for the child.

Most self-limited problems such as those related to an infection or to recent trauma do not require a visit to a specialist, and the PCP continues to make all of the care decisions. However, if the condition does not resolve itself as quickly or completely as was first thought, the PCP may seek advice from the specialist about which additional tests or treatments may be most appropriate for the child over time. This interaction between the PCP and the specialist continues until the specific disorder is treated effectively and the family is satisfied with the course of care. In this case, the PCP was the case manager throughout the course of care, although the specialist was involved by providing expert advice and consultation.

Children with self-limited conditions are not the type of children specialists see on an on-going basis. Children followed by a specialist on a continuing basis often have a complex, chronic, and potentially serious condition. The specialist, because of his or her training and expertise, is best suited to provide case management in these cases, especially when the disease is being actively treated with frequent modifications in therapy. Part of the value of specialty care is that specialists often work with a multidisciplinary team that includes specially trained nurses, dieticians, social workers, and other health care providers (e.g., psychologists, physical and occupational therapists) needed in the care of specific conditions.

Specialists are able to work with such a team because they often work in hospital-based specialty clinics. While the specialist may be best suited to provide the medical/technical aspects of the case-management role, in truth, most specialty clinics are not a true medical home for the child because they do not provide routine primary care such as immunizations; they do not provide much of the routine anticipatory counseling provided by PCPs; and, most important, they do not care for the siblings of the affected child. Because of this division in the care of a CSHCN, to provide comprehensive, coordinated care for the child, there must be routine and regular interactions between the specialty care team and the PCP/medical home.

Communication, both verbal and written, between the specialist and the PCP is especially critical when the child requires complex and expensive diagnostic testing and treatments, and the PCP is required by the rules of managed care to be the one to obtain authorization for particular medications, tests, consultations, or admission to a hospital. If the PCP does not understand the reason for a particular test or treatment, there may be delays in the approval process that might not have occurred if the PCP were more knowledgeable about the course of care. And throughout the process, the opinions of the family must be taken into account.

What Drives Case-Management Decisions?

In the simplest of case-management situations, the PCP refers the child for a specialty consultation, and this referral is then approved by the payer of the consultation (e.g., medical group, health plan, insurance company, government payer). These routine referrals are rarely denied. The specialty consultant sees the child, advises the PCP on what should be done, and then no longer needs to be involved in the care of the child. However, in the case of a child with ongoing special health care needs, this process is not so simple. Multiple visits with the specialist are usually needed, and a list of sometimes expensive diagnostic tests is recommended. A variety of treatment regimens or care plans, sometimes expensive, may also be recommended. At this point in the child's care, case management is necessary to provide appropriate clinical care by managing the resources needed to do that. Factors that influence who and how case-management decisions are made include

- The background and training of the PCP and specialists involved

- The insurance type (if any) and the specific benefits provided

- The guidelines for case management in the contract between the payer and providers

- The family's ability to understand their child's problem and to be actively involved in deciding on and participating in the best course of treatment for the child (see Chapter 5)

The Primary Care Physician as Case Manager

Physicians in training learn about the costs of tests and treatments as well as how managed care organizations provide case management that consists mostly of resource utilization and management. Pediatricians in training further learn that CSHCN interact with and receive care and services from a large number of clinical professionals and social agencies. Due to an often complex web of insurance regulations and contracts, pediatricians in training learn that organizing and providing care in the way they would prefer often involves negotiations with the case manager. In this way, physicians in training begin the complicated process of learning the resource management component of case management. It is rare for a child not to ultimately receive the care and services he or she needs. The processes of getting those services can, however, be arduous and painstakingly slow for providers and families.

Once in practice, the physicians continue their education in the ways of managed care. The authorization process, which is controlled by the payer and not the direct provider, means that PCPs and specialty pediatricians can't order a test or medication—especially if it is unusual or very expensive—and assume that it will be approved. Drug formularies, and thus the availability of specific medications, often are limited by insurance type or the policies of the payer organization. Expensive tests, which often are part of routine care provided by specialists such as cardiologists or surgeons, usually require prior authorization. If the pace of the evaluation or treatment course is not critical, this is usually not a problem.

There also are ways to obtain rapid approval of essential tests, procedures, and medications, especially if the physician is personally involved in the approval process. However, because physicians have many patients and consequently limited time to be involved in these issues, the approval process places additional administrative burdens and costs on the providers and often on the family.

In their practices, PCPs and specialists quickly learn to make care decisions that are influenced by real or, at times, perceived limits of insurance coverage. If a test or medication is not approved by the payer organization, physicians vary in how diligently they will argue and appeal that decision. Sometimes the physician can successfully educate the case manager about the care of what might be to the case manager a rare condition that he or she knows little about. However, sometimes care plans are limited by the benefits covered in the particular insurance plan. Once again, families with a CSHCN must be vigilant in seeking, when possible, the insurance plan most likely to cover the needs of their child.

With complicated medical illnesses requiring ongoing and at times expensive treatments and testing, coordinated and comprehensive case management becomes even more necessary and difficult. After referral to a specialist, the PCP must decide whether to maintain an active role

in the child's care or relinquish the care decision making to the specialist. The role that the PCP chooses to play largely depends on his or her
training and comfort level with the particular condition. With common
conditions such as asthma, the PCP often stays very involved, whereas
he or she is not as actively involved with rare conditions. PCPs, however, like and need to stay aware of the child's treatment plan and
course. The role of the PCP also can be defined by the policies and
practices of the medical group or practice to which he or she belongs,
the role specified in the contract with the (insurance) payer, or the
wishes of the family.

In some contracts, the PCP maintains control of the primary decision making. For CSHCN, even when the PCP has primary responsibility for case management, he or she often will defer decision making to
the specialist. In other contractual situations, the control of care decisions and coordination is with the specialist. However control is arranged, regular communication between the PCP and the specialist is
essential. Because many CSHCN receive multidisciplinary team care, if
PCPs are to be fully engaged in case management, they must be in
regular communication with their team. This is one important advantage of the specialist case-management model, because the pediatric
specialist often is located with and meets frequently with the care team.
The decision as to who should lead the case-management process may
happen quickly or it may evolve slowly over time depending on the
disease and all of the above factors. Based on the success of the case
management, primarily assessed by the health and well-being of the
child, decisions concerning role can be maintained or changed over
time. Roles also change as the child gets older and makes more of his
or her own decisions.

The Specialist as Case Manager

A specialist enters into the child's care when the child is first seen in
consultation. A pediatric rheumatologist (cares for children with arthritis and other rheumatic diseases) may see a variety of children; some
are easy to manage and require few recommendations or return visits,
while others are more complicated and require a great deal of time to
manage. In general, for all specialties, the more complicated the child's
condition, the more likely it is that direction will come from the specialist. In many parts of the country, a pediatric rheumatologist (or other
pediatric specialist such as a neurologist or gastroenterologist) is not
available in the community, and, therefore, the pediatrician performs
the role of case manager by necessity. In that case, the specialist makes
most of the clinical care decisions in consultation with the PCP, and

the PCP, who knows the community better, plays a larger role in coordinating the other services needed by the child such as a plan for care in school. PCPs are thankful for the help they receive in managing a complex child, and the specialist appreciates the community involvement of the PCP. While some PCPs stay actively involved in decision making and the clinical care plan, most do not because they do not have the time or training to become deeply involved in the complex medical issues of just a few of their many patients.

The types of chronic conditions that PCPs will stay involved with is dictated by their experience, how they choose to focus their time and practice, and the local availability and interest of particular specialists. For example, while most PCPs refer the majority of childhood arthritis complaints to a pediatric rheumatologist, this can vary depending on the complexity of the diagnosis, the availability of a pediatric rheumatologist, and the demands by the family that a specialist see their child. The less available a particular specialist, the more likely it is that the PCP will have greater experience with the condition and that he or she can take care of the problem. As an example, in some communities, children with migraine headaches or simple seizures may be referred to a pediatric neurologist, while in other communities, without the appropriate specialist, the primary care physician takes care of the child. Medically informed families tend to request specialty consultation sooner and more frequently. The number of informed families is increasing daily because of the Internet. While most specialists encourage their families to use the Internet, we caution families to recognize the risk of misinformation or assuming that their child is just like the children they may read about on the Internet.

Like other areas of pediatrics (e.g., neurology, genetics), pediatric rheumatologists see many complicated and relatively rare illnesses that are sometimes subtle in their initial presentation. In contrast, many conditions really are, and do remain, simple and actually require less testing and medication than the PCP might think. In these instances, the role of the specialist is to limit unnecessary medications or planned tests. However, even a patient who begins with mild symptoms at first may turn out later to have a quite complicated and serious illness and probably would require more involvement from the specialist. The challenge that specialists often face with patients like these is that the tests and medications needed are not routinely used by the PCP, who may not be familiar with all the potential complications of treatment. Therefore, the specialist's role, although seemingly routine and possibly unnecessary to an outside reviewer, is essential to the good care of the child.

For example, a typical child with a single swollen joint does not require extensive evaluation by the pediatric rheumatologist. These children are usually 1 to 5 years of age and present with painful swelling of a knee. They feel worse in the morning and usually limp. It is important to note, however—and sometimes most primary care providers don't know this—that these children also can have involvement of their eyes. Thus, referral to an ophthalmologist to screen routinely for uveitis (inflammation in the eye) is routine for pediatric rheumatologists. While other parts of the diagnostic evaluation are routine and easily done by the PCP, the involvement of the rheumatologist is essential because finding and treating uveitis early may well prevent blindness, the most serious complication of this disease. Because the PCP may not have known to do this, the critical role of the specialist is obvious. Another seemingly simple intervention routinely performed by the pediatric rheumatologist is injecting the child's inflamed joint with medications to alleviate the pain and swelling. This can rapidly improve the child's pain and makes the overall management of the child's arthritis easier. It also could result in fewer complications than would occur if the child had been treated with high-dose oral medications for a prolonged period of time.

Whoever most effectively case manages the child must know about critically important care issues (e.g., potential complications of a condition or its treatment) that can change over time. As our knowledge of a disease and its treatment increases over time, specialists are much more likely to keep up-to-date on the changes than a busy PCP. The role of specialist as case manager becomes even more apparent when one multiplies all the duties of a case manager by all the specialty conditions a PCP might see and be asked to care for. For many CSHCN, and especially the more severely affected children, the pediatric specialist, in close collaboration with the PCP, provides the most effective clinical case management.

As mentioned above, case management has three components: clinical care, resource management, and patient and family education and self-management. In routine practice, the specialist designs and often personally provides the clinical care. With most forms of commercial or governmental insurance, the entity financially responsible for the care will provide, or at least review, the resource management component of case management. The education of the children and their families, as well as support for their self-management (to the degree possible), requires the combined efforts of the PCP, the specialist, and the payer. The specialist is responsible for designing the appropriate educational materials and courses. Although the clinical care team does most of the education, that education must be consistent with what the PCP also is telling the family. Finally, the specialist and the payer must agree on, and provide the materials and equipment needed for, education and self-management.

Role of Specialist After Condition Is Diagnosed and Treatment Begins

What about the ongoing care of a child after the diagnosis and treatment is well established? What should be the role of the specialist at that point? How much of the clinical care or care coordination should the PCP resume? At a point when the child is in remission and doing well, it is reasonable and important for the family and the pediatrician to increasingly manage the child's care and decide with the specialist why and when a follow-up visit with the specialist is needed. However, as long as the child's care is still being actively managed, often with potentially toxic medications, the specialist has a much better understanding and feel for the course the disease might take and the complications that might develop from the disease or its treatment. It is this depth of relevant knowledge and experience that allows the specialist to actively manage severely ill children in the most effective and efficient manner. Complications resulting from the disease or its treatment may have significant long-term adverse consequences for the child. Even when managed by the specialist, complications such as a reaction to a medication will occur, and the specialist is best equipped to handle these complications when they do arise.

In all specialties, there are children who do not seem very ill during the early stages of their disease, yet they require aggressive and complex medical management to avoid later complications and significant morbidities. In situations like this, the specialist must be an assertive force in case management because PCPs and others not familiar with the condition may be lulled into a false sense of security by the child's initial apparent well-being. This became clear to the first author of this chapter only after changing from general pediatric practice to pediatric rheumatology. Unfortunately, most practitioners will not have the opportunity for such first-hand learning, underlining the need for the specialist's active, assertive participation.

The child's long-term health care needs are always better served by the comprehensive care that can be given by a pediatric rheumatologist and the entire care team. An experienced pediatric rheumatology nurse, social worker, or occupational and physical therapist can provide team care in a single setting with an expertise that provides optimum clinical outcomes for the child and the best education about the illness and its management for the family. Team care is prevalent throughout all pediatric specialties. Examples include endocrinologists with diabetic educators and gastroenterologists with registered dieticians and nurses expert in stoma care. Team care for a CSHCN often forms the basis of case management. The care team has the essential obligation to keep the PCP aware of all decisions being made and to allow that provider and the family to be as involved as is appropriate for optimizing the care of the child.

Specialist and Financial Issues

Case management, as we have been discussing it, has a clinical focus that should be the primary focus of all involved. However, case management also has a financial component. Fortunately, the best clinical care usually leads to the best financial outcomes as well. The short-term increase in expense due to referral to a specialist is most often offset by the long-term better health outcomes of the children and by the improved understanding and satisfaction of the families. An example of better financial outcomes achieved by the specialist in managing a complex child is that intensive, even frequent, outpatient care is more cost-efficient than an admission to the hospital.

Specialist and the Family

Besides clinical care and financial management of resource utilization, the final component of case management is patient and family education, including self-management. One of the most important things that a knowledgeable specialist provides to a family is good and useful information about the underlying disease as well as their child's prognosis. However, while textbooks, references, and the Internet can help provide some general information for pediatricians and families, parents often can get inadequate or incorrect advice over the Internet. Early referral to a specialist lessens the possibility that a PCP will have made an incorrect diagnosis or even started the child on a wrong course of treatment.

For example, pediatric rheumatologists see many patients who have been misdiagnosed as having one disease but who actually have a different disease. However, with Internet information availability, parents quickly become experts on the diagnosis given to them by the PCP and all of its potentially morbid complications. Trying to erase those worries while explaining the proper diagnosis without making the referring physician appear less than competent can sometimes be difficult. With early referral, the PCP need only explain to parents that their child has a complex group of symptoms or laboratory findings that might indicate some form of underlying disease and that they should get the opinion of an expert to help them sort things through.

The Insurance Company as Case Manager

As the health insurance industry and managed care have evolved in this country, decision making about the medical care of a patient can and often does include the payer of the health care services. At various levels of the health care system, payers and financially responsible organizations manage the care of children by, at times, restricting options for treatment and specialty consultation. In our experience, while the best thing for the child is usually done in the end, it can either be a very simple process with reasonable decisions or a complicated and contentious situation in which the PCP or specialist debates and appeals the recommendation of the payer.

Some of this contentiousness comes from the large variety of benefit plans that families have subscribed to and thus a huge variety in what they may actually have coverage for. It is so hard for practitioners to keep up with all the details of the insurance plans of their patients that most practices have had to hire additional staff just to keep up with insurance payment and approval polices. Despite the occasional hassles, it is important to remember that the interests and needs of the child, within the limits of coverage, are the goals of all involved.

The Family's Role in Case Management

In some insurance systems, the path of making referrals and managing a child with special health care needs is easy, which, of course, pleases families with CSHCN. With commercial health plans, the family usually has the option once per year through their employer to change insurance plans if they are not pleased with their child's care. Families with government-funded insurance, in most states, also have the option of seeking a provider who might give better care and service to their child. Where families of CSHCN often face limited choice is with regard to the specific specialist. This is due to the national shortage of pediatric specialists (Jewett, Anderson, & Gilchrist, 2005).

All insurance programs have ways for families to speak up and advocate for their child in demanding better care. Advocacy by the family on their child's behalf can create at times an adversarial feeling between the PCP and the family. For example, the physician and the family do not always agree about the need for a referral to a specialist. Families advocate for their child when demanding tests requested by the specialist but not approved by the payer. Families also may lobby their PCP, the specialist, and the payer for more expensive and less well-proven treatments when standard treatments have failed.

At times, families have created conflict by demanding services that their providers or the payers do not feel are necessary or appropriate. Conflict with or pressure from patients and families can raise the fear of malpractice litigation that in turn can lead some providers, both PCPs and specialists, to order tests and make referrals that they might not otherwise have done. Thankfully, these situations don't arise very often, and most referrals to and requests by providers are reasonable and the family is pleased with the resulting plan of care.

THE EVOLUTION OF CASE MANAGEMENT

How can we best provide a seamless system of case management for our sickest children—those with complex, chronic medical problems—when our medical care delivery system can be just as complex? One important action families can take is to work with regional or national groups supporting CSHCN (see Chapters 5 and 10) and lobby providers and payers to supply all necessary and appropriate care and services.

Families in some states are lucky in that there are public programs with a long and positive history of providing case-management services for CSHCN. In California, there is Children's Medical Services Branch, a 78-year-old program that coordinates and pays for clinical and case-management services for CSHCN on a categorical basis (www. dhs.ca.gov/pcfh/cms/). This system provides case management by nurses experienced in the needs of CSHCN who work collaboratively with the specialists and care team.

Ideally, a CSHCN would be co–case-managed by a primary care physician and a specialist with the payer involved as necessary. The involvement of the PCP, specialist, and payer allows for care and services to be coordinated, comprehensive, effective, efficiently delivered, and fully involving the child and family. This requires good and regular communication among all involved providers, the family, and the payer.

Excellent health care for children in this country dictates that all of the parties involved in caring for children work together for the good of the children, especially children with chronic health care problems. This includes payers that need to be mindful of which services are necessary for good care, as well as PCPs and specialists who must provide coordinated and comprehensive health care with an awareness of the utility and costs of tests and treatments. Families of CSHCN also have an important role to play in that they need to carefully evaluate and consider the insurance they choose, if they have a choice. If they have a child with complex needs, they need to know which services are covered by their plan and which are not. This is especially important when it comes to mental health services. Families need to know who pays for which services and whom to approach about how care decisions are made. They need to evaluate their PCPs and question them about their usual involvement in the care of their patients with special health care needs. If their child needs specialty care, the family needs to seek out and advocate for that care. And, most important, the family needs to work closely and collaboratively with their PCP and specialist to obtain the best care and services they can for their child.

REFERENCE

Jewett, E.A., Anderson, M.R., & Gilchrist, G.S. (2005, September 30). The pediatric subspecialty workforce: Public policy and forces for change. *Pediatrics, 116*(5), 1192–1202.

9

DISRUPTING DREAMS, MAKING DISCOVERIES, AND DECIPHERING SYSTEMS OF CARE:

THE LONG-RANGE VIEW OF THE DEVELOPMENTAL SPECIALIST

Laurel K. Leslie and Kristin Gist

A newborn with previously undiagnosed Down syndrome, a fetus with a visible heart deformity on ultrasound, a 6-month-old with persistent seizures of an unclear etiology and an uncertain prognosis, a 2-year-old girl with delayed language and social interactions suggestive of autism, a 5-year-old boy in a motor vehicle accident who sustains brain damage—all are examples of the types of children with special health care needs (CSHCN) cared for by health care and developmental/educational professionals and by early intervention specialists for children 0–5 years of age. The five children mentioned above were first identified as having special health care needs at different ages, had diverse types of impairment, and demonstrated unique prognostic trajectories. Yet, the experiences of their parents over time showed remarkable similarities. Each of the children's parents went through a three-phase process that included 1) confronting their dying dreams for a *healthy* child, 2) discovering anew what their child's future and their own might hold, and 3) deciphering among a complex array of care delivery systems which services they and their child would need.

In this chapter, we explore how health care and affiliated professionals can best work with families in regard to these three phases (dream disruption, discovery, and deciphering). In doing so, we draw on our own perspectives as a developmental–behavioral pediatrician and as a director of a developmental services division in a children's hospital. We discuss each of the three phases, providing clinicians with strategies they can pursue to best assist families as they experience the phases. Some of the suggested approaches focus on communicating and coaching parents; others address system-level efforts that clinicians can undertake to improve care for the children and their parents. Throughout, we highlight the role of clinicians in strengthening the relationship between a child and his or her parents, encouraging the parents' resilience and subsequent ability to function as advocates and case managers for their children, and serving as a bridge between complex care delivery systems and families. These efforts will ultimately play a large role in improving care for CSHCN.*

NOTE ON TERMINOLOY

In this chapter, we use the term *parents* throughout to indicate one (or more) primary caregiver for a child with special health care needs. While we generally use the term in the plural and refer to two parents, we are aware that CSHCN may be raised by a variety of caregivers including two parents, one parent, an extended family member or members, and a guardian or guardians. Further, even in a two-parent household, one individual may serve as the primary caregiver for the child. Similarly, because professionals working with CSHCN may be affiliated with a health care system, an early intervention or educational program, or a disabilities agency, we have elected to use the non-specific term *clinician* instead of health care providers.

Finally, where we include quotations from parents, we are drawing on written notes or e-mails that parents have sent us over the years. In addition, one parent privately published a series of letters written to her child at each of the child's birthdays, which she has shared with us. While this is not the same as drawing upon systematically collected research data, it does have the benefit of representing the real-world concerns of real parents we have known and whose children and families we have served. As such, the letters reflect the experiences of caring for CSHCN that we attempt to express in this chapter.

DISRUPTING DREAMS

"I once heard it said that when they tell you something is wrong with your child, it is as though time skips a beat, and when it begins beating again, nothing is ever the same. . . . We want to be assured that even though time has "skipped a beat," that is all it has done. We want to know time will right itself, and our world will again be a safe, predictable place, our hopes and dreams for our children will come to fruition, and we will stay secure within the unchanging constancy of hopes and dreams that parents since

* This chapter could not have been written without stories that parents, children, and other professionals have communicated to us over the years. In addition, we are indebted to the families and clinicians who read through this chapter in its various iterations and were willing to share their own perspectives with us. Lastly, we thank Amy Monn and Brenda Bantados for their editorial assistance.

Adam and Eve have dreamed for their children." —B.G., mother of a daughter with epilepsy and severe mental retardation (Giesecke, 2001, p. 133)

One of the commonalities of parenting is dreaming about their children's later lives. Often these dreams go unacknowledged verbally but include parents' core fantasies, desires, and projections into the future for their child. When parents first learn that their child may have a chronic condition or a special health care need, their dreams for their child's life are altered or even shattered. The alteration can be slow or abrupt, depending on the condition, the way the information has been communicated, and the parents' ability to absorb information and their normal coping habits.

Information about a child's condition may be shared in a primary care medical setting by an obstetrician, pediatrician, or family doctor, or it may be conveyed in a specialized medical clinic by a specialist who has completed a complex medical and/or developmental evaluation of the child. Alternatively, the information may be shared by a clinician at a state or community-funded disabilities agency or by an early interventionist or educational psychologist associated with programs specified under the Individuals with Disabilities Education Act (IDEA). Sometimes, this communication occurs acutely in an intensive care unit, labor and delivery suite, or emergency facility. Other times, families hear about a diagnosis after a prolonged series of evaluations, examinations, and laboratory tests conducted by an often bewildering series of professionals. In addition, some children's symptoms are never clearly identified, and families continue to live with an uncertain diagnosis and prognosis, searching—sometimes desperately—for a clinician or a page on the Internet that can provide some answers.

No matter who delivers the news, how immediately the message is conveyed, or what the content of the message is, the fact remains that the clinician conveying information about the child's condition directly and inevitably confronts and alters the parents' dreams for that child as they existed before the moment the information was first communicated. This initial phase of dream disruption is generally intense and difficult, and it can be fraught with conflict.

The clinician must conduct a thorough evaluation of the cause of the child's condition in a manner that both conforms to the guidelines of care developed by his or her professional organization and is respectful of the parents' needs for and readiness to have their child assessed for possible medical, developmental, educational, or psychological problems. The clinician must then communicate a diagnosis to the child and parents. And yet, a tension exists among the clinician's role to impart information, the parents' need to hear that information, and the parents' hold on what they had imagined for their child, sometimes only moments before.

During this time of disrupted dreams, a key task for the clinician is to communicate a diagnosis with thoughtfulness and respect for the parents' experience. However, many clinicians enter into this communication process without reflection on or skills-training in delivering a difficult diagnosis. Fortunately, the last several decades have seen the growth of a number of organizations whose membership includes clinicians and family members of CSHCN. These organizations have collaborated to provide materials to the public about the diagnostic process as well as guidelines for clinicians in how to communicate a difficult diagnosis to families (Autism Society of America, n.d.; Cooley & Graham, 1991; Garwick, Patterson, Bennett, & Blum, 1995; Kennell & Rolnick, 1960; National Down Syndrome Society, n.d.; Perlman et al., 1991; Sharp, Strauss, & Lorch, 1992). The specific suggestions below are drawn from our own clinical experience as well as from the resources developed by these organizations.

Our suggestions for clinicians working with parents at the stage of dream disruption fall into two general categories: 1) respectful communication that takes into account individual families' unique situations and perspectives and 2) self-knowledge regarding one's own attitudes toward the child's condition, one's diagnostic and treatment skills, and the potential conflict between what one may want for the child and what the child's parents may desire. Each of these areas is discussed below.

Respectful Communication

Parents have shared with us how important it is to let them know as soon as possible about their child's needs, and that the setting for this conversation must be chosen with care. Parents want to be talked to in person, with both parents together, if possible, and in a setting that is comfortable and private, away from disturbances and distractions so that all parties concerned can focus on the discussion at hand. Some families also like to have an additional support person present, such as extended family members, close friends, or religious leaders.

Communication style is important. In a seminal study whose results have been replicated, Cunningham and Sloper (1977) studied parents of children diagnosed with Down syndrome to try to better understand parents' needs regarding the clinician's communication style. Parents reported that they wanted to hear the information in a realistic, frank, and sympathetic but positive manner. They wanted their clinician to use straightforward and understandable language that didn't contain much jargon. They asked that clinicians be seated so that they didn't appear rushed and that they maintain close proximity and good eye contact with the parents. In our experience, parents also want their own concerns about their child's condition to be elicited straightforwardly by the clinician. Many parents are afraid to voice their concerns or perspectives on their child's condition, and therefore the gentle solicitation and acknowledgement of these may be important for both the clinician–parent relationship and parental participation in treatment over time.

To these ends, we have found it helpful to begin with simple questions. For example, in conducting an evaluation of a child with as yet undiagnosed problems, we ask, "What do you want to get out of this evaluation?" When sharing a diagnosis with a family, we state, "I've told you a lot about this disorder from my perspective as a clinician; I'd be interested in knowing what your questions and concerns are."

Parents' concerns may seem trivial, irrelevant, or unimportant to the clinician at first; for example, a parent of a newborn with a cleft palate may be wondering, "How will I breastfeed?" "Will he be mentally retarded?" "Will he be able to go on dates?" "Will he go to college?" and seem not at all interested in the careful facts the clinician is sharing about the etiology of the disorder or the surgical interventions to be scheduled. It is helpful for the clinician to remember that such questions are often manifestations of the disrupted dreams about this child that the parent is confronting. Parents we have served have shared with us the feeling that their disrupted dream for their child is on a direct collision course with the information the clinician is imparting.

Many parents, naturally, are consumed with these disrupted dreams and have reported that much of what a clinician says in a first meeting may not be heard or absorbed. One parent related a memory from the night after her premature son's birth: "I was asked what I wanted to do with the baby: donate it to science, give it to the hospital, or take it home for burial—to die. Although perhaps there were questions we needed to answer, it was very difficult to make this decision at such an emotional time" (T.L., personal communication, February 7, 2005). In fact, in two studies conducted with parents of children diagnosed with cancer, more than half reported difficulty recalling much information at all from their first meetings with their clinician (Eden, Black, MacKinlay, & Emery, 1994; Ford, Fallowfield, & Lewis, 1994).

We often suggest a second consultation after the first meeting, either in person or over the phone, to review the issues again with parents. Whether or not parents are ready to hear the information, it is helpful to provide them with up-to-date summary handouts, including related web sites, to take home to read later. We have had families ask us for written *to do* lists because the scope of information being presented can be so overwhelming. If clinicians can provide or direct parents toward reliable information, parents can begin to assimilate appropriate information in a time frame that works for them.

Family members have suggested that the clinician explore other possible life challenges that the family is contending with that might affect their ability to process the information provided. Families come into this devastation with challenges that are seemingly unrelated to their child's condition and that clinicians may have no idea about. One mother of a sick neonate commented:

> "When my son R. was transferred 30 miles to the nearest NICU with asphyxia and persistent fetal circulation, I was reluctant to call my parents. Although my dad was a pediatrician and would have provided much needed knowledge and support, he also had heart disease. . . . I was afraid if I sounded upset, he'd have a heart attack. I called anyway . . . and, sure enough, he arrested on the way to the airport. He remained on a respirator with irreversible brain damage as I tried to cope with the shock of a sick baby with a worrisome prognosis." — K.C., personal communication, January 21, 2005

Finally, in our experience, individual family members may respond differently and may actually have a great deal of conflict about the child's condition and how to manage it. For example, one family member may steep him- or herself in information regarding a disorder while another remains convinced everything will be fine and no interventions are needed. The clinician needs to be sensitive to where each of the family members is coming from and to the stress that different coping mechanisms among family members can have on marital, household, and family stability.

Self-Knowledge

Parental responses can be varied and include panic, anxiety, denial, shock, grief, depression, guilt, and anger at themselves, the other parent, the clinician, or the care system. Parents have consistently commented to us that they appreciate a clinician who can sit comfortably with them in all their emotions. In a seminal work often quoted in the patient–pediatrician communication literature, Kennell and Rolnick (1960) pointed out that the clinician who shrinks from sharing a difficult diagnosis with a family is not necessarily neglectful or callous but may be having difficulty coping with his or her own feelings. Clinicians need to make sure they are listening to their own feelings. Acknowledging his or her own perspectives and fears about a disorder may help the clinician serve as part of the healing process for a family.

Clinicians also need to be careful not to immediately assume that a family has the same perspective that they do about the child's disorder. Asking questions such as "What is your understanding of this disorder?" "How do or don't you see it fitting your child?" "Have you known anyone with this type of problem?" "What has this problem been like for that person?" "What else have you heard about this problem?" can help to elicit a family's explanation for the child's problem and their expectations for what will happen to the child over time (Kleinman, Eisenberg, & Good, 1978). Garwick and colleagues' study (1995) pointed out that families with a positive attitude regarding the disorder or with previous positive experiences generally cope better with the diagnostic process.

It is essential to learn how the family's cultural and/or religious background may affect their interpretation of the disorder. Through anthropologic and cross-cultural research, scholars have found that the illness experience and the expression of illness behavior are heavily influenced by cultural norms and processes (Gidwani, Sobo, Seid, & Kurtin, 2003). Religious beliefs can play a large role in driving care decisions. Although as clinicians we must safeguard the child's best interests, we also must take care not to project our own attitudes onto a family who may interpret a disorder in a different manner than we do (see Chapter 4 for more on cultural processes in relation to CSHCN).

As much as possible, clinicians need to incorporate a lifelong learning perspective into their work that allows them to provide up-to-date information on diagnostic and management strategies. In a situation where a clinician does not have current data regarding a condition, it is best to share that fact with a family and either learn more about the condition in concert with the family or refer the family to a clinician who has had more experience with that condition. The provision of obsolete information can inadvertently damage the child–parent relationship, the clinician–parent relationship, and the parents' future attitude toward treatment. For example, Garwick and colleagues' study (1995) of how families first learned about their child's chronic conditions provided examples of parents of children with Down syndrome who received outdated information from the hospital regarding the role of institutionalization, and the significant damage done to their relationship with interventionists and their child following receipt of that information.

Similarly, clinicians need to take an evidence-based approach during the diagnostic process. Unfortunately, some parents have relayed to us experiences with clinicians who "blew off" the parents' concerns or did not respond with evidence-based guidance and direction. There is good evidence from studies to suggest that parental concerns are strong markers for developmental and/or behavioral problems (Glascoe & Dworkin, 1995). Telling a family of the child with health or developmental concerns that their child will outgrow the problem may not make the family feel better, and it may deprive the child of important early intervention services available to them through the medical system, the early intervention/special education system, or state or locally funded disability agencies. For example, the parents of an 18-month-old toddler, who was later diagnosed with an autistic spectrum disorder, express their frustration and fury; they had been asking their pediatrician since their child turned 8 months about her very abnormal social interactions and odd behaviors.

"Each time we raised an issue and tried to communicate our concerns, the pediatrician told us our daughter's behavior was normal, that different children develop at different rates, and that we shouldn't compare her development to that of our older child. We were made to feel like paranoid, neurotic parents, which made us increasingly more reluctant to discuss our concerns with him. We found ourselves begging for information that we knew we didn't want to hear. In the end, when we sought help elsewhere, we were actually relieved to get the bad news, because at least we knew it was real. . . . Up until that point, all we had were unanswered questions. The unrealistic prospect that everything was going to be OK was more damning than the reality of the problem. It's been nearly 8 years since her diagnosis and I still feel angry that we lost a critical 9 months in working with her."
—K.N., personal communication, September 21, 2004

Finally, sometimes parents present concerns to a clinician and there is no clear diagnosis available at that time. For children at very high risk, and without a diagnosis, parents prefer to have a clinician conduct developmental surveillance and give parents connections and tools to monitor their child rather than do nothing. Similarly, children with symptoms of autism or those who were severely premature and/or ill as newborns elicit parental anxiety due to the ambiguity of the prognosis and outcome. Parents want to hold onto their dreams and yet they are watchful and worried that normal development may not evolve. These children require ongoing assessment in a respectful manner, and their parents require ongoing communication to determine the right time for their children to be referred to and linked with available systems of intervention and support.

DISCOVERING A CHILD ANEW

"You are floating along in your little sailboat of life. You suddenly hit a rock that was under the water (child with disability is born or you begin to have the idea something is not quite right). You are not sure what to do. . . . You discover you are off course and have no idea where you are or how to get home. After a while, realizing you are not getting any closer to home, you gather some supplies (resources) and plug up the hole in your boat and set sail again. Some days the sun shines and some days the clouds of depression blot out the joy of sailing. . . . After a while, you realize that even though the journey is hard, you have built up muscles and thick skin and that you have all the resources you need and that the sunset each night is beautiful and the stars are guiding you. You acknowledge that you have been affected but you are stronger and are surviving and thriving on your new journey: destination—still unknown." — K.L., mother of a child with cerebral palsy and hearing loss after birth asphyxia, personal communication, April 19, 2005

The second phase in the families' process of caring for a child with special health care needs is discovering their child anew. This stage begins with parents grieving for the loss of the dreams they had for their child. This is a draining, frightening, and consuming process and requires that parents let go of the lost dreams and generate new visions for their child. Importantly, families are not just discovering new dreams for their child. The child's special health care needs also may require reframing the parents' experiences with their child, their priorities and values, and even their day-to-day routines. Sometimes, the scope of needs of a CSHCN may be so significant that new dreams must be discovered for the life-course trajectories of the parents and, potentially, the siblings of the CSHCN. Some parents are unable to surmount the difficulties of this phase; others are unable to let go of their lost dreams. Both of these types of parents need support and thoughtful reflection from clinicians.

Clinicians can support families during this discovery phase in two ways: 1) by providing parents with an opportunity to work through the discovery process through discussions with the clinician and 2) by linking families with agencies and community organizations that also can help a family through this phase of discovery. Each of these strategies is discussed in more detail in this chapter.

Working Through the Discovery Process

Similar to the five stages of grief in response to death outlined by Elizabeth Kubler-Ross (1969), parents who are in the process of discovering
their child anew go through myriad emotions including shock, guilt,
anger, and bartering. Ultimately, most parents develop some strategy
for acknowledging their child's special needs.

However, parents differ vastly in how they manifest that acknowledgement. Some may respond to their child's newly discovered needs
with alacrity. As one father of a child with autistic spectrum disorder
features reported, "My main feelings of anxiety actually fell away after
the initial shock of the diagnosis, because it gave us something to work
toward; the diagnosis was liberating in that sense" (K.N., personal communication, September 21, 2004).

Another parent with a premature infant in a neonatal intensive
care nursery responded with a very different perspective.

> "I felt guilty that giving birth to a [so-called] defective baby had
> caused my father's death. I worried that my baby might have
> cerebral palsy, and I wondered if he would ever stop screaming
> and crying. I wondered if I would ever be able to love him. My
> pediatrician pointed out after one month that I wasn't even refer-
> ring to my baby by his name."—K.C., personal communication,
> January 21, 2005

Parents may become easily overwhelmed by the scope of work they
must undertake to care for their child with special needs, as the following newsletter excerpt written by a parent of a CSHCN shows:

> "For those doctors who deal with sick or *special needs* children, I
> would say to you: We are mothers and fathers just like you. We
> are trying to just keep our heads above water and we don't know
> when the next tidal wave is going to be hitting us. Some of us
> are drowning in a sea of uncontrollable sadness and work, and
> find it hard to get the strength to drag ourselves out of bed, to
> the hospital, appointments, or the ongoing and exhausting saga
> of letting therapists into our homes."— Rosen Cohen, 2002, p. 2

In fact, part of the discovery process for parents involves coming to
terms with the realities of caring for their child. Parents have a number
of immediate practicalities they must face; for example, they may ask
themselves, "What do I say to families and friends?" "Can I work?"
"How do I run errands if he uses a wheelchair?" For many, these practicalities are not insubstantial. The health care needs of the child may
affect one or more parent's ability to hold down a job and thus would

have a fiscal impact on the family. Structural changes or other renovations may need to be made to a house or apartment. Medications, special diets, and specialty clinician visits may need to be incorporated into already busy family lives. The child care center that was reserved may no longer be accessible, as most centers cannot accommodate CSHCN. Siblings' needs may also go unattended, and this may lead to behavioral problems in the sibling concurrently or at a later point in time. Even strong marital relationships may be substantially stressed by a child's special health care needs.

Clinician Support for Discovery

Clinicians can support families during this discovery phase by providing them with an opportunity to process these practical and relational challenges in a safe, nonjudgmental setting. Clinicians need to be comfortable with the different approaches families take to deal with their child's special needs, ranging from the father's quick embrace of an advocacy role described above to the overwhelmed parent who feels as if she or he is barely treading water. Knowing how to best support these parents in their personal ways of responding to their child's needs and when to consider suggesting an alternative strategy requires good listening and communication skills. Clinicians also need to be able to emotionally manage the divergent, seemingly contradictory feelings a single parent may voice. As one wise parent said,

> "[T]here is a fine line between denial and hope. Perhaps they are flip sides of the same coin, a coin named *reality*. I know that in my experience as the parent of children with disabilities, I have lived and still do live in both of these places, because the place called reality can be a painful, heartbreaking, disillusioning place. . . . It is difficult for professionals working with families to know how to temper reality for families. If one takes denial away from a parent, one runs the risk of taking hope away also. Without hope, we frail human beings cannot survive."—C.H., personal communication, April 11, 2005

Clinicians have an important role to play in assisting parents as they move through the process of reconceptualizing their dreams for their children. One mother of a child with cerebral palsy and hearing loss told us that the developmental evaluation report she received from our developmental clinic was the first report she encountered in which someone described her daughter as an adorable, blonde, blue-eyed little girl instead of labeling her with a medical diagnosis. We have found that, once a diagnosis is made, it is critical to move from a diagnostic framework that looks for pertinent signs and symptoms of a disorder to a more functionally focused, strength-based approach that sees the child as a person and not a disorder.

Similarly, clinicians also play an important role in helping parents learn to define their roles as case managers and advocates for their CSHCN and in supporting parents in that role. Depending on the type of special health care needs a child displays, the child and family may have to access a bewildering array of health, developmental, and educational specialists as well as face an equally overwhelming number of administrative hurdles. By explaining these systems, their eligibility criteria, and their procedures, clinicians can help parents move more easily into their new roles. The clinician can identify advocacy and support organizations in the community to assist parents who can't move into these roles for personal or functional reasons.

Linking Families to Agencies and Community Organizations

Besides supporting parents in the discovery process, clinicians can specifically help families by referring them to available agencies and community organizations. Details regarding the types of services provided by these groups are described in the section that follows. In general, though, agencies may provide a number of medical, developmental, and educational services to address each child's special health care needs. Some agencies also provide practical support (e.g., respite care). Community organizations, on the other hand, usually are not-for-profit groups that act to provide information, advocacy, and support for CSHCN and their families. Referrals to community organizations can help parents access up-to-date information regarding diagnostic and treatment strategies. Community organizations often have support groups that allow parents to find other families who may be experiencing similar types of emotions or may know how best to access local resources. Many community organizations are affiliated with national organizations, easily identified in this age of Internet information, that advocate for increasing research, diagnostic assistance, and treatment support for specific disorders. One mother's comment aptly captured how important these types of referrals can be.

> "Once R. was referred to the early intervention program under IDEA [Individuals with Disabilities Education Act], the focus changed. Instead of learning what was wrong, we spent all our time and energy on what to do. Here I was able to share my sadness with other parents, and along with them and R.'s teacher,

I began to find happiness and hope."—K.L., personal communication, April 19, 2005

Counseling may help families as they sort through these issues. Parents may need a safe space to discuss their often bewildering array of feelings about their children, including possible resentment that could, unfortunately, end in abuse. Many parents tend to ignore their own personal needs in the wake of so much demand on their time to care for CSHCN, and regular counseling can help them in that they will be setting aside a small amount of time on a regular basis to think through their own needs.

Unfortunately, clinicians have great difficulty knowing when to offer mental health support to parents and other family members, and even if they did know when to offer it, those who need services may be unable to access them for a variety of reasons. In addition, mental health plans may provide limited services without evidence of a psychiatric diagnosis. Some plans can be quite rigid about whom available services are meant to serve. For example, if a child's disorder triggers a mental health referral through the child's insurance, the mental health practitioner may be restricted to addressing only the child's needs and not the needs of the family members (e.g., their adjustment needs). As a result, such systems have particular challenges addressing the sometimes tenuous relationship between parents and their children with special needs.

Children with special health care needs whose areas of functional limitations span a variety of domains also can encounter difficulties accessing treatments. One school psychologist commented to us that it was difficult to access counseling and therapy for children with a wide range of cognitive and physical disabilities (e.g., cerebral palsy, spina bifida, osteogenesis imperfecta type III, Asperger syndrome), who suffer from low self-esteem and difficulty socializing with their general-education peers. While this partially reflects poor reimbursement to the mental health provider, she commented that there also is a lack of providers with expertise in treating children with disabilities, particularly those with cognitive or speech delays who may respond less well to verbally oriented therapy. Some of these children may suffer from serious behavioral issues, and their parents may need training in parent-mediated behavior modification techniques. A similar shortage of trained behavioral interventionists exists in many communities, especially interventionists who can modify their training to address the motor or verbal limitations some CSHCN face.

DECIPHERING THE SYSTEM: LINKAGES TO SERVICES

"When J. was 17 months old, and I was 9 months pregnant with my third daughter, we finally admitted to ourselves that some-

thing was not right with [her]. After many visits to our pediatrician, we found an ad for a free hearing consultation. So we made
an appointment and took J. to be evaluated. Looking back, I realize the woman doing the evaluation saw definite problems with
J., but instead of upsetting us with what she felt was the problem,
she directed us to the Developmental Evaluation Clinic at our
Children's Hospital. Once the evaluation was done and we learned
that J. was on the autistic spectrum, we came to appreciate that
we still had an immense amount of work to accomplish. My background was in civil engineering, but I suddenly realized I had
to become an expert on child development, and educate myself
quickly on how to get the best help for my daughter through the
state system, and our medical insurance. So while I was grieving
over the news about my daughter, I still had to move forward
and get her the best help as quickly as I could. At that evaluation,
we were thankfully connected to the infant program provided
locally under IDEA where I began to learn that therapy by a
professional would only be a couple of hours a week; the rest was
up to my husband and me. . . . This job was a full-time job: no
vacation time and no time off. It would not be easy or always
smooth going, but as a family, we would make the difference for
J."—N.M., mother of a child with an autistic spectrum disorder
feature; personal communication, September 21, 2004

Just as it is important to help the family through the diagnostic and
discovery processes, it is equally important to help them navigate
through a complex and often unclear series of systems of care for
CSHCN. Families of CSHCN often need assistance understanding the
differences among, and how to make connections with, the myriad
clinicians who may be involved in their child's care. Depending on the
specific type of special health care need, a child may receive care from
many different medical specialists, each with a particular expertise.
These specialists may include pediatric doctors with expertise in specific
organ systems (e.g., genetics, neurology, nephrology, cardiology). They
also may include intensive care physicians and staff, or surgeons if a
child's disorder requires hospitalization and/or interventional procedures. If the child's special health care needs appear to be affecting his
or her motor, language, or cognitive development, a similarly large
array of allied health professionals may be involved in the child's care,
including developmental psychologists, occupational therapists, physical therapists, speech pathologists, educational specialists, and behavioral modification experts. If a child or family develops mental health
needs, either as a direct complication of the disorder or as a consequence

of the challenges inherent in any chronic disease or developmental disorder, mental health professionals may be needed.

Not only may a family be overwhelmed by the sheer number of professionals involved in their child's care, but they also must navigate the fragmented systems of care currently in place. We have found it helpful to conceptualize this de facto service system for CSHCN in three broad categories: 1) medical programs; 2) intervention and educational programs, either in affiliation with a medical center or in a state or federally funded agency; and 3) community organizations. Medical programs are critical for identifying infants and children with special health care needs through screening and/or diagnostic evaluations and for providing any necessary ongoing medical and/or psychiatric care and supportive services. Intervention and educational programs usually employ developmental specialists—psychologists, occupational therapists, speech therapists, physical therapists, educational specialists, and behavior management specialists—and provide early intervention and special education services. As described above, community organizations play a critical role in helping clinicians and families understand available services in their community and offering important emotional and social support for families.

The De Facto System of Care

Available medical programs may be publicly or privately funded but are increasingly defined by covered benefits in a family's health plan. Several federally funded medical programs, including Medicaid, Medicare, and Title V programs, specifically fund services for CSHCN. For example, federal legislation with respect to Medicaid and the Early and Periodic Screening and Diagnosis Treatment (EPSDT) program within Medicaid mandates that any medical, developmental, and/or mental health condition identified during a Medicaid physical examination by a clinician must receive an appropriate diagnostic workup and treatment. Medicare covers children with renal disorders. The Title V statute, State Programs for Children with Special Health Care Needs, provides funds to states to design and implement direct care programs and services. The programs vary in the specific populations served because they are designed in response to the strengths and limits of the child health infrastructure in individual states. A directory of available programs, including eligibility criteria and scope of services, can be found online (Institute for Child Health Policy, 2003).

Accessing these federal programs may not be possible for some families because most of the programs require that a family meet financial eligibility criteria. Therapies may be covered for children with federally subsidized health insurance, but it may be difficult to access providers. Reimbursement is often far below cost and there are decreasing numbers of providers willing to accept Medicaid due to low reimbursement rates and high costs of care (Newacheck, Pearl, Hughes, & Halfon, 1998).

Accessing services is not easy for the many families who are not eligible for government-subsidized programs. Unfortunately, many commercial health plans are limiting covered benefits for children with chronic conditions through medical necessity clauses. These clauses have been described as problematic for patients of all ages, as they are often defined fiscally by which services are covered by a health plan and they do not take into account which services may be medically indicated (American Medical Association, 2005; Rosenbaum, Kamoie, Mauery, & Walitt, 2003). Medical necessity clauses are often based on adult definitions of *medical necessity*, which typically fail to take into account children's unique developmental needs and the importance of preventive therapeutic interventions, thereby severely restricting services for children. For children with certain health plans, services may be denied unless the condition is caused by illness, injury, or congenital defect—adult definitions of medical necessity. This excludes many childhood disabling conditions of unclear etiology and prognostic trajectory.

For example, developmental evaluations and services are frequently not covered benefits, and for children with an evolving disorder of unclear prognosis such as prematurity, autistic spectrum disorder, or developmental delay without a known etiology, intervention services may be inaccessible and unfunded, placing added stress on an already grieving family. Alternatively, parents may assume that if services aren't provided, they must not be needed, leading to a false sense of security and an assumption that the organization is providing the full range of services documented to be effective in the research literature. Physicians may find themselves in the unfortunate position of being ill-equipped to perform diagnostic screening, evaluation, or treatment services themselves (due to lack of time, training, or reimbursement) and also face the frustration of being unable to access services for a family either inside or outside a health plan or medical system of care.

Even if services are ultimately funded, the process of seeking coverage through one's health insurance plan can be arduous and difficult to navigate for both the family and the clinician. There are increasing numbers of providers who refuse both public and private reimbursement and are moving toward cash-pay for developmental services, as even those authorized by a health plan may not be reimbursed. Chapter 3 explores in more depth the financial issues that both public and private medical sector systems face in caring for children with special needs.

Despite the access problems for medical programs, some services can be obtained for families through programs mandated by federal IDEA legislation under the educational system of care in the United States. IDEA legislation requires states to provide services for all children ages 0 to 2 years, 11 months identified with a developmental delay. This legislation allows states the choice of providing services for children ages 0 to 2 years, 11 months who are found to be at risk for developmental delay but who do not yet meet criteria for the disorder (e.g., an infant exposed to drugs in utero whose motor, language, and cognitive milestones are age appropriate). Eight states include infants and toddlers at risk for developmental delay in their programs. In addition, Part B of IDEA requires states to provide services for children ages 3–5 (preschoolers) and for special education (school age and adolescents) services. Finally, some states have developed state-specific programs to address particular subcategories of CSHCN and associated disabilities. These programs are described in more detail in Chapter 2. Unfortunately, our experience shows that parents may be reluctant to immediately enroll in public special education programs for a number of reasons including denial of a possible disorder, fear of stigma associated with enrollment in services through the school system, or lack of sufficient intensity of services.

Community organizations can be conceptualized as a third system of care for families with CSHCN. These organizations can be effective mechanisms for sharing new diagnostic and treatment strategies with parents, providing social support, or raising funds for ground-breaking research. Particularly in this electronic age, community organizations may spread information regarding potential strategies before the health and educational systems are aware of them. Clearly, these organizations can be important partners for clinicians who care for CSHCN. Clinicians also can play a reciprocal role with organizations. Sometimes information that is dispensed may not be evidence-based, and informed clinicians can help community groups and parents sort out information as it becomes available. For example, in San Diego, the authors of this chapter have developed a web site, www.howkidsdevelop.com, which provides information on developmental milestones, developmental delay, available services, and links to respected community and national groups.

Other Complexities of the System

Besides the problems of eligibility, availability, and acceptability of services detailed above, service delivery for CSHCN is complicated by the fact that identification and intervention services often occur in one or more service sectors. For example, federal programs may utilize separate funding streams and yet have overlapping mandates; hence, what services are provided by a specific agency varies immensely in any given community. For example, services for a child with autism may be provided through the school system in one community and through the state developmental disabilities unit in another. Services for a child with special health care needs in any given locale are thus dependent on how federal legislation has been interpreted and implemented in that community. Paradoxically, overlap of agency services may actually lead to fragmentation of services, particularly if programs need to limit their scope of work. In some communities, the different types of services needed by a family of a child with autism (e.g., behavioral therapy, respite care, speech therapy) may be provided in an uncoordinated manner by different agencies where coordinated care would allow for synergies in service provision. In addition, programs may be mandated for some specific disorders and not others, leaving some children's special health care needs unaddressed.

Service and funding gaps may be particularly problematic for children at developmental transition points (e.g., toddlerhood to preschool, preschool to school-age, adolescence to adulthood). For example, in many states, funding streams for early intervention services shift from federal to state or local agencies at age 3 years, resulting in transition problems and changes in eligibility requirements that can affect who is eligible for what level of service. Also, because of this shift in funding, a child referred into the system at 2 years, 7 months to 3 years of age may have a delay in accessing services. It is critical that the clinician become educated about what services are available to whom and to direct accordingly. If a program is highly recommended to a family but is outside the school district in which a family resides, that family is set up for frustration.

Another potential set of challenges involves variation in types of services needed over time. These service needs may be driven by the child's developmental status. A child on the autistic spectrum may require services that focus on speech development and behavior modification in the preschool years; with successful interventions, the child may be able to be mainstreamed into elementary school but require a new type of service (e.g., social skills training) in the school-age years.

Variation in services needed over time may be a function of family members' readiness to accept a diagnosis. The parent who is reluctant to move into a public agency to access services for a possible autistic spectrum disorder may only be ready to move forward on obtaining speech therapy, depending on where he or she is in their process of acceptance and discovery. If a child is engaged in therapy either in addition to or instead of a publicly funded program for children with special needs, the therapist often becomes a critical support for the family and a point of communication and resource for the clinician. For example, therapists in these programs may know more about ongoing community services or newly approved treatments than the general or specialty pediatrician and thus be a good source of information for parents. It may be that this provider, by developing a relationship with the family, can move the family toward acceptance of services from available public systems. Unfortunately, for some health plans, this type of family centered pathway is inaccessible.

Access is another issue. Making strong recommendations for services that are actually inaccessible can set everyone (clinician, parents, and child) up for frustration and financial hardship. Stories of families moving just blocks away to access services that are available in one district and not another are not uncommon.

In addition to system problems, some sociodemographic characteristics of families appear to be related to delayed or limited care. Huang, Kogan, Yu, and Strickland (2005) examined the associations of sociodemographic characteristics with both the prevalence and the causes of delayed or forgone care in a nationally representative sample of CSHCN. The authors found that delayed or forgone health care was more problematic for adolescents, those with severe limitations, those who lived in the South or West, those without medical insurance, and those from families living near the federal poverty level. Families of Latino heritage also had more difficulty accessing medical specialists, experienced language barriers, and more often reported "provider not accessible."

The Clinician's Role in the Deciphering Process

Given the complexity and barriers to services inherent in the de facto system, what can a clinician utilize to assist families in deciphering systems of care? We have conceptualized our approach as falling within two areas: 1) care at the individual child and family level and 2) development of systems of care at the population level.

At the individual child and family level, we have found it particularly important to educate parents regarding the three previously discussed sectors of the de facto system of care: medical, interventional/educational, and community. We have found it helpful to partner with providers in other sectors to develop detailed flow charts—one for each age group (infant/toddler, preschool, and latency/adolescent)—delineating the pathways through which services can be accessed. This tool, which is updated annually by clerical office staff, includes eligibility guidelines, program possibilities, and phone numbers for accessing services. The age-appropriate flow chart, when shared with parents at a health care visit, provides a visual map of how the systems work and whom to call. When parents get home and think they have forgotten key information or need further information, they have a reference tool at hand. A simplified, generic template similar to our county-specific tool is shown in Figure 9.1.

Most important, we feel that the most positive change can occur when clinicians turn their focus toward affecting change at the population level. For example, to address the specific needs of CSHCN in foster care, we established an advisory board composed of representatives from the various public and private agencies and programs supporting CSHCN in our area. Representatives from the programs serving children ages 0–3 years; special education directors or clinical personnel from school districts serving children surrounding the practice; and exceptional family resource representatives, community college and other child development program directors or teachers, parent representatives and physicians can work together in forums like ours to better understand one another's perspectives, offerings, and barriers. Our experience shows that meetings can be as infrequent as quarterly and still result in improved communication, access, and support for families.

For the majority of CSHCN, interdisciplinary and intersystem partnerships are essential for appropriate case management, yet these partnerships present barriers related to different specialty languages, schedules, settings, and eligibility criteria. The state of Oklahoma has begun an important initiative called the Sooner SUCCESS Program specifically to address these barriers. Community care coordinators who are independent of a specific sector service system or agency have been hired in six pilot counties with the specific task of coordinating local departments of health, mental health, education, and disability services. Preliminary results suggest that families and clinicians benefit from developing explicit partnerships among these sectors.

Finally, advocacy at the local, state, and national levels to improve services for CSHCN and their families is critical. For example, in California, coalitions were developed to push for additional taxes on tobacco with the stipulation that funds acquired be used to assure school readiness for young children. With grant funding from this source, we have developed a screening and intervention program that targets young children ages 0–5 years with possible developmental and/or behavioral problems. Screening for delay occurs in physicians' offices, child care programs, and community settings (e.g., domestic violence shelters, migrant camps); intervention services are provided for children with

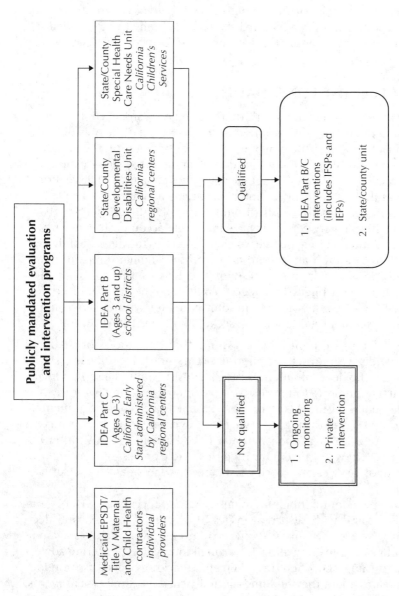

Figure 9.1. Referral template for children with special health care needs. (*Note:* Each community will need to determine what agencies provide publicly mandated and private services and operationalize this template for their community. Each of these prototypical public programs goes by different designations and is coordinated by different agencies. Italics indicate names of specific agencies in San Diego County. The San Diego forms also include specific eligibility requirements and contact information.)

severe enough problems to access categorical programs as well as for children with mild-to-moderate problems that may be resolved with less intensive intervention. At the national level, the American Academy of Pediatrics is partnering with national advocacy groups and the federal government to advocate for a medical home (e.g., specified setting to provide coordinated, comprehensive care) for CSHCN (see Chapter 6).

IN IT FOR THE LONG HAUL

"As the milestone of your thirtieth birthday approached, I anticipated mourning the loss of your youth. Not that thirty is old. It is just that this birthday would mark the passing from the decade of your twenties into another decade and all that usually means in the life of a young adult. One's twenties are a time of discovery and fulfillment—college, finding a career, perhaps marriage and beginning a family. With the milestone of your thirtieth birthday, the gap between your life's milestone accomplishments and those other young people celebrating their thirtieth birthdays widens . . . and I am face to face with the familiar old pain, the familiar old disappointment of the loss of the child—and woman—you might have been, could have been, should have been." —B.G., mother of an adult daughter with epilepsy and severe mental retardation (Giesecke, 2001, pp. 135–136)

Many health care professionals assume that the process of shattered dreams, discovery, and deciphering occurs once, in a linear fashion, following the determination of the diagnosis. Families also may make similar assumptions. Clinically, we have often heard families voice their reexperiences of these phases. For example, one parent commented, "I thought I was through grieving, but every year on his birthday, I found myself crying when I should have been happy." Another exclaimed, "But we just went through this whole process of working with the school last year; how come we need to negotiate these services again?"

We have found it helpful to describe the process for CSHCN families as a spiral with recurrent cycles of dreams, discovery, and deciphering systems. Dreams are often confronted over and over again at rites of passage (e.g., turning 3, starting kindergarten, entering adolescence, turning 21), when unspoken and unacknowledged assumptions and dreams about the child unexpectedly surface. Anniversary events, like the date of a child's near-drowning that caused cognitive and motor delays, can also spark a reexamination of dreams. These same types of events may trigger new discoveries about a child, including newfound strengths as well as challenges. Deciphering the system of care, unfortunately, continues for many families throughout the lifetime of the child even as the child moves into adulthood for a number of reasons. First, the types of problems related to the disorder may change over time. For example, the parents of an infant with Down syndrome may be dealing with issues such as hypotonia and cardiac abnormalities, while the parents of a kindergartener with Down syndrome may be more concerned about their child's social and academic skills. Second, the agencies where a CSHCN receives services may vary over time. Third, even within a single agency, providers working with a CSHCN change over time. The classic example is a school where teachers change each year and need to be reeducated regarding the needs of the CSHCN and how to best meet those needs in the classroom setting. Last, the CSHCN goes through the same developmental stages as other children, from infancy to young adulthood, and may be facing issues related to these transitions.

What can we then conclude about the role of the clinician over the long haul? Clearly, all clinicians have multiple roles to play in helping families decipher and access available services. By understanding the services available in a particular community for a certain disorder or under a specific health plan, clinicians can help families navigate these systems. Knowing whom to contact at what organization is equally important. Also essential for the clinician is the ability to monitor where the family is in the process of dream disruption and discovery and to help the family modulate the types of services they access over time so that the child's best interests are served.

Most important for the CSHCN and his or her parents will be identifying which clinician serves as the primary provider and medical home for the child. Whether or not the medical home is provided in a primary care or specialty office may vary, depending on the needs of the CSHCN and his or her parents as well as the skill sets and practice patterns of different clinicians in a community (see Chapter 6; see also Chapters 7 and 8). It is important to note that different clinicians bring unique skill sets and perspectives to their interactions with families. For example, specialty clinicians with expertise in specific diagnostic and treatment areas function as important repositories of information regarding evidence-based diagnostic and treatment services as well as service providers for both families and primary care clinicians in their communities. Some dedicated clinical nurse specialists perform important educational and support roles for CSHCN and their parents. The primary care clinician has a different skill set. While the clinician may or may not play a part in the diagnostic process, he or she often functions as the family's general physician and coach, addressing routine and complex medical questions and conditions that may arise, monitoring a family's coping strategies, and helping to link a family with appropriate services. With any child, the clinician in the primary care setting needs to determine if the child with special health care needs is growing, developing, and maturing emotionally at rates that are appropriate for children with their particular health needs. Primary health care professionals thus can play an important role in continuing to help families come to terms with their child's diagnosis, as its manifestation changes over time with the child's ongoing development.

CONCLUSION

In this chapter, we have outlined the three-stage parental process of confronting dreams, discovering one's child anew, and deciphering care systems we have found helpful in our work with CSHCN families. We have described some general approaches that can guide clinicians from diverse backgrounds who are involved in the care of CSHCN and their families. In the end, however, it is each clinician's compassion that is the most critical factor brought to encounters with these children and their families. When clinicians listen to the families they care for, they learn. And what they learn from the families will help them provide the most effective and individualized care possible.

REFERENCES

American Medical Association. (2005). *Model managed care contract supplement 1: Medical necessity.* Chicago: Author.

Autism Society of America. (n.d.). Retrieved May 6, 2005, from http://www.autism-society.org

Cooley, W.C., & Graham, J.M.J. (1991). Down syndrome—an update and review for the primary pediatrician. *Clinical Pediatrics, 30*(4), 233–253.

Cunningham, C.C., & Sloper, T. (1977). Parents of Down's syndrome babies: Their early needs. *Child: Care, Health and Development, 3*(5), 325–347.

Eden, O., Black, I., MacKinlay, G., & Emery, A. (1994). Communication with parents of children with cancer. *Palliative Medicine, 8*(2), 105–114.

Ford, S., Fallowfield, L., & Lewis, S. (1994). Can oncologists detect distress in their out-patients and how satisfied are they with their performance during bad news consultations? *British Journal of Cancer, 70,* 767–770.

Garwick, A.W., Patterson, J., Bennett, F.C., & Blum, R.W. (1995). Breaking the news: How families first learn about their child's chronic condition. *Archives of Pediatrics & Adolescent Medicine, 149*(9), 991–997.

Gidwani, P., Sobo, E.J., Seid, M., & Kurtin, P.S. (2003). Laying the foundation: Identifying major issues in applied child health services research. In E.J. Sobo & P.S. Kurtin (Eds.), *Child Health Services Research: Applications, Innovations, and Insights* (1st ed., pp. 25–63). San Francisco: Jossey-Bass.

Giesecke, B. (2001). *Letters to Sheri.* Albany, OR: Selah Publishing.

Glascoe, F., & Dworkin, P. (1995). The role of parents in the detection of developmental and behavioral problems. *Pediatrics, 95*(6), 829–836.

Huang, Z.J., Kogan, M.D., Yu, S.M., & Strickland, B. (2005). Delayed or forgone care among children with special health care needs: An analysis of the 2001 National Survey of Children with Special Health Care Needs. *Ambulatory Pediatrics, 5*(1), 60–67.

Individuals with Disabilities Education Act (IDEA) of 1990, PL 101-476, 20 U.S.C. §§ 1400 *et seq.*

Institute for Child Health Policy. (2003). *Directory of state Title V CSHCN programs: Eligibility criteria and scope of services.* Retrieved May 6, 2005, from http://cshcnleaders.ichp.edu/TitleVDirectory/directory.htm

Kennell, J.H., & Rolnick, A.R. (1960). Discussing problems in newborn babies with their parents. *Pediatrics, 26*, 832–838.

Kleinman, A.M., Eisenberg, L., & Good, B.J. (1978). Culture, illness and care: Clinical lessons from anthropologic and cross-cultural research. *Annals of Internal Medicine, 88*, 251–258.

Kubler-Ross, E. (1969). *On death and dying.* New York: Touchstone.

Medicaid Early and Periodic Screening, Diagnosis and Treatment Act Amendments of 1989, Omnibus Budget Reconciliation Act of 1989, PL 101-239, 42 U.S.C. §§ 1396 *et seq.*

National Down Syndrome Society. (n.d.). Retrieved May 6, 2005, from http://ndss.org/

Newacheck, P.W., Pearl, M., Hughes, D.C., & Halfon, N. (1998). The role of Medicaid in ensuring children's access to care. *Journal of the American Medical Association, 280*(20), 1789–1793.

Rosen Cohen, L. (2002). Bedside manner 101: A parent's perspective. *The Section on Developmental and Behavioral Pediatrics Newsletter, 11*(1), p. 2.

Rosenbaum, S., Kamoie, B., Mauery, D.R., & Walitt, B. (2003). *Medical necessity in private health plans: Implications for behavioral health care.* DHHS Pub. No. (SMA) 03-3790. Rockville, MD: Center for Mental Health Services, Substance Abuse and Mental Health Services Administration.

Sharp, M.C., Strauss, R.P., & Lorch, S.C. (1992). Communicating medical bad news: Parents' experiences and preferences. *Journal of Pediatrics, 121*(4), 539–546.

IV

PRESENT STRATEGIES, FUTURE DIRECTIONS

The complexity of the needs of children with special health care needs (CSHCN) and the opaqueness and nonresponsiveness of systems meant to serve them often mean that care coordination is left to already overburdened families. Recognizing the challenges families face, the American Academy of Pediatrics (AAP) Committee on Children with Disabilities has called on primary care physicians to play an active role and partner with families to help coordinate care (American Academy of Pediatrics Committee on Children with Disabilities, 1999). The AAP noted that care coordination is "the key to efficient management of the many complex issues surrounding the care of children with special health care needs" (p. 980), yet acknowledges that myriad barriers make care coordination difficult for both families and primary care pediatricians. Many of these barriers were discussed in the previous section (see also Seid, Sobo, Reyes, & Varni, 2004).

Notwithstanding the challenges outlined above and earlier in this book, most parents do learn to cope—some more, some less—with the systems through which they must work to secure appropriate care for their CSHCN (Sobo, Seid, & Gelhard, 2006). The process of acquiring the skills necessary to optimize services for one's CSHCN can be understood as what has been termed *functional biomedical acculturation* (Sobo & Seid, 2003), a process that leads a person to be at least minimally or functionally acculturated to the world of the health care system (i.e., biomedicine) in a way that allows him or her to function within the system and achieve desired ends.

For parents of CSHCN, these skills may include those needed for gaining timely access to specialty services, for expediting permissions for continued care, and for ensuring that one's questions are answered and that each specialist knows what the other specialists are doing for the child. In a nutshell, parents of CSHCN must learn how to act as extraordinarily skilled health care consumers if they are to realize the health-related goals that they have for their children (Prussing, Sobo, Walker, & Kurtin, 2005).

Yet, it has not been clear what type of resources and tools would be most effective in helping both families and health care providers learn more quickly how to effectively navigate and manage these systems. The literature reveals limited understanding of how interactions between families and systems, families and providers, providers and their organizations, or providers and providers evolve over time into a trajectory or trajectories leading toward the best possible care for the children in question. This book's significance stems from the fact that knowledge of these interactions and an in-depth understanding of the learning curves implicated are key to designing policies, programs, and practices that maximize the likelihood of positive outcomes for CSHCN—and possibly for all children.

CSHCN are perhaps most vulnerable to suboptimal care during the critical period of discovery that occurs before they are 5 years old—the time when most of their problems are first diagnosed or recognized—and when their parents are first thrust into the foreign world of the health care system. The preceding chapters have explored the reasons for this vulnerability and have asked what can be done to ensure the best possible care for CSHCN. They have summarized issues that cut across chronic or disabling childhood conditions and override specific diagnostic labels. The chapters have built upon the key contributions of earlier scholars; moreover, they have enhanced the existing knowledge base by identifying understudied areas as well as by tying together the results of disparate studies and differing viewpoints to provide coherent reviews of the topics assigned.

In Chapter 10, anthropologist E.J. Sobo summarizes and presents, in the form of a conceptual model, major aspects of the learning curves for parents and practitioners identified in the preceding chapters and through her own previous research. She then discusses ways to accelerate learning, identifying crucial moments at which this might be accomplished and methods for fostering the growth of knowledge and skills.

In Chapter 11, health services researchers Lisa A. Simpson and Denise Dougherty develop ideas for future directions in research and policy for CSHCN in their early years, setting CSHCN-specific research and policies into larger contexts. Research trends that are addressed include the growing constraints on research dollars, the increase in data sources to support research, the prospects for the use of information technology for the multicenter research needed for CSHCN (because of the relative rarity of these conditions), and the incorporation of children's issues in an implementation or translation-oriented research agenda. Larger forces in policy to be addressed include the push toward block granting of public programs, consumer choice in health care, use of quality measures within programs that increasingly link payment to quality outcomes, and the pressing need to move advances in science into actual care practices and processes. Exploring these trends while maintaining a sharp focus on their applicability to CSHCN enabled Simpson and Dougherty to identify gaps in research and policy structures for CSHCN and to recommend how these structures might be changed to better meet the needs of CSHCN and their families.

REFERENCES

American Academy of Pediatrics Committee on Children with Disabilities. (1999). Care coordination: Integrating health and related systems of care for children with special health care needs. *Pediatrics, 104*(4 Pt. 1), 978–981.

Prussing, E., Sobo, E.J., Walker, E., & Kurtin, P. (2005). Between "desperation" and disability rights: A narrative analysis of complementary/alternative medicine use by parents for children with Down syndrome. *Society Science & Medicine, 60,* 587–598.

Seid, M., Sobo, E.J., Reyes, L., & Varni, J.W. (2004). Parents' reports of barriers to care for children with special health care needs: Development and Validation of the Barriers to Care Questionnaire. *Ambulatory Pediatrics, 4*(4), 323–331.

Sobo, E.J., & Kurtin, P.S. (Eds.). (2003). *Child health services research: Applications, innovations, and insights.* San Francisco: Jossey-Bass.

Sobo, E.J., & Seid, M. (2003). Cultural issues in health services delivery: What kind of "competence" is needed, and from whom? *Annals of Behavioral Science & Medical Education, 9*(2), 97–100.

Sobo, E.J., Seid, M., & Gelhard, L. R. (2006). Parent-identified barriers to pediatric health care: A process-oriented model and method. *Health Services Research, 41*(1), 148–172.

10

MASTERING THE HEALTH CARE SYSTEM FOR CHILDREN WITH SPECIAL HEALTH CARE NEEDS

Elisa J. Sobo

With no true map, and no single point of entry, how do parents (or guardians) of children living with chronic or disabling conditions[1] gain access to and navigate through the various components of the health care system to optimize their children's health outcomes and potentials? How do they discover, chart, and master what is generally, for them, a strange new world? And how do health care workers trained within the curative biomedical paradigm and a system developed for short- and not long-term care grapple with the needs of families with children who have chronic conditions and who may never be *cured* no matter how hard anybody tries?

Building on ideas presented in the previous sections, and drawing on the literature as well as original research, this chapter proposes a noncategorical conceptual model of the learning curve experienced by many parents of children with special health care needs (CSHCN) as they gain mastery over their care-related roles, rights, and responsibilities.[2] While spotlighting the parent experience, the model identifies modifiable factors and programmatic changes that providers and policy makers as well as parents can work toward. It also suggests ways to accelerate parental acculturation to the health services system that will now be a part of their lives. Connections between parent and provider; provider and provider; and parents, providers, and the community also

---

[1] This chapter focuses on parents of children with disabilities and health conditions that, while sometimes profound, are nonetheless not life threatening in the near term. Death and dying entails additional layers of complication that this chapter and the model proposed (as well as this book as a whole) do not attempt to accommodate.

[2] This chapter grew out of a paper presented on April 13, 2003, at the Society for Psychological Anthropology Biennial Meeting. As part of its expansion, it draws on the final report from the final phase of a Down syndrome project prepared by project manager Kimberly Dennis. This project, for which Sobo was Principal Investigator, was funded by a grant from Sol and Ruth Gerber and administered by the Children's Hospital Foundation. Thanks are due to the Gerbers; to the DS Association of San Diego for assistance with study recruitment; to all project staff (Kimberly Dennis, Erica Prussing, and Elizabeth Walker); and to the parents who shared their experiences with us.

---

are discussed as the chapter explores how all aspects of care can be most effectively, efficiently, and consistently coordinated to optimize the health and developmental potential of the children involved, while easing the parental case management, knowledge management, and stigma management burdens.

The model holds great promise in relation to the goal of improving care for CSHCN through the role it may play in helping clinicians understand the parents' perspective. It provides parents with a general map of the territory and identifies particular aspects of the CSHCN journey that, when promptly and thoughtfully addressed, may lead to an acceleration or shortening of the learning curve that all who provide or manage care for CSHCN must matriculate through. It is organized around the parental point of view, which differs in sometimes subtle but always significant ways from the provider experience of caring for CSHCN. Moreover, although the *details* of the parental experience will vary with the child's condition and with a parent's age, gender, occupation, class, ethnicity, immigration status, and financial situation, for example, the *patterns* identified should be the same across categories. Knowledge of the patterns will provide a framework or scaffold for customizing care on a case-by-case basis. Such customization is seen as one of the cornerstones of high-quality health care service delivery (Institute of Medicine Committee on Quality of Health Care in America, 2001).

BACKGROUND

Although most people have at times faced barriers to care, some face more barriers than others. Children with special health care needs are particularly vulnerable, as they generally require ongoing interactions with the health care system, and with each interaction there is a chance of underperformance and a suboptimal outcome. Care often must be coordinated across several specialties, and with each layer of participation chances for dissatisfaction or problems with quality arise. Sometimes, chain reactions ensue, leading to otherwise preventable disasters. Parents and practitioners can learn to work together and communicate effectively, or they can learn dysfunctional interaction patterns that, conditioned as the patterns are by the sociocultural and policy contexts in which they emerge, may turn a child's care trajectory from one of healing to one of harm.

Each person is unique, and CSHCN are all the more so because their exceptionalities are expressed in a wide variety of configurations. Certainly, every family faces unique challenges and rewards in this respect. However, universal features in the experience of parenting and procuring care for CSHCN also seem to exist, and some generalizable lessons can be learned that can make these features more satisfying for parents of future generations of children and for providers.

Model-Building Methods

The noncategorical model proposed in this chapter draws not only on the information presented in the preceding chapters but also on a long-term, collaborative, interdisciplinary program of research carried out through Children's Hospital San Diego (Children's), in California. That research examined not only different organizational aspects of Children's and the professional groups within it but also the experiences of patients and families being served by Children's. It included work with parents of CSHCN, beginning with a federally funded study regarding barriers to care as they are experienced by the English- or Spanish-speaking parents of school-aged CSHCN (Seid, Sobo, Reyes, & Varni, 2004; Sobo, Seid, & Gelhard, 2006.[3] It also included pilot work undertaken in a weekly clubfoot clinic and a larger-scale interview study involving English-speaking parents of 30 children with Down syndrome (DS).[4]

Down syndrome is an exemplary special health care condition because it includes both physical and mental dimensions, demanding both developmental and medical attention. Further, it often entails numerous subsidiary diagnoses, such as heart, hearing, respiratory, and joint conditions (American Academy of Pediatrics, 2001), and it has no biomedical cure. Clubfoot is a generally discrete and usually treatable condition existing on the less intense end of the CSHCN spectrum.

Theory-building efforts related to the apparent overlap between the clubfoot and DS findings, and the ways in which they built on the barriers to care work, were supplemented with a longitudinal series of interviews in which the DS project team got to know four more families of children with the syndrome—in this case, new babies (Dennis,

---

[3] This project, "Barriers to Care for Chronically Ill Vulnerable Children," was funded by the Agency for Healthcare Research and Quality (R03 HS 013058). The principal investigator was Michael Seid. In addition to Seid and Sobo, Leticia Reyes Gelhard and Gabriela Hussong worked on the project.

[4] This project focused at first on the use of complementary and alternative medicine for children with Down syndrome (Walker, Sobo, & Kurtin, 2002). The project subsequently evolved to be more concerned with coping, specifically in terms of dealing with an initial diagnosis, coordination of care, and stigma management (Prussing, Sobo, Walker, Dennis, & Kurtin, 2004; Prussing, Sobo, Walker, & Kurtin, 2005). The sample was about two-thirds White and heavily female (see also Prussing et al., 2004, 2005).

2004).[5] However, in contrast to and building on findings from the original research, this was more directly focused on the emergent question of how one learns to navigate the so-called system of health care when graced with a high-needs child.

Previous Studies

Although much literature exists on disability, most work focuses on the social and cultural reception or the adjustment of the person with a disability him- or herself. The experiences of parents of children with disabilities have received little attention except in terms of parental coping and adjustment—for example, in relation to parents' own physical and mental health status or divorce rates. Perhaps parents' role as managers of care for children with disabilities generally has not been addressed because of a belief that the parental role in health care is passive. This could be related to faith in the health care system's ability to function or in the existence of good communication across the continuum of care, which research has shown does not always exist (see Institute of Medicine, Committee on Quality of Health Care in America, 2001). Similarly, for reasons having to do with the acute care focus of the health care system, which has until now left chronic care in a blind spot, and with misplaced faith in the systematized nature of the system, little attention has been given to where in the health care system to locate the medical home for CSHCN, and who from the medical side is best suited to case manage on their behalf (see Chapter 6). Nonspecialist providers, and even many specialists, are ill-prepared for the organizational aspects of chronic care that confront them at all levels. This includes one-on-one dealings with patients and parents as well as communicating across the continuum of care.

One way to shed light on how people gain competence in regard to CSHCN, whether in a parental or provider role, is to look at how people gain competence in clinical professions to begin with. Anthropologists have focused on the process of acculturation that accompanies professional training in medicine (Good & Good, 1993; Sinclair, 2000) or surgery (Cassell, 1991). Within nursing, Patricia Benner (2001) identified five levels of competency through which nurses progress. After the Dreyfus model of skill acquisition (Dreyfus & Dreyfus, 1986), Benner termed this a transition from *novice* to *expert*. Expertise emerges from practice and experience, not books. The chapters concerning provider experiences in Section III of this book confirm that this is how to ap-

---

[5] We conducted a series of five in-depth interviews with mothers from each of these families over the course of 6 months (October 2003 to April 2004). The resulting 20 interviews, like the 30 one-time interviews of parents of children living with DS, were audiotaped with the participants' permission. The interviews lasted, on average, $1\frac{1}{2}$ hours.

proach care for CSHCN. It is quite possible that parents, too, move through competency levels from novice to expert as they master the skills entailed in navigating or managing the health care system and ministering to their child's particular needs.

Another area from which to draw insight is the medical sociology and anthropology literature concerning how identities and futures must be revised in light of certain diagnoses (e.g., multiple sclerosis, HIV/AIDS). The manner in which chronic illness or disability interacts with identity in adults has received a great deal of scholarly attention (e.g., Bury, 1982, 1991; Corbin & Strauss, 1988; Goffman, 1963; Green & Sobo, 2000; Herzlich & Pierret, 1987; Murphy, 2001). The familial aspects of these practices and the related cultural marginalization of parents of CHSCN are now beginning to receive scrutiny (Gray, 2001; Landsman, 1998, 1999, 2003, 2004; Larson, 1998; Rapp, 1999; Skinner, Bailey, Correa, & Rodriguez, 1999; see also Chapter 4). All indications are that the essential qualities of identity-related experiences for CSHCN parents, such as the processes entailed in reframing one's sense of identity after a diagnosis, are not dramatically different from those for chronically ill adults, although they may be quite different in other ways. The relevance of parental identity adjustments for family well-being and for clinical care has been noted (see Chapters 4 and 9) and is accounted for in the model. All parents of and providers for CSHCN should be aware of this aspect of adjustment.

THE PRESENT MODEL

How can we combine insights from the literature with what we have learned in the preceding chapters regarding provider perspectives and the parent experience to devise a noncategorical model for mastering health care for CSHCN in the United States? We need a model that not only applies to care for children with any type of long-term special health care need, but one that also speaks to the needs of both parents and providers. The challenge posed here is to create a model that fosters communication between parents and providers by offering each an entrée into the other's worldview. Although it is true that a great deal of power and authority is ascribed to clinicians, parents are the ultimate decision makers for their children, so their viewpoint and their experiences must serve as the major organizing principle of the model.

When the project team analyzed the transcripts from the one-time interviews, a host of complex issues was revealed (Prussing, Sobo, Walker, Dennis, & Kurtin, 2004; Prussing, Sobo, Walker, & Kurtin, 2005). The longitudinal interviews helped to crystallize these and other issues into three categories of overriding concern: initial diagnosis or classification, care coordination, and stigma management. The model described here draws heavily on the final report that Kimberly Dennis generated to describe that work (Dennis, 2004). The content of the clubfoot clinic participant observations could be organized quite easily using these overarching categories. Further, much of the data from the barriers to care research fit squarely within the care coordination category of the longitudinal interviews. These added to the developing model's face validity (a common research term for something's common sense appearance or validity when taken at face value). Face validity also is supported by the fact that the model subsumes some of the issues discussed in Chapter 9.

After presenting a schematic representation of the trio of overarching categories that make up the model, this chapter discusses the categories in depth, describing the themes and the parental experiences that they encompass. The chapter concludes with recommendations for ways in which health care providers and local organizations can help new parents understand and learn to navigate the landscapes into which they are thrust upon the birth of their exceptional child. New parents also can use these recommendations to educate themselves on what to look out for and to demand to optimize the services that their child receives and the ways in which their family as a whole is cared for.

The model in Figure 10.1 is organized on a timeline because the disability first must be identified and classified or, in biomedical parlance, *diagnosed* for a care trajectory to commence in full. However, and most important, the model is dynamic. Classification is not an instant process. Diagnosis itself can take time, and the experience of being diagnosed or labeled informs the direction the care trajectory takes. Further, although chronically ill children or children with disabilities are perhaps most vulnerable to suboptimal care during the critical period of discovery that occurs before they are 5 years old—the time when most of their problems are first recognized—for some conditions, a number of subsequent, subsidiary diagnoses phases are entailed. So the timeline is not necessarily unilateral; the events it describes can be spiraling, with some experiences occurring more than once, or simultaneously. Finally, interactions in one sphere affect interactions in other spheres, and experiences build up interactively over time.

Initial Classification

Without being asked, many of the parents in the initial DS sample focused their comments on how communication surrounding their child's DS classification affected their adjustment to the condition and their attitude toward the health system. Thus, parents demonstrated

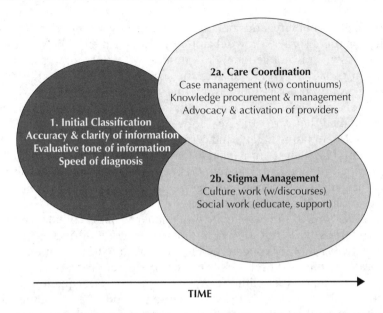

TIME

Figure 10.1. Noncategorical model of parental coping: Managing health care for the child with a chronic illness or disability. (*Note:* The model depicted is dynamic. For some conditions, a number of subsequent, subsidiary diagnosis phases are entailed. Also, interactions in one sphere affect interactions in the other spheres, and experiences accrete interactively over time. In 2a, the two continuums of care that must be coordinated are the developmental and physical care continuums.)

that this stage was important to them (see Chapter 9 for discussion from the clinician perspective).

Diagnosis can not only be disruptive of dreams parents might have for their child, but it also can be devastating if it is mishandled. Many parents have told of being presented a diagnosis—with all the disease-related connotations that the term *diagnosis* carries—in catastrophic terms. One parent said, "All they tell you is the bad stuff. They don't tell you any of the good stuff. . . . They don't tell you, 'Don't worry, your child will melt your heart and smile at you just like how all your other children did.' "

Often, parents described a sense of stigmatization, particularly regarding mental retardation, which many preferred to recast as *developmental delay* because of this term's implicit promise of progression. Upon diagnosis, several parents were provided with information about adoption options, which they found inappropriate.

The experiences of parents of children with clubfoot were different, demonstrating how important it is for noncategorical modeling to draw on a range of conditions. Although some of these parents were mortified by the sight of their child's foot or feet and the associated threat to the child's mobility, and some were troubled by attributions of causality for the disorder, they did not worry about their child's mental capacity, which is not generally in question with clubfoot. Also, clubfoot can usually be corrected over the span of 2 to 3 years, although many parents do not initially know this.

In cases of both DS and clubfoot, it is not until an official diagnosis is proclaimed that care can move forward. With clubfoot, it is ideal to start treatment immediately, and certain conditions associated with DS also should be seen to immediately. However, for the parents of children with clubfoot, as for many parents in the DS group who had to wait for genetic test results, getting a formal diagnosis could entail a chain of referrals and a good measure of waiting.

Just as for DS, and despite the visual salience of the clubfoot condition, referrals were not always automatic or system-driven. Parents who noticed cause for concern had to learn from that point on how to advocate for their children. As well, from the parent perspective, each time a new practice or clinician was brought into the equation, they were forced once again to explain themselves and to allow someone new to physically scrutinize and (at best) annoy their baby. In the case of clubfoot, the condition is visually obvious and the need to submit to yet another examination seemed senseless to some parents. For some DS parents, until genetic tests came back, there was still the possibility that nothing was wrong, and the extended uncertainty was distressing.

According to some parents, the speed and tenor of initial classification was crucial, because it was here that the foundations were laid for their enduring relationship with the health care system and for their adjustment to the addition of the exceptional child to their family circle (see Chapter 4). It was during the initial classification stage that various cultural frames or ideals were first activated regarding issues such as mental competence, physical prowess, blame for anomalous births, and role of the health care consumer (see also Prussing et al., 2004, 2005).

Care Coordination

Once a child had been diagnosed, care coordination began in earnest. The struggles of the parents from all groups were similar, but the struggles of the parents of children with DS were more intense and more extensive due to the larger number of services they had to coordinate for their children. Problems with referrals persisted. For example, "She's been referred to OT [occupational therapy] at two months old and she's almost six months old and I still have not heard anything from OT," said one mother. Parents' need to case manage was complicated by the need to manage knowledge for providers and for themselves.

The need for parents to act as care coordinators has partly to do with the fragmentation of the system, which is made more apparent by the variety of specialist care that needs to be organized and articulated. The more complex a child's condition, the harder the care coordination will be; but in any case, parents often are shocked at how much of this work is left up to them. For example, one mother of a child with DS explained how she could not exist simply as "just a mother" because she had to become what she called a "caseworker," devoting extensive time and energy to enforcing her entitlement to services and coordinating those that best served her daughter's needs.

Another reason that parents have to adopt the coordinator role has to do with the differential epidemiology of childhood disease and disability, in which only a few children generally suffer from any given condition (e.g., one in about 850 children have either clubfoot or DS; March of Dimes 2001a, 2001b) in comparison with adult epidemiology in which many suffer from just a few conditions (e.g., one in three adults has heart disease; American Heart Association, 2006.) This diffuseness makes it difficult for any one physician to have full knowledge of all possible conditions, and it is therefore imperative for parents both to case manage their child, assuring her or him access to all appropriate services, and to pass information or knowledge on to the providers. Thus, knowledge management entails not only amassing and digesting information on services, scientific advances, guidelines for care, and other options, but also passing this information on to providers and encouraging them to use the information as appropriate and to look for additional information on their own; that is, the parents need to *activate* the providers.

Parents of a DS child recognized the time and resource constraints that providers faced and tailored their expectations accordingly. They did, however, expect providers to show an interest in their child, ask questions, and take the initiative in learning a little more about DS. In talking about her child's first (and former) pediatrician, one parent remarked, with no admiration, "His office didn't even know that she's supposed to be on a different growth chart." An opposite problem was the tendency of some providers to ascribe all of the children's ills (e.g., rashes) to DS rather than to acknowledge that (or even explore whether) they were simply the typical ills of childhood.

In the case of clubfoot, this did not seem to be an issue, largely perhaps due to the nature of the condition. However, some parents did wish that the providers of care for children with clubfoot could advise them on other infant care issues such as a rash the child had or umbilical cleaning. They expressed frustration at having to make a separate appointment for that type of care, although in fact specialists may not actually know about basic health issues.

One other issue that was more salient for the DS parents was a perceived lack of awareness on the part of providers of the need for family-centered care. As one parent explained, "It would be nice to have them say, 'How are you guys doing?' and it wouldn't take that long to ask that. And if you say, 'I've been struggling,' they could reply, 'Well, there's some family counselors that are great and maybe you could go check that out.' Maybe something like that would make it a lot smoother and easier." Some parents suggested that a social worker or nurse be available either before or after the consultation with the physician to talk about emotional or social support issues. More than anything, it seemed that the parents—perhaps especially the new ones—just wanted providers to be aware that they might be having difficulties or experiencing a range of emotions.

For some parents, some of these difficulties came from having to coordinate both care and information. As one parent said, "My misconception . . . was that I wouldn't be the expert. That somebody else would know more than I did." Parents indicated that if they could find a primary care pediatrician who specialized in or had a passion for DS, they would switch with little hesitation. But they were at a loss regarding how to go about finding such a doctor. Another parent commented, "First and foremost, the best resource for a parent is to have a list of doctors that specialize in DS, because even when you go on the web trying to find a physician, it doesn't say, 'I specialize in DS or I know a lot about DS.' "

Partly because of this knowledge gap, and sometimes also because their primary care physician was also the physician for their other children, parents stayed with providers who did not know much about DS. Consequently, as one parent said, "I have to walk our general practitioner through things. You know I come with this information. . . . Please do this, please do the work for me, please have this test run. And . . . that's very awkward. And they don't like to be challenged that way." Here, ideals for active health care consumerism clashed with practitioner ideals regarding patient power.

The pressure to stay on top of everything is made worse by the fact that parents feel that they do not know all the right questions to ask to get the information they need. As one parent of a DS child put it:

"You just want to make sure you're doing everything you can do, because it's like walking into a foreign country and not knowing the language. You only know what people tell you or if you pick up the right book. . . . It's like the shuttle landing on Mars and they land here [in one little spot] and they're going to tell you what Mars is like, but really there's this big thing of water right over here, but if you never get to it, [you wouldn't know]. It's very similar to that."

Although empowered parents accept their care-coordination role, they do so with some trepidation, concerned that if they overlook or are not aware of a needed test or assessment their child will suffer. "I feel like the impetus for tests—Should we do this now?—comes from me," said one parent early in the interviews. "I'm not a doctor. I feel that I may miss something and it won't get done." Several months later, in her last interview, the parent reiterated that feeling with even more conviction: "One of the most important things is that I can't really abdicate responsibility to still be the overseer of her health care. . . . I still need to be relatively organized and think ahead and make sure that all the tests are getting done."

DS parents also cited the need for better, more coordinated communication among doctors, residents, fellows, and interns, and noted their frustration at having to answer the same set of questions over and over. "I understand they're a teaching hospital, but she's a frequent flyer," explained one of the mothers. "With every student or resident, I'm telling them the same story all the time. . . . Look it up or bring them all in at the same time, so I don't have to keep repeating myself." The clubfoot clinic was host to many trainees, and parents had similar experiences.

More important perhaps was the frustration over conflicting information given by the various clinicians. A DS parent provided an example, saying, "I have one resident telling me it's a small hole [in her heart], another resident telling me it's a medium-sized hole, another one telling me it's a large hole, the other one telling me, 'Don't worry about it, she'll be fine, she'll outgrow it.' "

Like the parent who mentioned Mars, many parents noted the need for some kind of map or guide to the territory. One parent said that it would have been useful in the early days to have "a 1-2-3 step thing" to guide her at different time points. She recalled, "I was at four or five months and, like, 'What do I do now?' " Another explained that you lose "the first year of their lives trying to figure out how the system works to get them the help they need. . . . If I had to ask for anything, that's what I'd want—someone to give me [an] owner's manual on how the system works." I'm learning the game now. . . . I finally figured out the rules after a year and now I'm, 'Okay, I can play this game.' "

Parents often provided one another with guidance. In addition to general information about the health system, specific strategies for getting the most out of the system were shared. One parent recalled an important strategic lesson she learned from talking to other parents: "I would have never known that if you put DS as a diagnosis for OT/PT, it's not going to get covered. I would have never known that. But knowing ahead of time that I need to put in *low tone* or *prematurity*, things like that that will actually get covered, I already have a heads up."

Stigma Management

In addition to the instrumental work of care coordination, there is extensive expressive (e.g., symbolic, emotional) work required in parenting a child with a disability. In the model, this is identified as *stigma management*, and it entails both culture work and social work. *Culture work* uses existing cultural frames or ideals to shed a positive light on a child's condition; *social work* shores up social relations, which can, especially with conditions like DS, be tremendously stressful. It also builds new social networks and finds new individuals to fill support and friendship roles.

Commenting on how much better she felt after talking to another parent of a child with DS a few weeks after coming home from the hospital with her own DS baby, one interviewee said, "She just talked about her own experiences . . . what life was like, and for her [child's] siblings, and the resources that are out there . . . her experiences with elementary school, starting kindergarten, and reality. . . . She made it seem not so bad."

The DS parents generally tried to reframe DS in positive terms, and they learned from one another some ways to do it. For example, we heard parents compare their experience to that of someone who'd planned a trip to Italy and ended up in Holland: different from what was expected, but joyous nonetheless. This motif is stock in most DS support media.

Original refigurations are not easy to create. Parents are in a complicated psycho-cultural bind in which love of and hope for their children compete with negative cultural views of the children's conditions—views shaped by U.S. ideals regarding physical and mental perfection, individual accomplishment, social adulthood, and so forth (see Table 10.1). These negative views (internalized to a greater or lesser extent by different parents) both fuel biomedicine's curative stance and compete with more positive disability rights movements and generic

Table 10.1. Competing cultural frames or ideals

On the one hand. . .	On the other. . .
Adherence, doctor knows best	Active health care consumer
Independence for social adulthood	Interdependence
Single ideal for physical and mental perfection	Diversity, individuality
Cure	Care, nonintervention

Judeo–Christian views about the value of every individual. The same challenging bind exists with clubfoot and, it would seem, with all conditions that disable, at least as they are experienced in the present U.S. context.

One strategy parents of children with DS used to deal with this issue involved framing their experiences as transformational opportunities to become better people through devoted parenting. They also deployed religious imagery, for example, by calling a child with DS "a gift from God." Disability rights rhetoric promoting the value of physical diversity also is used in this way. The label *exceptional child* has roots here.

Parents of children with clubfoot took a different tack. Clubfoot is relatively correctable, and because of this, it fits well with the curative stance of biomedicine, which was the discourse (set of ideas and related mode of speaking) often activated. Further, parents learned to engage this discourse in a way that tapped into all-American athletic imagery. For instance, on entering the clinic, new parents were told about famous athletes born with clubfoot. And when one baby broke his cast before it was fully dry by flexing too much after leaving the clinic, staff congratulated him for this and celebrated his physical vigor.

Clinic cultures are not monolithic, and this can be to the benefit of parents seeking to represent their children in a positive light. For instance, on viewing the Dennis-Browne splint that her baby would wear for several years after casting, one mother at the clubfoot clinic said that it looked to her like a snowboard. From then on, that was what the clinic staff called it too: Children did not get splints, they got *snowboards*. Activating the image of a healthy, athletic, snowboarding child diminished the splint's negative connotations of disability, ill health, and inactivity (see Figure 10.2).

The benefit of this type of imaging is not just protection against stigma. It also protects against the fatigue that the social work of educating others about disability can entail. To get around this, parents of children with clubfoot generally did not label their children as having clubfoot as such. They learned to say things such as "Little Johnny's

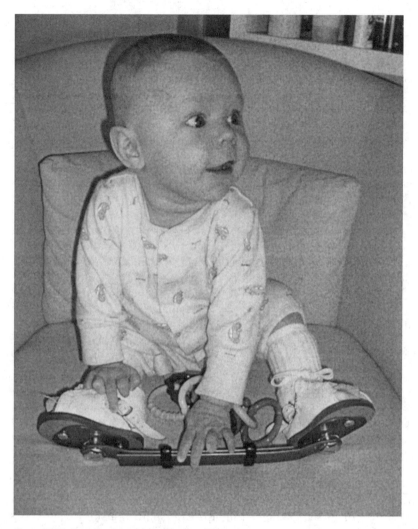

Figure 10.2. Example of a clubfoot "snowboard."

feet need a bit of straightening." In this declarative way, questions were deflected and activation of Dickensian imagery was bypassed.

In general, parents whose children had DS had a more difficult time with stigma. They offered many examples of having to cope with ignorant, panicked reactions to their children. These sometimes entailed rifts within the family due to attributions of blame, which took a huge amount of social work to handle. The parents made it clear that they had enough to cope with without having to help everyone else cope too.

APPLYING THE MODEL

By juxtaposing the experiences of two groups of parents of exceptional children, we have identified some commonalities and can begin to build a noncategorical model of parental coping—a model that can be understood and applied by health care workers (see Figure 10.1). Informed not only by focused interview and participant observation research but also by the information presented in the preceding chapters and, more broadly, by long-term, broader-based participant observation in a regional children's hospital's health outcomes unit, the model can serve to provide a map of the territory with which those involved in the care of CSHCN will contend. As such, the map will help its readers to orient themselves to the territory relatively rapidly and to enjoy earlier navigational success than those who must forge their own way in the dark.

A shortcoming of health service model building is that the imposition of a simplified heuristic leaves little room for the fine-grained details of real life. Even so, the mere existence of a model as such can help to guide action, underwrite research, and steer health care professionals toward at least some of the psychocultural complexities of parenting children with special health care needs. This is necessary because professionals otherwise may not realize the potentially harmful—or helpful—impact their individual responses may have on these exceptional children. They often labor in systems structured to fragment and bureaucratize care rather than to offer coordinated healing services to whole patients and families. Further, they may forget that for families of newborn or young children, the experience of seeking chronic health care or support for disabling conditions is new and confusing. They forget that they, too, once had to learn how to navigate the health care system.

Learning Curves and Leverage Points

The model points our attention toward three overriding activities that parents must endure or engage in: getting a diagnosis (initial classification), care coordination, and stigma management. It helps us focus within these areas on potentially modifiable factors and key variables with regard to the parent (and therefore the child's) experience. This enables us to make recommendations regarding ways to improve the quality of care that children with special health care needs receive.

Recommendations for demand-driven changes can be summed up as

1. Appreciate the child, acknowledge his or her condition, refer the case as needed, and otherwise provide fast diagnostic confirmation.

2. Inform and empower the parent and others involved in the child's care (i.e., communicate across the care continuum).

3. Participate as fully as possible in the child's care, including advocating for him or her when appropriate.

All of this should be done in the context of providing nonjudgmental, family-centered, case-managed care (see Table 10.2).

Policy's Role and System Articulations

Recommendations for enhanced care during the initial classification (diagnosis) phase can generally be met by single providers. Enhancing care once the child is engaged with the system (however tenuously) is harder because it depends less on individuals and more on policy and program arrangements for systems of care, such as existing arrangements for medical homes and formal case management as well as the developmental and physical health provision systems themselves. The articulation of these last two systems is essential, as the developmental needs of children (e.g., occupational therapy) must be considered an integral part of a child's overall health and well-being. Recommendations for providers are discussed in the following sections; in theory, federal policies would support all of them, but locally specific policy, program, and budget changes (as well as incentive alignment, where appropriate) must be made accordingly.

Discussion of the recommendations proceeds along the temporal or phase-based axis shown in Figure 10.1, beginning with activities that should be engaged in during the initial classification phase. The second half of the discussion concerns support for parents engaged in activities outlined in the care coordination and stigma management phases.

Appreciate, Acknowledge, and Refer

In general, parents' love for their child deserves to be appreciated before the child's exceptional health conditions are acknowledged and explored. Even when an infant's condition is terminal, incurable, or profoundly debilitating, every effort should be made to first express appreciation of and respect for the life at hand, and only after that should reference be made to the condition that is suspected or diagnosed. To immediately devalue a child or express low expectations for her or him sends a strong negative message to parents that can exacerbate initial parental hesitations regarding the child, or create a distance between parent and provider and foster distrust of the health care system as a whole.

When a child is born with or presented in the clinic with an impairment, the clinician who identifies it should deliver this information nonjudgmentally and with compassion. This can be difficult, especially

Table 10.2. Recommendations for providers

1. Appreciate, acknowledge, and serve or refer

- Welcome every child as a person before addressing possible health problems
- Make initial diagnosis and begin care without delay
- Keep and use a referral list for diagnosis of special conditions
- Make all necessary referrals for the parents
  - ○ Assist parents in understanding and determining who can help them understand their health plan options
  - ○ Decide how case management will be handled
  - ○ Continue to communicate across the continuum as needed
- Present initial information slowly and incrementally
  - ○ Ensure that information to be provided is accurate and up-to-date
  - ○ Provide adoption information only after appropriateness has been determined
  - ○ Provide timelines for care
  - ○ Provide information on older children and adults with the condition
- Keep and use a resource and referral list to help address families' emotional needs
- Conduct a series of follow-up calls with new parents

2a. Inform, empower, and communicate

- Self-educate
  - ○ Stay up-to-date on health care guidelines for CSHCN
  - ○ Research the literature regarding the types of CSHCN served
- Provide each parent with a notebook and calendar at the start
- Distribute and discuss appropriate health care guidelines with parents
- Keep and use a directory of providers with experience caring for CSHCN
- Keep and use a directory of organizations and agencies supporting families with CSHCN
- Keep and use a parent *buddy list* for linking new parents to experienced ones
- Encourage dialogue between parents and providers
  - ○ Encourage questions
  - ○ Encourage families to share knowledge and information
- Engage in and support provider–provider communication across the continuum of care for each CSHCN
  - ○ Know who is case managing for the child and where the child's medical home is and ensure that the parents have the same information
  - ○ Stay informed about health insurance coverage policies for CSHCN
- Encourage families to acknowledge the emotional and social aspects of having a CSHCN and refer to resources and referrals list as needed

2b. Participate and advocate

- Ask more questions of parents
- Realize (and remind parents as needed) that some conditions or behavioral situations are simply part of a normal childhood
- Model destigmatization by practicing nonjudgmental care
- Push for policy and program changes in support of provision of high-quality care
- Continue to model nonjudgmental acceptance of/for CSHCN and their families
- Use the power of one's privileged provider position to advocate for policies and programs that support high-quality care

for nonspecialist providers. Chronic or disabling conditions are not valued by the mainstream biomedical model, with its emphasis on cure, and certain disabilities or diseases are stigmatized by the sociocultural milieu of which providers are inevitably a part. Further, the average clinical curriculum does not include much teaching on communication of any kind, let alone the communication of what may be bad news (Vandekieft, 2001).

However, mentorship and role play can help providers master non-evaluative techniques for sharing diagnostic suspicions or news (Rabow & McPhee, 1999; Vandekieft, 2001). Also helpful are organizational and professional cultures that favor making case management roles and medical home assignments explicit, and that do not devalue noncurative care or socially disable nonnormative bodies (see Chapter 9) through sociocultural processes that make life harder for the children (e.g., the lack of universal design principles such as ramps or lever door handles in buildings, the idealization of independent living). Further, clear policies for the provision of adoption information can help alleviate inappropriate actions in regard to this option.

If tests must be run or further evaluation is required, response times should be as fast as possible. Days can seem like weeks to distressed parents, and the tests being done are far from routine as far as they are concerned. In addition, parents forced to secure their own referrals can easily become lost in the morass of the health care system. Its usual inefficiencies are exacerbated for parents who, in the case of newborns, are not only under the typical stress of new parenthood but also under the atypical stress of perhaps losing or not being allowed the child they had imagined would be added to their family. Efforts should be made to secure referrals on their behalf. Further, the need for follow-up once parents leave the hospital must be met, for example, with a series of follow-up calls. Policies should be developed and resources set aside for this and for the documented assignment of a case manager or medical home for the patient and family.

Service to the family at this point also involves the initial provision of information regarding the condition diagnosed. Information should be up-to-date and accurate and it should be concise. The parents do not yet have a firm foundational understanding of the condition or its ramifications and of the services they will need, so large amounts of what is sometimes contradictory and often complex information will not be helpful. Issues pertinent to the very initial stages of care should be highlighted. Also, parents should be provided some information on older children and adults with the condition, in preparation for taking a longer-term perspective.

To help reduce the feeling of being overwhelmed and confused, newly initiated parents might receive, as soon as possible, a notebook and calendar to help organize all the information and to keep track of all the doctors and other individuals they talk with about their child. Clear plastic binder inserts made for filing business cards can be very useful, providing parents with an easy way to store and reference contact information for every provider with whom they interact.

Inform and Empower

After the initial diagnosis has been confirmed, a new phase of information processing and management begins. Parents enter the second phase of activities shown in Figure 10.1, including care coordination, which entails both case management and knowledge procurement and management on the parents' part, complementing (at least ideally, although in reality sometimes substituting for) formal case and knowledge management systems. Like anyone past the initial, highly disorienting phase of acculturating to a new world, parents at this stage can take in more—and more complicated—information than they could at the start. Still, information needs will differ from parent to parent; providers should specifically ask parents about their perceived informational needs, as providers are generally quite inaccurate when guessing (Sobo, 2004).

The incremental approach to information provision implied above, in which parents are made aware of which concerns, issues, and tests they need to focus on immediately and which they might think about later, should still be the rule. However, for the incremental approach to work best, a chronic care model must be in place; the acute care model built around a one-time interaction will not support sequential information provision. One strategy is to provide resource or issue lists with items arranged in chronological order. On the same lists, providers may indicate which tests or procedures primary care pediatricians could do and which require referral to a specialist. Along these lines, directories of providers who specialize in various conditions can be assembled and made available to parents, empowering them to seek out those who are most experienced with their child's particular problems.

In addition to being offered on an incremental basis or in a chronologically ordered list, with the option for more if desired, the information provided should be accurate. It also should be up-to-date and nonjudgmental. Provider time must be set aside to update information sets periodically and to ensure the accuracy of all new information packages considered for dissemination.

Further, resource lists that are made available should include annotations aimed at giving parents a better understanding of how each organization can help their child; simply listing organization names and numbers is not enough. Also important is information on how the organizations interact and which (if any) can perform clearinghouse activities. If a central clearinghouse organization does not exist, providers might instigate the formation of a coalition, or nominate one specific resource organization for this activity.

Besides providing information, practitioners should take into account the knowledge that parents bring to the table and respect the fact that each parent knows his or her child best. At the same time, practitioners must empower parents to ask questions. Creating an atmosphere of openness during clinic visits is essential to fostering in parents the sense that their involvement is welcomed. Ways to do this include asking open-ended questions and refraining from interrupting parent statements, especially at a visit's start. Assisting parents in developing their skills as advocates for their children has a secondary benefit in that they also can help activate other providers involved in their child's care, thereby making the job of the primary provider that much easier.

More help should be provided at this time regarding what is increasingly referred to as health information literacy—that is, the ability to know when information is needed, how to locate it, how to evaluate its credibility, and how to effectively use (credible) information to solve or inform one's understanding of the problem at hand. Parents could be referred to existing resources, or tailored information could be provided. Some existing resources include *How to Evaluate Health Information on the Internet,* provided by the National Cancer Institute of the U.S. National Institutes of Health at http://cis.nci.nih.gov/fact/2_10.htm, and *Untangling the Web,* provided by the University of Washington Retirement Association at http://healthlinks.washington.edu/hsl/liaisons/schnall/UntanglingTheWeb.pdf. The Sheridan Library at Johns Hopkins University offers *Evaluating Information Found on the Internet* at http://www.library.jhu.edu/researchhelp/general/evaluating. Parents also can be referred to The Healthfinder web site (www.healthfinder. gov), the U.S. government's own gateway for reliable information. Parent membership in peer-to-peer education, support, and advocacy organizations should be promoted (see Chapter 5).

Parents also can learn from other parents. Sharing information is much more efficient than having each family reinvent the wheel. Parents can provide one another with guidance on navigating the new territory of health care for CSHCN as well as essential emotional support for parents of the newly diagnosed. A buddy system could be developed, so that in addition to referral to parent organizations such as Family Voices (http://www.familyvoices.org/), Mothers from Hell 2 (http://www.mothersfromhell2.org/), and condition-specific groups, parents of the newly diagnosed can meet personally with others in similar situations. Providers can maintain a list of parents who are willing to be contacted, along with the age(s) of their child(ren). Because numbers may be small in any one practice, networks for buddy referrals should be created. Also, because parents seem to enter the system at different vantage points and access information in different ways, such a resource might be produced and available from several different entities, including local condition-specific organizations, obstetric units, health insurance plans, pediatricians' offices, and regional centers. In California, 21 regional centers exist to assist persons with developmental disabilities and their families in locating and developing services and programs within their communities.

Throughout the process of informing and supporting parents, providers should bear in mind that the developmental needs of children are considered by parents to be an integral part of a child's overall health and well-being. Too often, developmental issues are treated in isolation, and parents therefore have to navigate two often fairly disconnected systems of care. Provider advocacy for linkage would be most welcomed here.

Participate and Advocate

Providers should not—and clearly many do not—leave all the work of care coordination to parents, although it seems to many parents as though they have. To offset this perception, providers can explicitly discuss their coordination work with parents so that parents know what goes on behind the scenes. Moreover, providers could do more behind the scenes than they have done, knowing how important that backstage work is to the harried families they serve.

Providers also can assist families by reminding them of their right to case management and their responsibility to remain aware of and in full contact with their child's medical home. Similar parental awareness-raising regarding their right and responsibility to know about their health insurance policies as well as how to lobby for reimbursement approvals is suggested.

In support of this, providers have their own self-educational and advocacy responsibilities. They must do more to educate themselves regarding their options in the care of the CSHCN. They must advocate for these families and children in the broader service community and even in policy settings. When policy is in line with what a provider wants to do, doing it is that much easier.

According to the Chronic Care Model (Wagner 1998; Wagner, Austin, Davis, Hindmarsh, Schaefer, & Bonomi, 2001), the best quality care is offered by a "prepared, proactive practice team." Providers can do more to ensure that they are a part of such a team (see Chapter 6). Indeed, that is crucial, for it is not all right for providers to demand that parents be advocates for and active participants in their children's care if providers are not willing to respond in kind. Further, this is as ineffective as it is unfair. Placing the entire burden on the shoulders of parents virtually ensures that crucial aspects of care will be left out. In fact, the program of research cited in the development of the model described in this chapter showed that most parents would like to alleviate this sense of having sole responsibility, and they are looking to their child's providers for relief. As influential as parents are in the lives of their children, they are not health care professionals, and they should not be forced to take responsibility as though they were providers to oversee their children's care.

Related to this is the finding that, although it is true that parents want providers to be forthcoming about their limitations, they also want these limitations mitigated. Providers should take the initiative to learn more—and do more—about the conditions of the children they serve, for example, through continuing medical education and involvement in community advocacy (see Table 10.2 for recommendations for providers).

Parents also suggested that providers ask more questions about how a child is doing both in general and with regard to specific health issues. This not only gives parents more confidence that providers know what to look for in a child of a particular age with a particular condition, but it also demonstrates explicit interest on the part of the provider. Although providers may conduct consultation work in their minds (i.e., thinking silently about what they see in a child), explicit interaction and discourse with the parents in which these thoughts are narrated helps parents know concretely that the visit was productive. Further, concrete knowledge that providers also are looking out for the children takes some of the perceived burden of care management off of the parents.

Besides child health matters, providers (at least those in a child's medical home; see Chapter 6) also should ask about overall family function. One of the reasons that providers may not do this is because they do not know what to do if people report problems. Pediatricians and other doctors should have a resource or referral list of support groups, counselors, and local organizations that a family can contact.

Beyond what has already been mentioned, participation in a child's care entails understanding the sociocultural barriers to care that a child and his or her parents encounter. These barriers have a major impact on family adjustment and also affect policy and program decisions because of the assumptions they may entail regarding preferred outcomes.

Parents have a great deal of cultural work to do; that is, they must make sense of their new situation using resources that their culture(s) offer them. Providers can help in several ways by participating in these processes. For example, they can help parents locate and latch onto the most productive disability related discourses (modes of thinking and speaking) that are available for those with similar cultural backgrounds. They can do this overtly by directing parents to various advocacy web sites, community groups, or literature in an act of empowerment. Celebrating each child as a person prior to performing medical services or consultations also is a way to subvert the power of stigma, explicitly participating in and communicating the attitude of acceptance and implicitly modeling the cultural practice of such.

Another part of this participatory destigmatizing stance includes having and projecting the knowledge that all children eventually experience certain problems (e.g., rashes, colds, fevers). A child's chronic or disabling condition should not be held responsible for all of his or her ills, and calling a condition a *typical childhood illness* can have a normalizing effect that parents will value.

Concurrent with the cultural work of resisting and revising stigma is the social work that parents must do. First, they must cope with the reactions of other members of their social circles regarding their child's condition; second, they must cope with society's culture-driven discriminatory response to their child and even to them, the parents. Much social work in the early phase entails educating others, mobilizing support, and maintaining distance from those who would undermine one's adjustment efforts. Providers should acknowledge the toll that this takes, and encourage parents in their efforts. Sometimes, in the style of family-based care, this will involve suggesting or agreeing to a meeting with a recalcitrant relative to explain the medical etiology of the condition and exculpate the parents from having *caused* it. Other times, providing the link to support groups or the names of potential buddy parents or families will be sufficient. But in all cases, continual self-education regarding the cultural and social battles parents face, as well as participation in relevant advocacy efforts, goes a long way toward achieving high-quality, satisfying care.

ACCELERATING LEARNING

The American Academy of Pediatrics, Committee on Children with Disabilities (1997) recognizes that "individuals with genetic and other chronic health conditions and their families confront a seemingly endless series of stressors in their daily lives. . . . These stresses may burden families emotionally, socially, and financially and may involve them with complex and often bureaucratic health, habilitation, education, and health insurance requirements'' (p. 643). The model proposed here can help to familiarize and sensitize care providers, parents, program developers, and policy makers to the health-seeking challenges of parenting a child with a chronic illness or disability. This may, in turn, support efforts to improve parent–health system interactions and increase the quality of health care trajectory for all children with special health care needs. At the least, it will accelerate the speed and increase the angle at which parents and providers traverse the CSHCN health care learning curve.

REFERENCES

American Academy of Pediatrics, Committee on Genetics. (2001). Health supervision for children with Down syndrome. *Pediatrics, 107*, 442–449.
American Academy of Pediatrics, Committee on Children with Disabilities. (1997). General principles in the care of children and adolescents with genetic disorders and other chronic health conditions. *Pediatrics, 99*, 643–644.
American Heart Association. (2006). *Heart disease and stroke statistics—2006 update.* Dallas, TX: Author.
Benner, P. (2001). *From novice to expert: Excellence and power in clinical nursing practice (commemorative edition).* Upper Saddle River, NJ: Prentice Hall.
Bury, M. (1982). Chronic illness as biographical disruption. *Sociology of Health and Illness 4*, 167–182.
Bury, M. (1991). The sociology of chronic illness: A review of research and prospects. *Sociology of Health and Illness, 13*, 451–468.
Cassell, J. (1991). *Expected miracles: Surgeons at work.* Philadelphia: Temple University Press.
Corbin, J.M., & Strauss, A. (1988). *Unending work and care: Managing chronic illness at home.* San Francisco: Jossey-Bass.
Dennis, K. (2004). *Helping families with children with Down syndrome navigate the health care system: Findings from an exploratory study.* San Diego: Center for Child Health Outcomes; Children's Hospital and Healthcare Center.
Dreyfus, H., & Dreyfus, S.E. (1986). *Mind over machine: The power of human intuition and expertise in the era of the computer.* New York: Free Press.
Goffman, E. (1963). *Stigma: Notes on the management of spoiled identity.* New York: Simon and Schuster.
Good, B., & Good, M.-J.D. (1993). Learning medicine: The constructing of medical knowledge at Harvard Medical School. In M. Lock (Ed.), *Knowledge, power, and practice* (pp. 81–107). Los Angeles: University of California Press.
Gray, D.E. (2001). Accommodation, resistance and transcendence: Three narratives of autism. *Social Science & Medicine, 53*, 1247–1257.
Green, G., & Sobo, E.J. (2000). *The endangered self: Managing the social risk of HIV.* London: Routledge.
Herzlich, C., & Pierret, J. (1987). *Illness and self in society.* Baltimore: The Johns Hopkins University Press.
Institute of Medicine, Committee on Quality of Health Care in America. (2001). *Crossing the quality chasm: A new health system for the 21st century.* Washington, DC: National Academies Press.

Landsman, G. (1998). Reconstructing motherhood in the age of "perfect" babies: Mothers of infants and toddlers with disabilities. *Signs: Journal of Women in Culture and Society,* 2469–2499.

Landsman, G. (1999). Does God give special kids to special parents?: Personhood and the child with disabilities as gift and as giver. In L. Layne (Ed.), *Transformative motherhood* (pp. 133–166). New York: NYU Press.

Landsman, G. (2003). Emplotting children's lives: Developmental delay vs. disability. *Social Science & Medicine, 56,* 1947–1960.

Landsman, G. (2004). "Too bad you got a lemon": Peter Singer, mothers of children with disabilities, and the critique of consumer culture. In J. Taylor, L. Layne, & D. Wozniak (Eds.), *Consuming motherhood* (pp. 100–121). New Brunswick: Rutgers University Press.

Larson, E. (1998). Reframing the meaning of disability to families: The embrace of paradox. *Social Science & Medicine, 47,* 865–875.

March of Dimes (2001a). *Quick references and fact sheets 09-269-00 1/01: Clubfoot and other foot deformities.* Retrieved January 4, 2006, at http://www.march ofdimes.com/pnhec/4439_1211.asp

March of Dimes (2001b). *Quick references and fact sheets 09-174-00 8/01 (R 12/ 04): Down syndrome.* Retrieved January 4, 2006, at http://www.marchof dimes.com/pnhec/4439_1214.asp

Murphy, R.F. (2001). *The body silent: The different world of the disabled* (Reissue ed.). New York: W.W. Norton & Company.

Prussing, E., Sobo, E.J., Walker, E., Dennis, K., & Kurtin, P.S. (2004). Communicating about complementary/alternative medicine: Perspectives from parents of children with Down syndrome. *Ambulatory Pediatrics, 4*(6), 488–494.

Prussing, E., Sobo, E.J., Walker, E., & Kurtin, P.S. (2005). Between "desperation" and disability rights: A narrative analysis of complementary/alternative medicine use by parents for children with Down syndrome. *Social Science & Medicine, 60*(3), 587–598.

Rabow, M.W., & McPhee, S.J. (1999). Beyond breaking bad news: How to help patients who suffer. *Western Journal of Medicine, 171*(4), 260–263.

Rapp, R. (1999). *Testing women, testing the fetus: The social impact of amniocentesis in America.* New York: Routledge.

Seid, M., Sobo, E.J., Reyes, L., & Varni, J. W. (2004). Barriers to care for children with special health care needs: Development and validation of the Barriers to Care Questionnaire. *Ambulatory Pediatrics, 4*(4), 323–331.

Sinclair, S. (2000). Disease narratives: Constituting doctors. *Anthropology & Medicine, 7*(1), 115–134.

Skinner, D., Bailey, D.B., Correa, V., & Rodriguez, P. (1999). Narrating self and disability: Latino mothers' constructions of identities vis-à-vis their child with special needs. *Exceptional Children, 65,* 481–495.

Sobo, E.J. (2004). Nurses' knowledge of parent or patient communication needs in a pediatric cancer unit: Room for improvement. *Journal of Nursing Care Quality, 19*(3), 253–262.

Sobo, E.J., Seid, M., & Gelhard, L.R. (2006). Parent-identified barriers to pediatric health care: A process-oriented model and method. *Health Services Research, 41*(1), 148–172.

Vandekieft, G.K. (2001). Breaking bad news. *American Family Physician, 64*(12), 1975–1978.

Wagner, E.H. (1998). Chronic disease management: What will it take to improve care for chronic illness? *Effective Clinical Practice, 1,* 2–4.

Wagner, E.H., Austin, B., Davis, C., Hindmarsh, M., Schaefer, J., & Bonomi, A. (2001). Improving chronic illness care: Translating evidence into action. *Health Affairs, 20*(6), 64–78.

Walker, E., Sobo, E.J., & Kurtin, P.S. (2002). Complementary and alternative medicine for Down syndrome: What do pediatricians need to know? *California Pediatrician, 18*(1), 34–35.

11

ACCESSING QUALITY CARE FOR CHILDREN WITH SPECIAL HEALTH CARE NEEDS:

THE FUTURE OF POLICY AND RESEARCH

Lisa A. Simpson and Denise Dougherty

T
he preceding chapters in this volume have demonstrated that children with special health care needs (CSHCN) require effective access to high-quality health care services, and that federal and state policy makers and research entities have taken a special interest in CSHCN (Perrin, 2002). However, the burgeoning numbers of such children, and a greater understanding of their needs and the needs of their families, mean that in many instances research and the policies they should inform have not kept up with the needs of these children. In this chapter, we suggest future directions for policy and research to bridge the gap between the health care that CSHCN and their families receive today and the health care that they need.*

We do this in the context of current discussions on policy and research, and we focus on what we consider two priority issues: access to care and quality of care received. Within each issue we focus on how the disparities in access to quality care and good outcomes—evident throughout our health care system—affect CSHCN. For each of these topics, we briefly review what is known about the issue (drawing on earlier chapters where appropriate), discuss the current policy issues that shape care for CSHCN, propose strategies that could improve care, and summarize the research needed to support further improvements in care. We conclude with thoughts about how families of CSHCN and health care professionals might be involved in the improvements.

*The research for this chapter was supported in part by the Pediatric Clinical Research Center of all Children's Hospital, the University of South Florida, and the Maternal and Child Health Bureau, R60 MC 00003-01, Department of Health and Human Services, Health Resources and Services Administration.

The views expressed in this chapter are those of the authors and not necessarily the U.S. Department of Health and Human Services, Agency for Healthcare Research and Quality.

ACCESS TO CARE

Effective access to care is the result of three basic factors: 1) predisposing factors, 2) need factors, and 3) enabling factors (Aday & Andersen, 1974). Although predisposing factors such as attitudes about insurance coverage and medical care are theoretically important, need and enabling factors appear to be the most critical determinants of effective access for CSHCN. Need factors include the type and severity of the child's condition or illness and the types of health care that ameliorate them. Enabling factors are programs and policies and their implementation that enable CSHCN to use effective services.

Policy Considerations

Access to high-quality health care often is presented as a relatively simple issue that can be accomplished by simply expanding access to health insurance coverage. However, effective access requires more than just having an insurance card. Chung and Schuster applied the Eisenberg and Power framework of *voltage drops* to health care access for children. In this framework, voltage drops are resistance points at which patients drop from the system like voltage from an electrical current (Chung & Schuster, 2004; Eisenberg & Power, 2000). The 5 voltage drops related to access are 1) access to insurance coverage, 2) enrollment in available insurance plans, 3) access to services and providers, 4) access to a consistent source of primary care, and 5) access to referral services. In this chapter, we further refine the voltage drops approach of access for CSHCN.

The previous chapters and the findings summarized here clearly indicate that for several reasons CSHCN's access to care is more likely to be affected by the concept of voltage drops than other children and their families. First, CSHCN typically have higher needs for health care (Simpson et al., 2005; U.S. Department of Health and Human Services, Health Resources and Services Administration, Maternal and Child Health Bureau [USDHHS HRSA MCHB, 2004]). For example, one study found that CSHCN had four times the number of hospitalizations and spent seven times as many days in the hospital as other children, and accounted for 52.5% of all child hospitalizations (Newacheck & Kim, 2005). In addition, CSHCN had twice as many physician visits and seven times as many nonphysician visits as other children. Further, parents of CSHCN appear to be less likely to have access to private employer-sponsored health insurance (Davidoff, Yemane, & Hill, 2004), which may be more generous than public coverage, and access to employer-sponsored health insurance may be lower because parents of CSHCN are less likely to work full-time (USDHHS HRSA MCHB, 2004). Research indicates that the degree to which each voltage drop prevents receipt of high-quality care by CSHCN is greater for CSHCN from racial and ethnic minorities and/or low-income families (Huang, Kogan, Yu, & Strickland, 2005; Leatherman & McCarthy 2004; Mayer, Skinner, & Slifkin, 2004; USDHHS HRSA MCHB, 2004; Yu, Huang, Schwalberg, & Kogan, 2005).

Reducing Voltage Drop 1: Access to Health Insurance Coverage

Access to health insurance has been a major focus of policy change for children, including CSHCN (Davidoff et al., 2004; Simpson et al., 2005). Early and recent efforts to increase the proportions of children with coverage have proven effective (Hudson, 2005). According to one estimate, between 1999 and 2002, the number of children overall without any health insurance coverage declined to 7.8 million children, a decline of 2.8 percentage points at a time when the rates of uninsured nonelderly adults (ages 18–64 years) were rising. However, all is not well for CSHCN. The uninsured rate for CSHCN is about equal that of all children (Davidoff et al., 2004), despite their greater needs. In addition, CSHCN in families with incomes less than 200% of the federal poverty level (FPL) were three times as likely to be uninsured as CSHCN with family incomes above 200% FPL (Davidoff et al., 2004). Data drawn from the 2001 National Survey of Children with Special Health Care Needs (National Survey of Children with Special Health Care Needs Data Resource Center, 2004; van Dyck, Kogan, McPherson, Weissman, & Newacheck, 2004) specific to CSHCN showed that almost one of out seven CSHCN were without health insurance coverage at some point during the 12 months preceding response to the survey, with Hispanic, poor, and near-poor CHSCN more likely to have been uninsured at some point in time (see Table 11.1). The general consequences of a lack of insurance are well known, but the consequences of breaks in coverage are just beginning to be examined and can be serious. In a study of discontinuous coverage for children (not specific to CSHCN), researchers found that 20% of children with breaks in coverage experienced delays in care, 13% had unmet needs for medical care, and 10% had unfilled prescriptions (Olson, Tang, & Newacheck, 2005).

Looking forward, there are four trends in the overall policy environment that, although not necessarily intended to reduce coverage and access to care for CSHCN, may inadvertently adversely affect this population. These trends are

Table 11.1. Access to care and disparities in care for young children (0–5 years) with special health care needs

DIMENSIONS OF ACCESS	KEY FINDINGS (%)
INSURANCE COVERAGE	
Ever uninsured in the past 12 months	13.7
<100% Federal poverty level	18.8
100–< 200% Federal poverty level ("working poor")	21.0
Hispanic	25.6
Black, non-Hispanic	14.7
% Current coverage NOT adequate	33.7
<100% Federal poverty level	41.3
100–<200% Federal poverty level	36.0
Hispanic	49.3
Black, non-Hispanic	30.4
1 or more unmet needs for specific health care services	15.9
<100% Federal poverty level	24.3
100–<200% Federal poverty level	23.2
Hispanic	22.1
Black, non-Hispanic	16.9
PROGRAM PARTICIPATION	
Participated in Special Education (ages 3–5 only)	23.0
<100% Federal poverty level	23.6
100–<200% Federal poverty level	
Hispanic	20.1
Black, non-Hispanic	18.4
ACCESS TO SERVICES AND UNMET NEEDS	
Difficulty getting a referral for specialty care*	19.7
<100% Federal poverty level	30.3
100–<200% Federal poverty level	21.9
Hispanic	27.7
Black, non-Hispanic	18.1

* Note: Denominator includes only CSHCN ages 0–5 years who needed specialist during past 12 months (56% of all CSHCN).

CYSHCN whose families needed support services and had one or more unmet needs for such services**	21.7
<100% Federal poverty level	27.2
100–<200% Federal poverty level	18.8
Hispanic	22.5
Black, non-Hispanic	26.0

** Note: Denominator includes only the CYSHCN whose families indicated needing one or more of the 3 family support services asked about in the survey.

From National Survey of Children with Special Health Care Needs, 2001. Special analyses conducted by the Child and Adolescent Health Measurement Initiative (CAHMI), Data Resource Center for Child and Adolescent Health, August 2005. www.childhealthdata.org; www.cahmi.org

1. Proposed changes to the Medicaid program

2. Reauthorization of the State Child Health Insurance Program

3. Reductions in Title V grants

4. Trends in the private market, including "consumer directed health care"

Medicaid Reform

A Medicaid Commission was established by the secretary of the U.S. Department of Health and Human Services in 2005 to make recommendations at two points in time on "ways to modernize the Medicaid program so that it can provide high-quality health care to its beneficiaries in a financially sustainable way" (U.S. Department of Health and Human Services Medicaid Commission, 2005). The first set of commission recommendations was released in September 2005 and was intended to provide a road map for Congress on how to reduce Medicaid expenditures by $10 billion over the next decade. The second set of recommendations is due in December 2006 and will focus on strategies to reduce Medicaid expenditures by another $50 billion while strengthening the program overall. None of the September 2005 recommendations focused directly on children's eligibility for coverage, but at least one could affect access by CSHCN; that is, the commission recommended 1) moving back the start date of the penalty period for persons transferring assets to enable them to become eligible for Medicaid coverage and 2) increasing the *look-back* period for determining assets from three years to five years. Both of these changes could make it harder for families with CSHCN to access Medicaid coverage. By December 31, 2006, the commission is tasked with making longer-term recommendations for the future of the Medicaid program that may have implications for CSHCN, as these proposals are to address the following issues: eligibility, expanding the number of people covered by quality care while recognizing budget constraints, choice, and other topics that the secretary may submit to the commission.

SCHIP Reauthorization

The State Children's Health Insurance Program (SCHIP) expires in 2007 unless reauthorized. (See Chapters 2 and 3 for more on this program.) Although SCHIP was not designed specifically for children with special health care needs, one out of six children eligible for SCHIP are estimated to be CSHCN (Peters, 2005). In some states, the prevalence of children with special health care needs in SCHIP is equal to or greater than that of the general population (Szilagyi et al., 2003). The precise number of CSHCN enrolled in the program nationally is not known, nor is the impact of SCHIP on access to care for CSHCN. In one study of the implementation of SCHIP in three states (Florida, Kansas, and New York), Dick and colleagues found that CSHCN in all three states experienced large improvements in their ratings of care; however, the impact of SCHIP on access to care for CSHCN was variable depending on the measure and the state (Dick et al., 2004). CSHCN had greater unmet needs after SCHIP enrollment than other SCHIP enrollees (except in Florida), but were better off than other enrollees on other measures (e.g., usual source of care in Kansas).

Features of the program relevant to the ability of CSHCN to get access to health insurance may be open to debate during SCHIP reauthorization. These include the substantial flexibility that states have—and will likely seek to increase—in setting eligibility criteria, making rules for verifying insurance coverage, and implementing waiting periods before children can be insured. All of these provisions were enacted to ensure that families would not disenroll from employer-sponsored coverage, and that employers would not cancel dependent coverage to take advantage of the public program (the so-called crowd-out or substitution effect) (Lutsky & Hill, 2001; National Conference of State Legislatures, 2003).

Eligibility for SCHIP is a major factor affecting access to coverage. States that remove asset tests and implement presumptive eligibility and self-declaration of income have higher enrollment levels than programs that don't, according to scholars at Yale University (Kronebusch & Elbel, 2004). However, these researchers found that continuous eligibility and adoption of mail-in applications had no effect on overall enrollment. Waiting periods may remain in place if SCHIP is reauthorized because they have been shown to prevent substitution (Lo Sasso & Buchmueller, 2004). Unfortunately, waiting periods also dampen enrollment rates (Kronebusch & Elbel, 2004; Lo Sasso & Buchmueller). Recognizing that one size may not fit all, some states waive waiting periods in cases of medical need (National Conference of State Legislatures, 2003), and this policy could be emulated by other states.

Maternal and Child Health (MCH) Title V Block Grants

Federal grants to states for MCH block grants were cut in fiscal years 2004 and 2005 and were threatened with additional cuts in fiscal year 2006 (Association of Maternal and Child Health Programs, 2005). Perhaps as a result, the number of CSHCN served by Title V programs declined more than 20%, from 1.3 million in 2002 to 1.1 million in 2003, after a period of steady increases from 1999 through 2002 (USDHHS HRSA MCHB, 2005a). Since 1981, states have had considerable flexibility in their use of block grant funds, so advocacy efforts are typically aimed at state personnel responsible for particular programs (Association of Maternal and Child Health Programs, 2003). A point for those responsible for CSHCN to consider may be that the responsibilities of these programs have grown enormously since their origins as *crippled children's* programs, and there is now some overlap with the responsibilities of other entities such as the Centers for Disease Control and Prevention's Nationwide Immunization Program and Medicaid (Centers for Disease Control and Prevention [CDC; n.d.]; Centers for Medicare and Medicaid Services [CMM; n.d.]). The responsibilities of Title V grantees cover all women and children and include infrastructure building, enabling services, and filling gaps in direct health services. States are required to report on 18 national performance measures, including six relevant to CSHCN (USDHHS HRSA MCHB[b]). With increasing demands on the programs and a tightening budget, there may be a need to refocus. On the other hand, the MCH program is the only one focused on the overall health of all women and children, and the only one with specific responsibility for coordinating services.

Consumer-Directed Health Care and Other Private Sector Initiatives

Consumer-Directed Health Care (CDHC) has emerged as the latest policy and market strategy to address rising health care costs (American Association on Health and Disability, 2004; Gauthier & Clancy, 2004). As CDHC is explored, employers and insurers are proceeding with other strategies, within traditional employer-sponsored insurance (ESI), to reduce costs to employers of health insurance, primarily by increasing consumer cost sharing (Robinson, 2002).

In theory, CDHC would reduce consumers' use of health services by making them better informed and giving them a greater financial stake in their medical care choices (American Association on Health and Disability, 2004; Davis, 2004). Definitions of what constitutes CDHC vary greatly, and the evidence to date on its effectiveness is limited (Davis). One major variant of CDHC is the health savings account (HSA), which is a high-deductible health plan with low premiums. HSAs are attractive to healthy, low-health-care-user populations because consumers can use the money in their HSAs to cover health insurance deductibles, copayments for medical services, over-the-counter drugs, and long-term care insurance and to pay health insurance premiums if they become unemployed. In addition, HSA contributions are tax free, holders can get interest and investment earnings, and HSAs are portable from one job to another. However, HSAs and other forms of CDHC are likely to result in increased insurance costs for people with chronic illnesses and other high users of health care, as they segment the risk pool by attracting younger, healthier, low-health-care users, leaving sicker, higher cost individuals in traditional insurance plans, thus concentrating the costs within a smaller group of people (Robinson, 2004).

The implications of CDHC for CSHCN have not been fully explored. Most of the research on CDHC has focused on commercial and adult populations and none on publicly insured families and/or CSHCN (Rosenthal & Milstein, 2004). A key assumption of CDHC is that health care services are overused and that giving financial incentives to patients, together with information on the quality of the services available from different providers, will reduce services that are of marginal or no value. This framework contains several assumptions that may not apply to CSHCN: 1) that families will act on financial incentives, 2) that information on quality is available, 3) that the services that are of marginal or no value is known, and 4) that families should be and are willing to change providers. Few, if any, of these assumptions is likely to apply to care for CSHCN, when more than 40% of families of CSHCN are already experiencing financial problems associated with having a CSHCN (see Chapter 3). First, providing financial incentives to these families, as long as they *reduce* and not *increase* costs, might be effective. A more likely outcome would be that relatively high users of health services could be forced into insurance plans with higher premiums and cost sharing or forced out of the insurance market altogether, resulting in a greater burden on Title V programs (Davis, 2004; Gabel & Rice, 2003). CDHC could be attractive to CSHCN if it were defined in disability terms, where the cost is not burdensome and the coverage options are flexible, broad, and deep. Second, the availability of information on quality and effectiveness to help consumers choose among providers and care options, an underlying premise of CDHC, is generally insufficient (see Quality of Care section for an expanded discussion of this point). Third, changing providers may be even more difficult for families of CSHCN, as it runs counter to the very definition of continuous healing relationships contained within the concept of a medical home.

A constant burden that proposals to enhance access to care must face is the apparently inexorable rise in health care costs. The reasons for these increases are complex and include the aging of the population, the development of new medical technologies, the identification of additional chronic diseases amenable to treatment, and a general rise in inflation (Lubitz, 2005; Thorpe, Florence, Howard, & Joski, 2005). Although expenditures for children overall represent a decreasing percentage of the nation's health care expenses from an estimated 13% in 1987 to 11% in 1999 (Simpson et al., 2004), the fact that a significant and growing proportion of these costs is paid for by public programs makes them the subject of considerable scrutiny by policy makers at the state and federal levels.

Reducing Voltage Drop 2: Enrollment in Available Insurance Plans

Being eligible for programs does not guarantee enrollment. Enrollment depends on eligibility, affordability, and—particularly important for public programs—knowledge of coverage availability.

First, eligibility criteria for public programs are extremely complicated (Davidoff et al., 2004). Employer-sponsored insurance (ESI) also has eligibility criteria that may preclude coverage for certain workers (e.g., part-time employees, contract workers; Stanton, 2004). Alan Weil, an expert in coverage issues, suggests that "layering SCHIP on top of Medicaid on top of a fragile employer-based system of coverage can only get us so far. . . . A better approach would begin with the premise that all children will be covered and then challenge ourselves to design a system that gives meaning to that goal" (Weil, 2004). Such a system would be state-based and value universality over precision, according to Weil. States would have an incentive to collect data in real time on the private and public coverage status of every child, to streamline eligibility for public programs, and to seek matching funds for gap-filling coverage.

Second, affordability of health care coverage has become a critical issue. According to analyses by the Kaiser Family Foundation, ESI premiums for family coverage have risen 59% since 2000 to an average of $10,217 annually in 2004 (Kaiser Family Foundation and Health Research Educational Trust, n.d.). States are considering increasing premiums for SCHIP (Kaiser Family Foundation, 2005), and the National Governors Association is recommending premiums as a cost-sharing mechanism for Medicaid-covered children, with exceptions for those who are provided mandatory coverage (National Governors Association, 2005).

Third, knowledge of the availability of coverage is a critical determinant of SCHIP coverage. When SCHIP was first passed, focused federal efforts, including policy changes in school lunch programs, supported numerous efforts to reach out to potentially eligible families and to simplify enrollment (White House, 1999). In addition, valuable private sector programs such as Covering Kids® were launched to focus on enrolling eligible children; however, the extent to which these focused on CSHCN as a target population is unclear (Robert Wood Johnson Foundation, 2005). Some states, as they faced budget problems, increased the administrative burden on applicants and the frequency of reapplication (Chung & Schuster, 2004).

To prevent this voltage drop and to preserve the availability of affordable coverage options, it is clear that more work is needed to ensure that CSHCN enroll and stay enrolled in available programs. Thanks to groups such as Family Voices, to funding for case managers, and to an increase in true *medical homes* (see Chapter 6), families of CSHCN enjoy access to a relatively good network of advice about insurance coverage and other critical determinants of care. However, research suggests that enrollment is neither easy nor universal (Davidoff et al., 2004; see Table 11.1).

Reducing Voltage Drop 3: Access to Covered Services and Providers

Enrollment in an insurance plan does not guarantee access to services (Chung & Schuster, 2004). As shown in Table 11.1, one third of parents of CSHCN do not believe they have adequate insurance coverage, with higher rates among poor and Hispanic CSHCN, a belief borne out by parents' reports that 15.9% of CSHCN had one or more unmet needs for specific health care services. Honberg and colleagues reported that only 59.6% of CSHCN in the 2001 National Survey of Children with Special Health Care Needs (NSCSHCN) met a health insurance core outcome consisting of three components (presence of insurance coverage, continuity of coverage, and adequacy of coverage; Honberg, McPherson, Strickland, Gage, & Newacheck, 2005). Policies that affect adequacy of insurance include range of covered services, cost sharing, medical necessity, and preferred drug lists.

Covered Services

Organizational policies regarding the coverage of treatments for populations of patients with similar conditions determines the types of services and providers who can receive any type of reimbursement (Singer & Bergthold, 2001). Policy makers are urging that states be given more flexibility to tailor benefits coverage to specific populations (National Governors Association, 2005), and in December 2006, the Medicaid Commission (USDHHS MC, 2005) is to make additional recommendations regarding benefits, design, and delivery. In addition, some states have suggested that the Medicaid Early Periodic Screening, Diagnosis and Treatment (EPSDT) benefit for children be narrowed or eliminated. The EPSDT benefit is critical in providing children, particularly CSHCN, with coverage for the wide range of services needed. For example, in seven states, the number of physician visits is limited to 15 a year, and 23 states do not cover physical therapy by an independent therapist. Getting benefits specific to CSHCN may be easier once an MCHB-funded project to develop a model benefit package is completed

(American Academy of Pediatrics, n.d.). Szilagyi and colleagues have suggested that SCHIP benefit packages need to adequately cover services required by CSHCN such as prescription medications and specialty, mental health, developmental, and home services (Szilagyi et al., 2003). There also is considerable lack of clarity about who covers what, and some traditional plans (including Medicaid and SCHIP) might assume that many services are covered by other programs (e.g., schools, early intervention programs) or that CSHCN with Supplemental Security Income (SSI) can self-pay.

Cost Sharing

Family cost sharing comes in the form of both insurance premiums and copayments at the time of services. For CSHCN who need a variety of services from a range of providers, copayments may add up to an unbearable financial burden, cause delays in treatment or unmet needs, or give rise to people disenrolling from an insurance program (Wright et al., 2005). Despite their better financial protection against out-of-pocket expenses relative to total health care expenditures (due to hospital and home health benefits), CSHCN on average pay 15% of total health care expenditures out of pocket (Newacheck & Kim, 2005). Some of the services most needed by CSHCN (e.g., prescription drugs, mental health services, dental care, hospital care) are the services with the highest cost-sharing burdens in private plans (see Chapter 3). Because copayments impede access at the point at which care is needed, the National Governors Association recommended implementation of premiums in Medicaid rather than impose copayments (National Governors Association, 2005). A September 2005 Medicaid Commission (USDHHS MC, 2005) recommendation would provide states the flexibility to increase copayments on nonpreferred drugs beyond nominal amounts regardless of beneficiaries' income. Fortunately, the commission noted that by federal statute, Medicaid-enrolled children under 18 cannot be charged copayments. The American Academy of Pediatrics recently stated its opposition to imposing copayments, especially for preventive services (American Academy of Pediatrics, 2005).

Medical Necessity

The term *medical necessity* is the fundamental underpinning of insurance coverage and is at the center of all decisions about whether specific services will be covered. Medical necessity became the focus of increasing controversy with the advent of managed care, and managed care organizations' interpretations caused much of the managed care backlash (Singer & Bergthold, 2001). Although most of the cases reported in the media and those subject to judicial review focused on care for adults, experts have called for a pediatric standard for medical necessity (American Academy of Pediatrics Committee on Child Health Financing, 2005; Fox & McManus, 2001; Markus, Rosenbaum, Stewart, & Cox, 2005; Wehr, 2001; Wehr & Jameson, 1994). Other recommendations have included providing greater clarity and uniformity in medical-necessity language (Fox & McManus, 2001; Singer & Bergthold, 2001), revising the Health Insurance Portability and Accountability Act of 1996 to allow states to customize payment coding to their unique coverage standards (Markus et al., 2005), widely adopting a number of best practices for health plans and legislation (e.g., keeping patients and providers informed in a timely manner, tracking numbers and types of denials, fully disclosing contractual information) (Singer & Bergthold, 2001), and moving slowly on efforts to make medical-necessity decisions entirely evidence based (Wehr, 2001). The American Academy of Pediatrics' Committee on Child Health Financing has proposed model contract language for medical necessity for children (American Academy of Pediatrics Committee on Child Health Financing, 2005) that calls for defining medical necessity to include interventions intended to promote typical growth and development appropriate for the age and developmental status of the child, taking into account the appropriateness of the intervention setting, evidence of effectiveness where such evidence is available, and placing the value on the children rather than on the lowest price. They also recommend that health insurers describe the processes by which health care professionals can provide justification for the medical necessity of health interventions. Parents of CSHCN also may want to participate in helping insurance plans make medical necessity decisions; several state chapters of Family Voices provide training and technical assistance on this topic (Family Voices of Colorado, n.d.; Family Voices of Tennessee, n.d.).

Restrictions on Prescription Drugs

In addition to other cost-control policies, state Medicaid programs are reacting to increased Medicaid drug costs by adopting preferred drug lists, prior authorization before reimbursement of specific drugs, limits on the number of prescriptions that can be filled without prior authorization, *fail first* requirements (patient failure to respond to an initial, cheaper drug), and drug category reimbursement exclusions (Soumerai, 2004). Limits such as these could reduce appropriate care, adversely affect health status, and cause shifts to more costly types of care (Soumerai). To prevent or ameliorate these consequences, they recommend steps such as assessing inappropriate use of high-cost drugs before implementing changes and instituting simple mechanisms to exempt high-risk patients (Soumerai).

Reducing Voltage Drop 4: Access to a Consistent Source of Primary Care

Despite the heavy reliance of CSHCN on specialty care and various therapies, families report that primary care also is important to them (Krauss & Wells, 2000). Although CSHCN are more likely to report having a usual source of care and a personal doctor or nurse (Tu & Cunningham, 2005; USDHHS HRSA MCHB, 2004), whether these sources provide primary care is unclear. Barbara Starfield, a leading expert in primary care, says that with few exceptions "Little or nothing has been done to ensure that 'regular sources of care' fulfill the criteria for good primary care" (Starfield, Shi, & Macinko, 2005). Current efforts to increase the use of primary care by CSHCN include medical home initiatives and hospital outpatient-based comprehensive care. In addition, Medicaid managed care programs for people with disabilities may automatically assign beneficiaries to a primary care provider. State Medicaid programs vary in whom they include in their definitions of primary care provider (American Academy of Physician Assistants, 1997; New York State Department of Health, 2006). According to focus group sessions held by Family Voices with parents enrolled in Medicaid managed care plans, some plans permit families to make a special request that a pediatric specialist be their child's primary care provider, and some have developed policies to pay primary care providers higher rates for providing care to CSHCN (Johnston & Wells, 2002). Starfield and colleagues have suggested several policy changes to increase the numbers and quality of primary care providers in the United States. These include higher reimbursement for primary care providers, changes in reimbursement for the elements of good primary care (e.g., the full medical home), improved coordination between primary care providers and specialists, state policies encouraging a better distribution of physicians, expanded training and loan forgiveness for primary care providers, reduction in the amount of paperwork, and encouragement of the creation and use of electronic health care records (Berman, Dolins, Tang, & Yudkowsky, 2002; Starfield et al., 2005).

Reducing Voltage Drop 5: Access to Referral Services

Of all the voltage drops, access to referral services may be the most important to CSHCN (Chung & Schuster, 2004; Krauss & Wells, 2000). One out of five CSHCN are reported to have experienced difficulty getting a referral for specialty care or needing, but not getting, all support services (see Table 11.1). For CSHCN of all ages, reported problems concerning obtaining referrals were most common among children who were uninsured. One third of these children had a reported problem receiving referrals compared with about one fifth of those with private coverage. In a study of access to outpatient specialty care, Black children were half as likely as White children to have access to specialty services (Shenkman, Tian, Nackashi, & Schatz, 2005). That same study found that certain characteristics of managed care (e.g., lower percentages of primary care providers paid on a fee-for-service basis, higher percentages of pediatricians in the primary care provider network, financial incentives for meeting quality of care standards) were associated with a greater likelihood of use of outpatient physician specialists.

A critical dimension of effective specialty access for CSHCN is coordination of care. In general, primary care providers often have no systematic ties with providers of specialty services, which makes referral, feedback, and tracking of care received challenging (Chung & Schuster, 2004; Forrest et al., 2000). Health information technology (HIT) may provide at least a partial solution. If HIT is developed correctly across systems of care for children (and not just within mainstream pediatric care), primary care providers should be able to identify and interact more easily with a range of specialty providers and settings where CSHCN receive care (e.g., public mental health services, school health), thus reducing the burden of coordination with specialists and therapy services (Chung & Schuster). In turn, specialists and therapists (e.g., mental health therapists, physical therapists, occupational therapists, speech therapists, school nurses) should be able to communicate in real time with the CSHCN's most important care provider, whether a primary care provider or other specialist (Krauss & Wells, 2000).

State and local agencies are responsible for promoting care coordination, and they have sometimes been criticized for their care coordination activities and policies (Rosenberg et al., 2005). For example, state Maternal and Child Health agencies, whose CSHCN programs are responsible for ensuring that SSI beneficiaries receive rehabilitative services, sometimes take issue with this responsibility on the grounds that the services are covered by Medicaid (USDHHS HRSA MCHB [b; n.d.]). A report on New York State concluded that "the 'system' for serving CSHCN lacks coherence" and that the state does not have an overarching 'systemic' approach to providing care" (Bauer, Duitch, & Birenbaum, 2003). Rather, New York State's coordination programs often were found to be inadequate and limited to coordination of services within one program.

Research on Access to Care for CSHCN

It is evident throughout this volume that, with a few exceptions, there is little research specifically on health care access for CSHCN. Even the data provided in Table 11.1 required a special request of the MCHB Data Resource Center managed by the Child and Adolescent Health Measurement Initiative to generate data specific to *young* CSHCN. There is clearly a great need for access research specifically on this population, and policy-relevant access research is critical for guiding the numerous policies and programs that affect access for CSHCN. Research on CSHCN was greatly advanced by the development of a "screener," a set of standardized questions that are used in multiple national surveys and research projects to consistently identify CSHCN (Bethell et al., 2002). The screener has made possible the National Survey of Children with Special Health Care Needs (NSCSHCN) from which the data in this chapter's three tables have been derived (van Dyck et al., 2004), stratification of data from the Medical Expenditure Panel Survey (MEPS) by CSHCN (Agency for Healthcare Research and Quality, 2005a; Newacheck & Kim, 2005), and analysis of data for military dependents (Williams, Schone, Archibald, & Thompson, 2004). One of the reasons for development of the CSHCN screener was that information on children with chronic illnesses and disabilities was only available condition by condition, a factor that made sample sizes in many settings too small (Bethell et al.). Some state agencies have used the CSHCN screener and other tools to identify CSHCN in their programs and to make recommendations for integrating them into health care delivery programs (Texas Health and Human Services Commission Medicaid/CHIP Division, 2003). However, for individual providers and health plans, the number of CSHCN may still be too small for meaningful analysis.

Many policy-relevant questions on CSHCN emerge from the review in this section. Some questions are specific to certain programs, but there also is a need for research on the combination of programs that are now theoretically available to CSHCN. Policy makers considering changes in Medicaid might benefit from research on the overall impact of potential cost controls as well as the impact of cost sharing (premiums and copayments) and prescription drug policy changes. Policy makers considering SCHIP reauthorization also could benefit from research on the impact of variations in

- Eligibility criteria and their implementation

- Premiums and copayments

- Covered benefits

- Approaches to preventing crowd-out (e.g., waiting periods)

- Outreach strategies

- Policies specific to services and providers that are particularly important to CSHCN (e.g., primary care, medical and nursing specialty care, variations in cost sharing and coverage for prescription drugs, mental health and other therapies, telehealth and telemedicine)

Policy makers considering MCH programs could use research on how cuts in block grants in the context of the expanded scope of Title V programs affect CSHCN, as well as on ways to improve the effectiveness of MCH efforts to coordinate and integrate care for CSHCN. Policy makers considering whether to implement consumer-directed health care, and other efforts to increase consumer involvement in health care payment and decision making, need research on how these changes may affect CSHCN as well as children in general. Many of the access questions relevant to Medicaid and SCHIP can and should be asked about private insurance, in addition to questions about the impact of declining coverage for dependents and families with part-time workers. Modeling research that examines the impacts of a policy of presumptive universal coverage (Weil, 2004), combined with other forms of access for CSHCN (e.g., early intervention, Title V, SSI), could be extremely valuable in reducing the diffusion of responsibility and accountability that may be partly responsible for the current fragmented *nonsystem* of care for CSHCN.

To ensure that data focused on CSHCN are brought to bear, a research center specifically focused on answering access questions critical to CSHCN could be organized to conduct or contract for quick-turn-around analyses. Finally, if policy changes get ahead of the research, as happened with many SCHIP questions in 1997, a *learn-as-we-go approach* could be developed modeled on the Child Health Insurance and Research Initiative (CHIRI) and other SCHIP evaluations (Agency for Healthcare Research and Quality, [a; n.d.]).

QUALITY OF CARE

Access to care has been the mainstay of advocacy among children's groups for decades, with many successes (e.g., Medicaid expansions, SCHIP). Less attention has been paid, however, to an equally important aspect of care—its quality—although there is new and hopeful movement on this topic (Agency for Healthcare Research and Quality, 2005a; Dougherty, Meikle, Owens, Kelley, & Moy, 2005; Leatherman & McCarthy, 2004). Since the release of a landmark report from the Institute of Medicine in 2001 called *Crossing the Quality Chasm: A New Health System for the 21st Century,* quality of care is now understood to be made up of six dimensions (Institute of Medicine, Committee on the Quality of Health Care in America, 2001). Health care is of high quality when it is safe, effective, patient centered, timely, efficient, and equitable (see

Table 11.2. Dimensions of quality of care

Safe	Care that is free from error and does not result in harm to the patient
Effective	Matching care to science, avoiding overuse of ineffective care and underuse of effective care
Patient centered	Honoring the individual and respecting choice
Timely	Less waiting for both patients and those who give care
Efficient	Reducing waste
Equitable	Closing racial and ethnic gaps in health status

From Institute of Medicine & Committee on the Quality of Health Care in America. (2001). *Crossing the quality chasm: A new health system for the 21st century.* Washington, DC: National Academy Press.

Table 11.2). Arguably, having access to the highest-quality care is most important for CSHCN for several reasons; for example, these children may be the most vulnerable to the effects of poor care, they experience and rely on health care services more than most children, and poor quality can have the most long-lasting adverse effects. As noted in the earlier chapters of this volume, high-quality care for CSHCN is often defined as care delivered through a medical home. Little attention has been focused on CSHCN within the overall field of research on quality, but the available data suggest cause for concern and policy action.

State of Current Quality of Care

Several publications have included important data that point to gaps in quality of care for CSHCN. The Commonwealth Fund released a chartbook in 2004 that represented the first and most comprehensive compilation of research findings and data on quality of care for children in general and included several results on CSHCN (Leatherman & McCarthy, 2004). Specific examples of poor quality of care in this report were found to exist among children with cystic fibrosis, sickle cell disease, asthma, and attention-deficit/hyperactivity disorder (ADHD). In addition, 39% to 59% of CSHCN (all ages) did not receive coordinated, ongoing, comprehensive, family-centered care in a medical home. Beginning in 2003, the U.S. Department of Health and Human Services began releasing annual National Healthcare Quality and Disparities Reports, which also drove home the message that quality of care for all children, including CSHCN, is too often suboptimal (Agency for Healthcare Research and Quality, 2004, 2005a; Dougherty et al., 2005). Finally, the 2001 national survey of CSHCN highlighted many dimensions of quality where opportunities to improve exist. All of the reports noted disparities in health care quality in the categories of race, ethnicity, and income. Disparity findings for CSHCN from the 2001 survey are noted in Table 11.3.

Within the context of growing information on quality of care, it is important to note that there are two areas where relatively less is known about quality: the safety of care for CSHCN and the role that organizational factors play in determining quality of care for CSHCN. The dearth of patient safety research involving CSHCN is surprising given the fact that patient safety has become the dominant focus of Agency for Healthcare Research and Quality (AHRQ) sponsored health services research. Studies that do exist clearly point to increased safety problems. In one study of hospitalized children (all ages), having a special medical need and being discharged to home health care were associated with an up to 12-fold or 8-fold increase in medical errors, respectively (Slonim, Lafleur, Ahmed, & Joseph, 2003). Given the complex nature of many of these children's conditions, error may occur due to a variety of mechanisms, including 1) a CSHCN whose condition has yet to be diagnosed presenting for another acute problem, 2) a young CSHCN requiring atypical management for her known condition, 3) a young CSHCN whose baseline status is unknown to that particular provider (e.g., an emergency department), 4) a CSHCN with a rare condition, and 5) a CSHCN who is technology dependent (Sacchetti, Sacchetti, Carraccio, & Gerardi, 2000). Most of the potential for medical error in these scenarios centers on missing patient information due to systems problems and/or communication difficulty with the child's parents. There is growing literature on the association between medical error and missing information (Cohen, Rivara, Marcuse, McPhillips, & Davis, 2005; Flores et al., 2003; Gandhi et al., 2000; Leape et al., 1995). Finally, in a recent study of missing clinical information during primary care visits among children and adults, the presence of more than two active medical problems was associated with an increase in missing information (15.9% of those with two to five problems and 19.1% of those with greater than five problems, compared with 13.6% overall; Smith et al., 2005).

Similarly, a small but growing body of work is revealing the impact that managed care and public program policies can have on the quality of care for CSHCN (Dick et al., 2004; Shenkman, Tian, Nackashi, & Schatz, 2005; Shenkman et al., 2003). In the study on the impact of SCHIP involving three states mentioned earlier, Dick and colleagues found that the disparities in the quality of care reported by parents of children with special needs (all ages) that existed prior to SCHIP enrollment disappeared after enrollment.

As we begin to understand the scope and nature of the problems involved with quality of care for CSHCN, we also begin to learn how

Table 11.3. Quality of care and disparities in quality for children (0–5 years) with special health care needs

Dimension of Quality	Key Findings (%)
MCHB Core Outcomes	
CSHCN with families who are partners in decision making and satisfied with services	61.6
<100% Federal poverty level	46.2
Hispanic	47.8
Black, non-Hispanic	54.9
CSHCN have medical homes	53.6
<100% Federal poverty level	40.1
Hispanic	43.2
Black, non-Hispanic	47.8
Community-based service systems are organized for easy use	77.5
<100% Federal poverty level	70.0
Hispanic	68.5
Black, non-Hispanic	67.6
Family Centered Care	
CSHCN lacking one or more components of family centered care	31.5
<100% Federal poverty level	46.3
Hispanic	41.8
Black, non-Hispanic	37.6
	% Sometimes/Never
How often CSHCN's doctors and other health providers spend enough time with them	15.8
<100% Federal poverty level	26.0
Hispanic	21.4
African American	23.1
	% Sometimes/Never
How often CSHCN's doctors and other health providers listen carefully to parents	12.9
<100% Federal poverty level	19.5
Hispanic	16.6
African American	14.2
	% Sometimes/Never
How often CSHCN's doctors and other health providers are sensitive to families' values and customs	13.5
<100% Federal poverty level	24.8
Hispanic	18.3
African American	20.2
	% Sometimes/Never
How often CSHCN's doctors and other health providers make parents feel like partners in caring for child	12.8
<100% Federal poverty level	19.6
Hispanic	19.6
African American	13.7

From National Survey of Children with Special Health Care Needs (2001). Special analyses conducted by the Child and Adolescent Health Measurement Initiative (CAHMI), Data Resource Center for Child and Adolescent Health, August 2005. www.childhealthdata.org; www.cahmi.org

to *improve* the quality of care for this population. The application of quality improvement methods to pediatric practice is not new. In 2001, Ferris and colleagues published a review of improvement strategies reported in the medical literature and concluded that several approaches were effective, most notably reminder systems for office-based preventive services and inpatient pathways for complex care (Ferris, Dougherty, Blumenthal, & Perrin, 2001). Since then, numerous additional reports have been published on both successful and unsuccessful efforts to improve quality of care for children with chronic conditions—usually asthma or ADHD (Homer et al., 2004, 2005; Leslie, Weckerly, Plemmons, Landsverk, & Eastman, 2004; Lieu et al., 2004; Lozano et al., 2004; Mangione-Smith et al., 2005; Olson, Rosenbaum, Dosa, & Roizen, 2005). Efforts have moved toward applying improvement strategies to overall improvement of the medical home for all CSHCN (Cooley & McAllister, 2004). The National Initiative for Children's Healthcare Quality (NICHQ) has been sponsoring Medical Home Learning Collaboratives in partnership with states.

Policy Considerations

The persistent and pervasive nature of problems with health care quality in general in the face of increased efforts on the part of providers, purchasers, and regulators to address the quality and safety of care is changing the scope and nature of the policy strategies being proposed and adopted. During the 1990s, the primary problem with quality of care was perceived to be unwanted variation. A tremendous amount of effort went into producing and disseminating clinical practice guidelines to promote the use of evidence-based medicine by clinicians. As the decade (and indeed the millennium) came to a close, policy makers in the public and private sectors were recognizing that such an approach was insufficient to address the problem. The release of the 1999 Institute of Medicine report on patient safety was critical in reshaping the policy dialogue, and it has resulted in significant shifts in public and private investments to improve quality (Kohn, Corrigan, & Donaldson, 1999).

An emphasis on the organizational and environmental context is now dominating the policy environment, as we begin to recognize that even the most committed practitioners have a limited ability to improve quality without changes in organizing and financing health care. Five aspects of the current policy dialogue are discussed in relation to their likely impact on CSHCN: 1) evidence-based practice, 2) quality measurement and improvement, 3) the public release of quality information, 4) pay-for-performance programs, and 5) health information technology. Little is known about the applicability or potential impact on CSHCN for most of these proposed strategies.

Policy Issue 1: Evidence-Based Practice

The concept of evidence-based practice (EBP) grew out of the focus on evidence-based medicine as it became clear that multiple practitioners—not just physicians—needed to use evidence in their practice. Evidence-based medicine is defined as "the explicit use of the best available evidence to inform decisions about the care of individual patients" (Sackett, Rosenberg, Gray, Haynes, & Richardson, 1996; Shojania & Grimshaw, 2005). One of the primary mechanisms to promote EBP has been the development of evidence-based guidelines that rely on systematic reviews (also known as evidence reports) to consolidate and synthesize the most recent research. However, very few of these evidence reports have been focused on children and even fewer on CSHCN. Similarly, until recently, the guidelines developed by the American Academy of Pediatrics (AAP) focused only on acute conditions. This changed with the publication in 2001 of the guidelines on the diagnosis, treatment, and long-term management of children with ADHD (Subcommittee on Attention-Deficit/Hyperactivity Disorder and Committee on Quality Improvement, 2001). A final issue in the promotion of evidence-based practice is the need for evidence not just of *clinical* interventions but also of *organizational* interventions, as we learn more about how critical they are to determining the quality of care children receive (Simpson & Fraser, 1999). Thus, to improve outcomes for children, we need not only evidence-based practice but also evidence-based management and evidence-based policy.

Policy Issue 2: Quality Measurement and Improvement

Measurement is a key first step in understanding where quality falls short for CSHCN and is a prerequisite to any improvement efforts (Dougherty & Simpson, 2004). The last decade has witnessed significant progress in our understanding of how to measure and improve the quality of care for children (Agency for Healthcare Research and Quality [b; n.d.]; Beal et al., 2004; Ferris et al., 2001; Miller, Gergen, Honour, & Zhan, 2005; Simpson, 2001; Simpson & Lawless, 2005). Many of these new measures are for CSHCN. Quality measurement research is not easy, but perhaps a bigger challenge is the development and continued use of measures (Dougherty & Simpson, 2004; National Quality Forum, 2004; Shaller, 2004). Quality measures can be used in multiple ways; for example, by

- Physicians and other health care professional offices to track their progress in caring for CSHCN

- Families of CSHCN to support their choices in care and a real partnership with the medical home

- The general public when choosing health plans or providers

- Private health plans, public insurers, and health care delivery systems to identify problem areas that need assistance with quality improvement

- Health plans and purchasers to select and reward higher performing providers and institutions (Hibbard, Stockard, & Tusler, 2003; McGlynn & Malin, 2002)

Quality measurement for CSHCN faces challenges because of the small numbers of such children in any one health plan or provider practice. Attempts to encourage health plans to measure patient satisfaction, patient centeredness, and timeliness for the CSHCN population has encountered resistance because these measures require new data collection (survey) efforts, which health plans view as costly (Zhan, Sangl, Meyer, & Zaslavsky, 2002).

Efforts to improve quality continue to be hampered by two key issues: the cost of these activities and the inconsistent evidence base supporting their effectiveness. In looking at the business case for quality for all children, Homer and his colleagues found that, in general, investments by practitioners and their offices to improve care did not generate any return on their investment in terms of practice income (Homer & the Child Health Business Case Working Group, 2004). In another example, researchers estimated that a medium-sized U.S. pediatric practice committed to improving the care of CSHCN by providing care coordination would spend between $22,809 and $33,048 annually, costs not reimbursed by insurance (Stille & Antonelli, 2004). Turning to the evidence base for quality improvement, a recent article summarized the challenge of the existing weak evidence base for improvement approaches overall, not just for children, and concluded that "evaluations of specific [improvement] interventions often fail to meet basic standards for the conduct and reporting of research" and that "the choices of particular [improvement] interventions lack compelling theories predicting their success" (Shojania & Grimshaw, 2005).

Policy Issue 3: Public Release of Quality Information

Making performance data available to health plan members could potentially give parents the information they need to make decisions based on provider quality, and this could lead to providers investing in improvement. However, there is little, if any, evidence that consumers overall are using performance information to select higher-quality providers and thereby forcing improvement actions on the part of providers (Hibbard, Slovic, Peters, & Finucane, 2002). Indeed, the most recent national survey by Blendon and colleagues at Harvard of consumers exposed to information on quality who used the information to make a health provider choice showed only the slightest increase in use over a 10-year period with fewer than 50% choosing a health plan, surgeon, or hospital based on reports on quality (Kaiser Family Foundation, 2004). When improvement has occurred after a public release of quality information, it has been due to the quality improvement efforts of the health care organizations themselves, not as a result of patients abandoning the poorer performers (Hibbard et al., 2003).

The publication of quality information in a report card format for CSHCN raises a host of complicated issues (Davies et al., 2002; Zasvlasky et al., 2000). Vulnerable patient groups such as the poor, the less educated, the chronically sick, and members of ethnic or linguistic minorities may find issues of importance to them largely absent from these reports. In addition, the way report card data are collected, analyzed, and presented may further marginalize the experiences of these groups who are already underserved by the health system. First, current report card efforts cover a limited range of clinical conditions and rarely report on issues of coordination or availability of specialized services, making their relevance to families with CSHCN questionable. Second, to the extent that the report does not take into account the characteristics of the patient population, it risks unfairly comparing one plan or provider to another. For CSHCN this could have at least two impacts. Plans or providers that delivered superior quality of care to CSHCN might find their proportion of enrollees with CSHCN growing due to parent selection. In an environment where the added costs of care to this population are rarely covered adequately, this could be financially devastating to a provider or plan. Alternatively, a provider or plan that demonstrated a poor performance on a report card, and that did not take into account the complexity of the patients served, would appear to be failing and might be shunned by families. This observation also has important implications for health care providers who serve primarily large numbers of vulnerable patients. The differential impacts of report card data on vulnerable patient groups (and their providers) need to be addressed by researchers and policy makers so that patient access is not reduced further by the providers' pursuit of quality and value.

Policy Issue 4: Pay-for-Performance (PFP) Programs

Building on the growing availability of provider and plan performance information, purchasers are addressing the misalignment between how care is paid for and the quality of that care by proposing or implementing pay-for-performance programs—that is, by linking reimbursement for care to payment (Endsley, Kirkegaard, Baker, & Murcko, 2004). To date, health care providers, whether hospitals or practitioners, have largely been paid based on productivity or utilization measures (i.e., how many patients they see) rather than on the quality of care they provide the patients. One national study in 2004 found 84 PFP programs covering 39 million enrollees, and this number was estimated to grow to 160 programs by 2006 (Baker & Carter, 2005). Whether these programs will result in improved quality of care remains to be seen. A systematic review by AHRQ was inconclusive, and a more recent report entitled *Early Experience with Pay-for-Performance: From Concept to Practice* found that in adults, care only improved for one of three areas (mammography, cervical cancer screening, and hemoglobin A1c) and that those physician groups who were already performing at a higher level of quality received more of the total additional reimbursements (Rosenthal, Frank, Li, & Epstein, 2005).

Policy Issue 5: Health Information Technology

Efforts to promote the adoption of Health Information Technology (HIT) have been long-standing, but the last two years have seen a dramatic increase in the amount of attention to HIT from the public and private sectors. Health care and policy leaders have recognized that efforts to improve quality and contain costs cannot proceed without a functional health information infrastructure. However, most Americans still have little or no idea how electronic health records (EHRs) could improve their health care and are very concerned about the privacy and security of their personal health information (PHI).

Although most of the recent national attention on HIT has not included a specific focus on children's needs, that is changing thanks to efforts by leading pediatric organizations, the Maternal and Child Health Bureau, and AHRQ, among others (AHRQ, 2000). These efforts have focused on immunizations (Hinman, Saarlas, & Ross, 2004), newborn screening, the pediatric standards to be included in the EHR (Russell & Spooner, 2004), and the exchange of health information through state-based regional health information organizations.

The question of whether HIT will improve the quality of care for CSHCN any time soon remains, however. At this point, we do know that health care providers for children are among the slowest to adopt

HIT, and that the unique characteristics of childhood raise specific issues for developing interoperable HIT systems, such as the need for age-specific norms for lab values, growth charting, and weight-based dosing functionality for electronic prescribing (Shiffman, Spooner, Kwiatkowski, & Brennan 2001). A recent study among health providers for children in Florida found that pediatricians were the least likely to routinely use an EHR: 13.7% of pediatricians as opposed to 26.1% of family practitioners with at least 20% of their practice under age 18 years, 29.6% of pediatric specialists, and 24.8% of all other ambulatory providers (Menachemi, Ettel, Brooks, & Simpson, 2006). Another application of HIT that could promote the quality of care for CSHCN is the clinical decision support system (CDSS). These are computer applications that use evidence-based guidelines and other sources of the latest effectiveness research to assist and prompt practitioners during the clinical process of care. Given the low incidence of most CSHCN conditions and diagnoses, pediatricians often are confronted with having only one or two children in their practice with a given genetic or congenital disorder, and keeping abreast of the latest management strategies is simply not possible. Properly designed CDSSs could give primary care practitioners the ability to provide up-to-date care for even the rarest condition.

In the study by Menachemi et al., even practitioners who did use an EHR often did not have functions that were important to the care of CSHCN, such as the ability to communicate electronically with public health providers or schools. Although most users had an EHR that provided patient medication lists (84.7%) and electronically available lab and X-ray results (62.4% and 57.9%, respectively), most did not have the ability to do weight-based dosing calculations (35.5%), electronic order entry (47.7%), clinical decision support (24.9%), or preventive service reminders (29.4%). Finally, although much attention is being spent on the development of EHRs, and health care organizations such as children's hospitals (where CSHCN receive a disproportionately large amount of care) are investing millions in purchasing and deploying EHRs, we also are witnessing a move to develop *personal health records*. A personal health record (PHR) differs from an electronic health record in a fundamental way: The patient/family are the owners and guardians of the data. They control which data come into the PHR, who can enter and view the data, and how the data are shared (Markle Foundation, 2003). As efforts move ahead, the capabilities of a PHR are particularly attractive to families of CSHCN and could support family empowerment and family-centered care if deployed appropriately and linked to the provider-based EHR.

We propose that the development and adoption of the interoperable health information systems necessary to improve quality of care for CSHCN address the following components:

1. Incorporation of pediatric-specific functionalities (e.g., weight-based dosing, decision support) in EHR and PHR applications

2. Interoperability that links clinical, public health, school, and other data, especially for children with developmental delays

3. Standardization of data elements and their underlying definitions

4. Incentives that reward pediatricians, other providers, and even families for using HIT

5. Sufficient funding to develop and test model systems of interoperable health information systems for CSHCN

Research to Improve the Quality of Care for CSHCN

Given the many problems in quality outlined in this chapter, it is clear that significant research gaps exist in our understanding of how to ensure high-quality care for CSHCN. We focus on four priority areas where additional research could go a long way toward improving care for CSHCN: 1) effectiveness of clinical services, 2) effectiveness of organizational and financial models for care delivery, 3) quality measurement and improvement research, and 4) translating research into improved care for CSHCN.

Effectiveness of Clinical Services

Inherent in the very formulation of the term *evidence-based practice* is the assumption that evidence exists as to the effectiveness of the myriad interventions and services received by CSHCN. Unfortunately, this assumption is false for much of the care that CSHCN receive (Perrin, 2002). Indeed, the gaps in the evidence base for children's services are pervasive, from many components of well-child care to palliative services for chronically ill and dying children as well as services in between. For example, the United States Preventive Services Task Force found insufficient evidence to recommend either for or against hearing screenings for newborns, causing a firestorm of protest (Atkins, Siegel, & Slutsky, 2005). The Advisory Committee on Heritable Disorders and Genetic Diseases in Newborns and Children struggled with the evidence base for treatment of hundreds of conditions for which screening tests had become available. Many of the recommended clinical preventive services for children are lacking a sufficient evidence base (Moyer, 2004). Well-designed efficacy studies for many of the specialized therapies that CSHCN receive (e.g., physical therapy, occupational therapy, speech therapy) have not been conducted (Perrin, 2002; Piper & Pless, 1980).

The dearth of research studies is due to many factors including the overall relative lack of pediatric research compared with adults (Schuster et al., 1997), the characteristics of children's health care and the epidemiology of childhood disability in particular (Forrest, Simpson & Clancy, 1997; Kuhlthau et al., 1998), the fact that the National Institutes of Health (NIH) policy on including children in research was established less than a decade ago (in 1997), and legitimate concerns about the ethics of conducting research on children, especially children with special health care needs (Field & Berman, 2004).

As the NIH budget more than doubled in the last decade or so (from $10.3 billion in 1993 to $28.7 in 2005) and the policy of including children took hold, one hoped that the lack of research on CSHCN would be rectified. A recent analysis found, however, that pediatric spending increased at an average annual rate of 12.8% compared with 14.7% for the overall NIH budget, and that the proportion of the NIH budget devoted to the pediatric portfolio declined from 12.3% to 11.3% (Gitterman, Greenwood, Kocis, Mayes, & McKethan, 2004). This growth takes into account the expansion of pediatric research through the Children's Health Act of 2000, which established the Pediatric Research Initiative (PRI) and directed the National Institutes for Child Health and Human Development to plan and conduct the National Children's Study (NCS). This act authorized $50 million for the PRI, but no funds have been made available to date. (Planning for the NCS has advanced despite insufficient funding.) If fully funded, this landmark study would follow 100,000 children from preconception through adulthood (to at least 20 years of age) and cost between 2 and 3 billion dollars over the life of the study (National Children's Study, 2005). The lack of evidence supporting many of the services provided to CSHCN may be an underlying reason for not including benefits for CSHCN. A now perennial theme in health care reform proposals is evidence-based coverage (Silow-Carroll & Alteras, 2004). In essence, evidence-based coverage is the idea that it is inefficient to pay for services that have not been demonstrated to make a difference in health outcomes (Wehr, 2001). A major problem preventing a move to more evidence-based coverage for children is the paucity of research demonstrating the value of many services delivered to children as described above.

Effectiveness of Organizational and Financing Models

The fragmented care system for CSHCN stymies access, likely impedes clinical quality, and causes parental dissatisfaction. Challenges include the coordination of care within the traditional medical system and the integration of services across the various *systems* relevant to CSHCN (e.g., health care, early intervention, education, behavioral health). Although there is promising evidence for the *medical home* as defined by the AAP (see Chapter 6), more research is needed to demonstrate the effectiveness of proposals to restructure care. Berman and colleagues in Denver found that a hospital-based comprehensive primary care program was associated with a decreased length of stay for nonintensive care hospitalizations (Berman et al., 2005). However, the overall rate of hospitalizations and emergency department visits did not decline, and surgical services did increase. Whether these rates can be reduced for medically fragile children such as those described in the Berman study remains to be determined. Most studies of *systems of care* have focused only on nonmedical aspects of systems for emotionally disturbed children. To our knowledge there has been no comparison of the impacts of state efforts to organize financing and care through the variety of programs and policies designed to serve CSHCN. We recommend a complementary set of approaches to enhance the evidence base for services for CSHCN. First, we propose a reexamination of the effectiveness research paradigm to make it more suitable to questions relevant to CSHCN (and other children). Standards such as those used by the U.S. Preventive Services Task Force for making decisions and other standards for inclusion and exclusion of research based on study quality criteria are rarely suitable for children's topics (Cramer et al, 2005). For example, the traditional *gold standard* is the patient-level randomized controlled trial (RCT). For the most part, funding for RCTs is limited to relatively short time spans and measures outcomes such as clinical morbidity or death. In addition, funding for RCTs has typically been awarded to individual academic settings; for adult topics, these settings often have sufficient populations to test specific clinical interventions. In contrast, research on the effectiveness of children's services often requires a long time horizon to detect improvements (or not) in health outcomes; important health outcomes for children go well beyond mortality and include functioning and quality of life for children and their families. Outcomes may be affected by care provided (or not) in multiple settings, ambulatory and inpatient, traditional medical and nonmedical. Fortunately, efforts are now under way to rethink effectiveness and evaluation research paradigms for clinical, organizational, and quality improvement questions, including how to enhance the toolkit of designs to fit children's needs.

Quality Measurement and Improvement

At the same time that investments in the clinical and organizational evidence base are needed, it is critical to continue to develop and use quality measures and improve the science base for quality improvement. Although overall measures of quality for CSHCN are growing in number and quality, numerous gaps remain (Miller et al., 2005). For example, there are no standardized quality measures for neonatal intensive care (Rogowski, Staiger, & Horbar, 2004), and inpatient measures for pediatric asthma—the most prevalent chronic disease of children—are only now being finalized by the Joint Commission for Accreditation of Health Care Organizations (E. Schwallenstocker, personal communication, December 7, 2005). Other needs include pediatric inpatient and provider-level quality measures that can be applied across different hospitals and clinics. Quality measures for therapy services such as mental health and occupational and physical therapy are almost nonexistent. AHRQ sponsored an effort to build a set of Quality Indicators specifically for children's care. The AHRQ Quality Indicators use hospital discharge data set to measure potentially preventable hospitalizations, inpatient care (e.g., survival after surgery for congenital heart disease), and medical errors (e.g., infections due to medical care; Agency for Healthcare Research and Quality, 2005b). Since an AHRQ initiative in 1998, there has been relatively little research support for building valid and reliable quality measures. This has slowed the growth of measures for children as well.

In many respects, the field of quality improvement research is in its infancy (Shojania & Grimshaw, 2005). A September 2005 symposium sponsored by multiple federal agencies and a philanthropic organization identified numerous challenges—and several solutions—to improving the science base for quality improvement interventions. A primary problem is that the current research funding and dissemination environment is not well structured for quality improvement evaluation. Symposium participants noted that we could learn more about what works in quality improvement if evaluations of quality improvement would use methods suitable to the questions being asked (e.g., what kinds of health information technology improve timeliness and patient centeredness of care?), to the patients of interest, and to the settings of care. In addition, researchers should work closely with the organizations that actually implement quality improvement strategies (e.g., states, health plans, practices). Under-resourced organizations should get more support for engaging in quality improvement and for evaluation. Methods should be found for disseminating critical details about the nature of the quality improvement interventions, so that others can learn and not reinvent the wheel (especially if the wheel was found to be broken). Consumer advocates at the symposium also noted that quality improvement funders and evaluation researchers should always keep the end in mind; that is, studies of care improvement should focus on benefits to patients and then on academic advancement and cost reductions.

Translating Research into Practice

The tremendous growth in the NIH budget has led to a growing emphasis on challenges in the clinical research infrastructure and the blocks to the translation of research into practice that exist (Sung et al., 2003). Although the NIH has responded with the development of various initiatives to promote translational research, few if any are focused specifically on CSHCN. Attention to the challenges inherent in translating research into practice has grown, and new models have emerged that build on the seminal work of Rogers on the diffusion of innovations (Bero et al., 1995; Dash, Gowman, & Traynor, 2003; Lavis, 2003; Lomas, 1993, 2000; Rogers, 2003). However, this focus—at least in the United States—has been too long dichotomized into two communities: those who worry about research to inform public policy and those who worry about research to improve clinical practice. These research communities differ in their traditions, training, and disciplinary biases and languages. Efforts to translate research into public policy are dominated by social scientists with extensive grounding in theoretical frameworks to guide their work. On the other hand, efforts to translate research into clinical practice have been largely led by clinician researchers in a relatively theory-free environment. The end result is that the lessons learned and conclusions of each are published in separate journals and discussed at different meetings, which leads to missed opportunities for each to inform the other. Fortunately, that appears to be changing as child health services research grows as a multidisciplinary field (Sobo & Kurtin, 2003).

A second constraint to the translation of research into practice that is specific to children and that affects CSHCN acutely is the complex patchwork of services and programs—detailed earlier in this book—with which these children and their families must interact to receive the care they need (Simpson, 2004). Newer models of research translation call for a process whereby users and researchers interact at multiple points in the process, rather than a single, unidirectional trajectory from researcher to user, to maximize the probability that the right questions are addressed and that the results are in fact used by the intended audience (Lomas, 1993, 2000). Although achieving this interaction is never easy, the complexity of the task increases exponentially when one considers the patchwork of programs and services delivered to children through more than 50 Medicaid programs, 35 standalone SCHIP programs, and numerous categorical programs for CSHCN including Title V programs, the Social Security and Disability Income

(SSDI) program, and foster care and rehabilitation programs (Simpson, 2004).

CONCLUSION

In the United States, a rich but complicated range of policies and programs have been developed and implemented to improve the life chances of CSHCN and to reduce burdens on their families. Nonetheless, many gaps in access and quality remain. In an era of increasing national health care expenditures and an aging population, efforts to fill access and quality gaps to the satisfaction of families of CSHCN and the health care professionals they work with may face challenges.

Although it may seem unfair to expect the families and health care professionals who work so hard to care for individual CSHCN to deal with these challenges, parents and health care providers often have proven to be the children's most effective intermediaries. As insurance coverage—a primary determinant of access to care—is being reexamined by employers and public entities, and quality measurement and improvement efforts focus on high-cost, high-prevalence chronic conditions experienced primarily by adults, parents and health care professionals will have significant roles to play to ensure that CSHCN get timely access to effective, safe, patient-centered, and equitable care. These roles can be at the policy level (e.g., working with employers and public policy makers, encouraging information technology) and at the clinical level. Joining with parents in similar circumstances can provide both psychosocial support to families and opportunities to learn about important policy decisions and engage in the democratic process to influence such decisions. Medical home efforts that have engaged parents as advisors for clinical practices are a model for parents and health care professionals to emulate.

Caring for CSHCN can be an all-consuming challenge for parents and professionals, and frustration can mount if these children do not seem to be a major focus of policy initiatives in access and quality. Worse, the implications of policy changes for CSHCN may not even appear to be on the radar screen. It may be that only those who care deeply about CSHCN can provide the combination of compelling personal stories and research evidence of the needs of CSHCN that can influence policy makers. When evidence is lacking, the committed can make an argument for more research. The potential for dramatic improvements in health care for CSHCN is palpable. Future achievements in genomic medicine and other technologies must be matched by improvements in access and quality if CSHCN are to receive the full benefit of what access to high-quality health care could provide.

REFERENCES

Aday L.A., & Andersen R. (1974). A framework for the study of access to medical care. *Health Services Research, 9*(3), 208–220.

Agency for Healthcare Quality and Research (AHRQ) (2000, September). *Information technology and children's health care* (Fact Sheet No. 00-P074). Rockville, MD: Author. Retrieved November 9, 2005, from http://www.ahrq.gov/child/itchild.htm

Agency for Healthcare Research and Quality. (2004). *National Healthcare Disparities Report.* Rockville, MD: Author. Retrieved November 18, 2005, from http://www.qualitytools.ahrq.gov/disparitiesreport/browse/browse.aspx

Agency for Healthcare Research and Quality. (2005a). *Selected findings on child and adolescent health care from the 2004 National Healthcare Quality/Disparities Reports* (Fact Sheet). Retrieved December 6, 2005, from http://www.ahrq.gov/qual/nhqrchild/nhqrchild.htm

Agency for Healthcare Research and Quality. (2005b). *The AHRQ quality indicators.* Retrieved December 11, 2005, from http://www.qualityindicators.ahrq.gov/introduction.htm

Agency for Healthcare Research and Quality. (a; n.d.). *Child health insurance and research initiative (CHIRI).*, Rockville, MD: Retrieved November 1, 2005, from http://www.ahrq.gov/chiri/

Agency for Healthcare Research and Quality. (b; n.d.). *Measuring health care quality: Quality and Disparities Reports.* Rockville, MD: Author. Retrieved December 8, 2005, from http://www.ahrq.gov/qual/measurix.htm

American Academy of Pediatrics. (2005). *AAP president appointed to Medicaid Commission.* Retrieved October 31, 2005, from http://www.aap.org/advocacy/washing/medicaid_commission.htm

American Academy of Pediatrics Committee on Child Health Financing. (2005). Policy statement: Model contractual language for medical necessity for children. *Pediatrics, 116*(1), 261–262.

American Academy of Physician Assistants. (1997, June). Physician Assistants as Medicaid Managed Care Providers. Retrieved August 9, 2006, from http://www.aapa.org/gandp/medman.html

American Association on Health and Disability. (2004). Health care trends: Consumer-directed health care. *Health and Disability News, 2*(4). Retrieved October 30, 2005, from http://www.aahd.us/newsletterarchive/Fall2004/researchCorner1.htm

Association of Maternal and Child Health Programs. (2003). *Title V leaders guide.* Retrieved October 30, 2005, from http://www.amchp.org/titlevguide/

Atkins, D., Siegel, J., & Slutsky, J. (2005). Making policy when the evidence is in dispute. *Health Affairs (Millwood), 24*(1), 102–113.

Baker, G., & Carter, B. (2005, First Quarter). *Provider pay-for-performance incentive programs: 2004 national study results.* Retrieved December 5, 2005, from http://www.medvantageinc.com/Pdf/MV_2004_P4P_National_Study_Results-Exec_Summary.pdf

Bauer, T., Duitch, S., & Birenbaum, A. (2003, October). Children with special health care needs: Next steps for New York. *New York Forum for Child Health.* New York: The New York Academy of Medicine. Retrieved November 10, 2005, from http://www.nyam.org/news/research.shtml

Beal, A.C., Co, J.P., Dougherty, D., Jorsling, T., Kam, J., Perrin, J., & Palmer, R.H. (2004). Quality measures for children's health care. *Pediatrics, 113*,(1, Pt. 2), 199–209.

Berman, S., Dolins, J., Tang, S.F., & Yudkowsky, B. (2002). Factors that influence the willingness of private primary care pediatricians to accept more Medicaid patients. *Pediatrics, 110*(2, Pt. 1), 239–248.

Berman, S., Rannie, M., Moore, L., Elias, E., Dryer, L.J., & Jones, M.D. (2005). Utilization and costs for children who have special health care needs and are enrolled in a hospital-based comprehensive primary care clinic. *Pediatrics, 115*, e37–e642.

Bero, L.A., Grilli, R., Grimshaw, J.M., Harvey, E., Oxman, A.D., & Thomson, M.A. (1995). Closing the gap between research and practice: An overview of systematic reviews of interventions to promote the implementation of research findings. *British Medical Journal, 317*(7156), 465–468.

Bethell, C.D., Read, D., Stein, R.E., Blumberg, S.J., Wells, N., & Newacheck, P.W. (2002). Identifying children with special health care needs: Development and evaluation of a short screening instrument. *Ambulatory Pediatrics, 2002, 2*(1), 38–48.

Centers for Disease Control and Prevention. (n.d.). *About NIP.* Retrieved October 30, 2005, from http://www.cdc.gov/nip/webutil/about/default.htm

Centers for Medicare and Medicaid Services (n.d.). *Medicaid Information Resource.* Retrieved October. 30, 2005, from http://www.cms.hhs.gov/medicaid/

Children's Health Act of 2000, PL 106-310. Retrieved December 11, 2005, from http://thomas.loc.gov/cgi-bin/bdquery/z?d106:HR04365:@@@D&summ1&|TOM:/bss/d106query.html|

Chung, P.J., & Schuster, M.A. (2004). Access and quality of child health services: Voltage drops. *Health Affairs (Millwood), 23*(5), 77–87.

Cohen, A.L., Rivara, F., Marcuse, E.K., McPhillips, H., & Davis, R. (2005). Are language barriers associated with serious medical events in hospitalized pediatric patients? *Pediatrics, 116*(3), 575–579.

Cooley, W.C., & McAllister, J.W. (2004). Building medical homes: Improvement strategies in primary care for children with special health care needs. *Pediatrics, 113*(Suppl. 5), 1499–1506.

Dash, P., Gowman, N., & Traynor, M. (2003). Increasing the impact of health services research. *British Medical Journal, 327*(7427), 1339–1341.

Davidoff, A.J., Yemane, A., & Hill, I. (2004). Public insurance eligibility and enrollment for special health care needs children. *Health Care Financing Review, 26*(1), 119–135.

Davies, H.T., Washington, A.E., & Bindman, A.B. (2002). Health care report cards: Implications for vulnerable patient groups and the organizations providing them care. *Journal of Health Politics, Policy and Law, 27*(3), 379–399.

Davis, K. (2004, August). *Will consumer-directed health care improve system performance?* New York: The Commonwealth Fund. Retrieved November 10, 1999, from http://www.cmwf.org/publications/publications_show.htm?doc_id=235864

Dick, A., Brach, C., Allison, R., Shenkman, E., Shone, L., Szilagyi. M., et al. (2004). SCHIP's impact in three states: How do the most vulnerable children fare? *Health Affairs (Millwood), 2*(5), 63–75.

Dougherty, D., Meikle, S.F., Owens, P., Kelley, E., & Moy, E. (2005). Children's health care in the first National Healthcare Quality Report and National Healthcare Disparities Report. *Medical Care, 43*(Suppl. 3), 158–163.

Dougherty, D., & Simpson, L.A. (2004). Measuring the quality of children's health care: A prerequisite to action. *Pediatrics, 113*(1, Pt 2), 185–198.

Eisenberg, J., & Power, E. (2000). Transforming insurance coverage into quality health care: Voltage drops from potential to delivered quality. *Journal of the American Medical Association, 284*(16), 2100–2107.

Endsley, S., Kirkegaard, M., Baker, G., & Murcko, A.C. (2004). Getting rewards for your results: Pay-for-performance programs. *Family Practice Management, 11*(3), 45–50.

Family Voices of Colorado. (n.d.). *Training/presentation request application.* Retrieved October 31, 2005, from http://www.familyvoicesco.org/Training.htm

Family Voices of Tennessee. (n.d.). *Tennessee (State Chapter) Family Voices of Tennessee at Tennessee Disability Coalition.* Retrieved October 31, 2005, from http://www.familyvoices.org/st/TN.htm

Ferris, T.G., Dougherty, D., Blumenthal, D., & Perrin, J.M. (2001). A report card on quality improvement for children's health care. *Pediatrics, 107*(1), 143–155.

Field, M.J., & Berman, R.E. (Eds.) & Committee on Clinical Research Involving Children (2004). *The ethical conduct of clinical research involving children.* Washington, DC: National Academies Press.

Flores, G., Laws, M.B., Mayo, S.J., Zuckerman, B., Abreu, M., Medina, L., & Hardt, E.J. (2003). Errors in medical interpretation and their potential clinical consequences in pediatric encounters. *Pediatrics, 111*(1), 6–14.

Forrest, C.B., Glade, G., Baker, A., Bocian, A., von Schrader, S., & Starfield, B. (2000). Coordination of specialty referrals and physician satisfaction with referral care. *Archives of Pediatrics & Adolescent Medicine, 154*(5), 499–506.

Forrest, C.B., Simpson, L., & Clancy, C. (1997). Child health services research: Challenges and opportunities. *Journal of the American Medical Association, 277*(22), 1787–1793.

Fox, H.B., & McManus, M.A. (2001). A national study of commercial health insurance and Medicaid definitions of medical necessity: What do they mean for children? *Ambulatory Pediatrics, 1*(1), 16–22.

Gabel, J., & Rice, T. (2003). *Insurance markets: Understanding consumer-directed health care in California.* Oakland, CA: California HealthCare Foundation.

Gandhi, T.K., Sittig, D.F., Franklin, M., Sussman, A.J., Fairchild, D.G., & Bates, D.W. (2000). Communication breakdown in the outpatient referral process. *Journal of General Internal Medicine, 15*(9), 626–631.

Gauthier, A.K., & Clancy, C.M. (2004). Consumer-driven health care: Beyond rhetoric with research and experience. *Health Services Research, 39*(4, Pt. II), 1049–1054.

Gitterman, D.P., Greenwood, R.S., Kocis, K.C., Mayes, B.R., & McKethan, A.N. (2004). Did a rising tide lift all boats? The NIH budget and pediatric research portfolio. *Health Affairs (Millwood), 23*(5), 113–124.

Health Insurance Portability and Accountability Act of 1996, PL 104-191.

Hibbard, J.H., Slovic, P., Peters, E., & Finucane, M.L. (2002). Strategies for reporting health plan performance information to consumers: Evidence from controlled studies. *Health Services Research, 37*(1), 43–63.

Hibbard, J.H., Stockard, J., & Tusler, M. (2003). Does publicizing hospital performance stimulate quality improvement efforts? *Health Affairs (Millwood), 22*(2), 84–94.

Hinman, A.R., Saarlas, K.N., & Ross, D.A. (2004, November). A vision for child health information systems: Developing child health information systems to meet medical care and public health needs. *Journal of Public Health Management and Practice* (Suppl. S91–98).

Homer, C.J., & Child Health Business Case Working Group. (2004). Exploring the business case for improving the quality of health care for children. *Health Affairs (Millwood), 23*(4), 159–166.

Homer, C.J., Forbes, P., Horvitz, L., Peterson, L.E, Wypij, D., & Heinrich, P. (2005). Impact of a quality improvement program on care and outcomes for children with asthma. *Archives of Pediatrics & Adolescent Medicine, 159*(5), 464–469.

Homer, C.J., Horvitz, L., Heinrich, P., Forbes, P., Lesneski, C., & Phillips, J. (2004). Improving care for children with attention deficit hyperactivity disorder: Assessing the impact of self-assessment and targeted training on practice performance. *Ambulatory Pediatrics, 4*(5), 436–441.

Honberg, L., McPherson, M., Strickland, B., Gage, J.C., & Newacheck, P.W. (2005). Assuring adequate health insurance: Results of the National Survey of Children with Special Health Care Needs. *Pediatrics, 115*(5), 1233–1239.

Huang, Z.J., Kogan, M.D., Yu, S.M., & Strickland, B. (2005). Delayed or forgone care among children with special health care needs: An analysis of the 2001 National Survey of Children with Special Health Care Needs. *Ambulatory Pediatrics, 5*(1), 60–67.

Hudson, J. (2005). *Trends in children's health insurance coverage: 1996–2002 (half-year).* Retrieved Nov. 1, 2005, from http://www.meps.ahrq.gov/Print Products/PrintProd_Detail.asp?ID = 712&TABLE = 'Statistical%20Brief% 20#99'&PPTYPE =

Institute of Medicine, Committee on the Quality of Health Care in America. (2001). *Crossing the quality chasm: A new health system for the 21st century.* Washington, DC: National Academies Press.

Johnston, C., & Wells, N. (2002, April 17). *Serving persons with disabilities in Medicaid* (Managed Care Conference). Retrieved November 10, 2005, from http://www.hrsa.gov/financeMC/disability/ppt7/default.htm

Kaiser Family Foundation (2005, August 8). *State watch: Indiana considers doubling SCHIP premiums* (Daily Health Policy Report). Retrieved November 3, 2005, from http://www.kaisernetwork.org/daily_reports/rep_index.cfm? hint = 3&DR_ID = 31884

Kaiser Family Foundation, Agency for Healthcare Research and Quality, & Harvard School of Public Health (2004, November). *National survey on consumers' experiences with patient safety and quality information: Summary and chart pack.* Retrieved November 9, 2005, from http://www.kff.org/kaiserpolls/ 7209.cfm

Kaiser Family Foundation & Health Research and Educational Trust. (n.d.). *Employer health benefits: 2004 summary of findings.* Menlo Park, CA, and Washington, DC: The Kaiser Family Foundation.

Kohn L.T, Corrigan J.M., & Donaldson, M. (Eds.). (1999). Institute of Medicine (IOM) Report *To Err is Human: Building a safer health system*. Washington, DC: National Academy of Sciences.

Krauss, M., & Wells, N. (2000). *The Family Partners Project: Summary of findings and conclusions*. Waltham, MA: Brandeis University.

Kronebusch, K., & Elbel, B. (2004). Enrolling children in public insurance: SCHIP, Medicaid, and state implementation. *Journal of Health Politics, Policy and Law, 29*(3), 451–489.

Kuhlthau, K., Walker, D.K., Perrin, J.M., Bauman, L., Gortmaker, S.L., Newacheck, P.W., & Stein, R.E. (1998). Assessing managed care for children with chronic conditions. *Health Affairs (Millwood), 17*(4), 42–52.

Lavis, J.N. (2003). How can research organizations more effectively transfer research knowledge to decision makers? *Milbank Quarterly, 81*(2), 171–172, 221–248.

Leape, L.L., Bates, D.W., Cullen, D.J., Cooper, J., Demonaco, H.J., Gallivan, T., et al. (1995). Systems analysis of adverse drug events. ADE Prevention Study Group. *Journal of the American Medical Association, 274*(1), 35–43.

Leatherman, S., & McCarthy, D. (2004). *Quality of health care for children and adolescents: A chartbook*. New York: The Commonwealth Fund.

Leslie, L.K., Weckerly, J., Plemmons, D., Landsverk, J., & Eastman, S. (2004). Implementing the American Academy of Pediatrics attention-deficit/hyperactivity disorder diagnostic guidelines in primary care settings. *Pediatrics, 114*(1), 129–40.

Lieu, T.A., Finkelstein, J.A., Lozano, P., Capra, A.M., Chi, F.W., Jensvold, N., et al. (2004). Cultural competence policies and other predictors of asthma care quality for Medicaid-insured children. *Pediatrics, 114*(1), e102–110.

Lo Sasso, A., & Buchmueller, T. (2004). The effect of the State Children's Health Insurance Program on health insurance coverage. *Journal of Health Economics, 23*(5), 1059–1082.

Lomas, J. (1993). Diffusion, dissemination and implementation: Who should do what? *Annals of the New York Academy of Sciences, 703*, 226–241.

Lomas, J. (2000). Using "linkage and exchange" to move research into policy at a Canadian foundation. *Health Affairs (Millwood): 19*(3), 236–240.

Lozano, P., Finkelstein, J.A., Carey, V.J., Wagner, E.H., Inui, T.S., Fuhlbrigge, A.L., et al. (2004). A multisite randomized trial of the effects of physician education and organizational change in chronic-asthma care: Health outcomes of the Pediatric Asthma Care Patient Outcomes Research Team II Study. *Archives of Pediatric & Adolescent Medicine, 158*(9), 875–883.

Lubitz, J. (2005, September 26). Health, technology, and medical care spending. *Health Affairs (Millwood)*, w5, 81–85. Retrieved November 1, 2005, from www.healthaffairs.org

Lutzky, A.W., & Hill, I. (2001). *Has the jury reached a verdict? States' early experiences with crowd-out under SCHIP* (Occasional Paper). Washington, DC: Urban Institute. Retrieved November 1, 2005, from http://www.urban.org/publications/310218.html

Mangione-Smith, R., Schonlau, M., Chan, K.S., Keesey, J., Rosen, M., Louis, T.A., & Keeler, E. (2005). Measuring the effectiveness of a collaborative for quality improvement in pediatric asthma care: Does implementing the chronic care model improve processes and outcomes of care? *Ambulatory Pediatrics, 5*(2), 75–82.

Markle Foundation (2003). *The Personal Health Working Group Final Report.* Retrieved January 4, 2006, from http://www.markle.org/downloadable_assets_final_phwg_report1.pdf

Markus, A., Rosenbaum, S., Stewart, A., & Cox, M. (2005). *How medical claims simplification can impede delivery of child developmental services.* New York: The Commonwealth Fund.

Mayer, M.L., Skinner, A.C., & Slifkin, R.T. (2004). Unmet need for routine and specialty care: Data from the National Survey of Children with Special Health Care Needs. *Pediatrics, 113*(2), e109–e115.

McGlynn, E.A., & Malin, J.L. (2002, August 21), *Selecting national goals and core measures of cancer care quality (*Background Paper #2). National Cancer Institute Contract, No. 282-00-0005_TO6.

Menachemi, N., Ettel, D.L., Brooks, R.G., & Simpson, L. (2006). Charting the use of electronic health records and other information technologies among child health providers. *BMC Pediatrics, 6,* 21.

Miller, M.R., Gergen, P., Honour, M., & Zhan, C. (2005). Burden of illness for children and where we stand in measuring the quality of this health care *Ambulatory Pediatrics, 5*(5), 268–278.

Moyer V. (2004). Evidence based medicine: Is it practical? *Archives of Disease in Childhood, 89*(5), 399–400.

National Childrens' Study. (2005). *What is the National Children's Study?* Retrieved November 18, 2005, from http://nationalchildrensstudy.gov/about/mission/overview.cfm

National Conference of State Legislatures. (2003, September). *Crowd-out provisions in non-Medicaid SCHIP plans.* Retrieved October 30, 2005, from http://www.ncsl.org/programs/health/schiptable09.htm

National Governors Association. (2005, August). *Short-run Medicaid reform.* Washington, DC: National Governors Association. Retrieved November 10, 2005, from http://www.aapd-dc.org/News/commission/indexmedcomm.php

National Quality Forum. (2004). *Child health quality measurement and reporting.* Washington, DC: National Quality Forum.

National Survey of Children with Special Health Care Needs Data Resource Center. (2004). *National Survey of Children with Special Health Care Needs.* Retrieved October 18, 2005, from http://cshcndata.org/DesktopDefault.aspx

Newacheck, P.W., & Kim, S. (2005). A national profile of health care utilization and expenditures for children with special health care needs. *Archives of Pediatrics & Adolescent Medicine, 159*(1), 10–17.

New York State Department of Health. (2006). Medicaid Managed Care, Model Contracts, Medicaid Managed Care Family Health Plus. (2006, April 1). Retrieved August 9, 2006, from http://www.health.state.ny.us/health_care/managed_care/mamctext.htm

Olson, B.G., Rosenbaum, P.F., Dosa, N.P., & Roizen, N.J. (2005). Improving guideline adherence for the diagnosis of ADHD in an ambulatory pediatric setting. *Ambulatory Pediatrics, 5*(3), 138–142.

Olson, L.M., Tang, S.F., & Newacheck, P.W. (2005). Children in the United States with discontinuous health insurance coverage. *New England Journal of Medicine, 353*(4), 382–391.

Perrin, J. (2002). Health services research for children with disabilities. *Milbank Quarterly, 80*(2), 303–324.

Peters, C.P. (2005, June 27). *Children with special health care needs: Minding the gaps* (Background Paper). Washington, DC: National Health Policy Forum and George Washington University.

Piper, M., & Pless, L. (1980). Early intervention for infants with Down syndrome: A controlled trial. *Pediatrics, 65,* 463–468.

Robert Wood Johnson Foundation. (2005). *Covering Kids®: A National health initiative for low income uninsured children.* Retrieved January 4, 2006, from http://www.rwjf.org/reports/npreports/coveringkids.htm

Robinson, J. (2002). Renewed emphasis on consumer cost sharing in health insurance benefit design. *Health Affairs (Millwood),* W 139–154.

Rogers, E.M. (2003). *Diffusion of innovations* (5th ed.). New York: Free Press.

Rogowski, J.A., Staiger, D.O., & Horbar, J.D. (2004). Variations in the quality of care for very-low-birthweight infants: Implications for policy. *Health Affairs (Millwood), 23*(5), 88–97.

Rosenberg, D., Onufer, C., Clark, G., Wilkin, T., Rankin, K., & Gupta, K. (2005). The need for care coordination among children with special health care needs in Illinois. *Maternal and Child Health Journal, 9*(Suppl. 2), 41–47.

Rosenthal, M., & Milstein, A. (2004). Awakening consumer stewardship of health benefits: Prevalence and differentiation of new health plan models. *Health Service Research, 39*(4, Pt. 2), 1055–1070.

Rosenthal, M.D., Frank, R.G., Li, Z., & Epstein, A.M. (2005). Early experience with pay-for-performance: From concept to practice. *Journal of the American Medical Association, 294,*1788–1793.

Russell, S.C., & Spooner, S.A. (2004). Barriers to EMR adoption in internal medicine and pediatric outpatient practices. *Tennessee Medicine, 97*(10), 457–460.

Schuster, M.A., Asch, S.M., McGlynn, E.A., Kerr, E.A., Hardy, A.M., & Gifford, D.S. (1997). Development of a quality of care measurement system for children and adolescents. Methodological considerations and comparisons with a system for adult women. *Archives of Pediatrics & Adolescent Medicine, 151*(11), 1085–1092.

Shaller, D. (2004). Implementing and using quality measures for children's health care: Perspectives on the state of the practice. *Pediatrics, 113,* 217–227.

Shenkman, E., Tian, L., Nackashi, J., & Schatz, D. (2005). Managed care organization characteristics and outpatient specialty care use among children with chronic illness. *Pediatrics, 115*(6), 1547–1554.

Shiffman, R.N., Spooner, S.A., Kwiatkowski, K., & Brennan, P.F. (2001). Information technology for children's health and health care: Report on the Information Technology in Children's Health Care Expert Meeting, September 21–22, 2000. *Journal of the American Medical Informatics Association, 8*(6), 546–551.

Shojania, K.G., & Grimshaw, J.M. (2005). Evidence-based quality improvement: The state of the science. *Health Affairs (Millwood), 24*(1), 138–150.

Silow-Carroll, S., & Alteras, T. (2004, October). *Stretching state health care dollars during difficult economic times: Overview* (No. 777). New York: The Commonwealth Fund.

Simpson, L. (2001). Quality of care: Time to make the grade. *Pediatrics, 107,*171.

Simpson, L. (2004). Lost in translation? Reflections on the role of research in improving health care for children. *Health Affairs (Millwood), 23*(5), 125–130.

Simpson, L., & Fraser, I. (1999). Children and managed care: What research can, can't, and should tell us about impact. *Medical Care Research & Review, 56* (Suppl. 2), 13–36.

Simpson, L., & Lawless, S. (2005). Quality measurement: Is the glass half full yet? *Ambulatory Pediatrics, 5*(5), 279–280.

Simpson, L., Owens, P.L., Zodet, M.W., Chevarley, F.M., Dougherty, D., Elixhauser, A., & McCormick, M.C. (2005). Health care for children and youth in the United States: Annual report on patterns of coverage, utilization, quality, and expenditures by income. *Ambulatory Pediatrics, 5*(1), 6–44.

Simpson, L., Zodet, M.W., Chevarley, F.M., Owens, P.L., Dougherty, D., & McCormick, M.C. (2004). Health care for children and youth in the United States: 2002 report on trends in access, utilization, quality, and expenditures. *Ambulatory Pediatrics, 4*(2), 131–153.

Singer, S.J., & Bergthold, L.A. (2001). Prospects for improved decision making about medical necessity. *Health Affairs (Millwood), 20*(1), 200–206.

Slonim, A.D., LaFleur, B.J., Ahmed, W., & Joseph, J.G. (2003). Hospital-reported medical errors in children. *Pediatrics, 111*(3), 617–621.

Smith, P.C., Araya-Guerra, R., Bublitz, C., Parnes, B., Dickinson, L.M., Van Vorst, R., et al. (2005). Missing clinical information during primary care visits. *JAMA, 293*(5), 565–571.

Sobo, E.S., & Kurtin, P.S. (Eds.). (2003). *Child health services research: Applications, innovations, and insights.* Hoboken, NJ: Jossey-Bass-Wiley.

Soumerai, S.B. (2004). Benefits and risks of increasing restrictions on access to costly drugs in Medicaid. *Health Affairs (Millwood), 23*(1), 135–146.

Stanton, M. (2004). *Employer-sponsored health insurance: Trends in cost and access* (No. 04-0085). Retrieved October 31, 2005, from http://www.meps.ahrq.gov/PrintProducts/PrintProd_Detail.asp?ID=635&TABLE='Research%20in%20Action%20#17'&PPTYPE=

Starfield, B., Shi, L., & Macinko, J. (2005). Contribution of primary care to health systems and health. *Milbank Quarterly, 83*(3), 457–502.

Stille, C.J., & Antonelli, R.C. (2004). Coordination of care for children with special health care needs. *Current Opinion in Pediatrics, 16*(6), 700–705.

Subcommittee on Attention-Deficit/Hyperactivity Disorder and Committee on Quality Improvement. (2001). Clinical practice guideline: Treatment of the school-aged child with attention-deficit/hyperactivity disorder. *Pediatrics, 108,* 1033–1044.

Sung, N.S., Crowley, W.F., Jr., Genel, M., Salber, P., Sandy, L., Sherwood, L.M., et al. (2003). Central challenges facing the national clinical research enterprise. *Journal of the American Medical Association, 289*(10), 1278–1287.

Szilagyi, P.G., Shenkman, E., Brach, C., LaClair, B., Swigonski, N., Dick, A., et al. (2003). Children with special health care needs enrolled in the State Children's Health Insurance Program (SCHIP): Patient characteristics and health care needs. *Pediatrics, 112*(6), e508–e520.

Texas Health and Human Services Commission Medicaid/CHIP Division. (2003, April). *Final report: A model for integrating children with special health care needs into Medicaid managed care* (Executive summary). Retrieved November 1, 2005, from http://www.hhsc.state.tx.us/Medicaid/reports/120202_CSHCNintoMMC_ExecSum.html

Thorpe, K.E., Florence, C.S., Howard, D.H., & Joski, P. (2005). The rising prevalence of treated disease: Effects on private health insurance spending. *Health
Affairs (Millwood)*, 5, 317–325. Retrieved November 1, 2005, from www.
healthaffairs.org

Tu, H.T., & Cunningham, P.J. (2005, September). *Public coverage provides vital
safety net for children with special health care needs* (Issue Brief No. 98). Washington, DC: The Center for Studying Health System Change.

U.S. Department of Health and Human Services Assistant Secretary for Planning
and Evaluation. Public Law 104-191 Health Insurance Portability and Accountability Act of 1996 (1996, August 21). Retrieved on August 9, 2006,
from http://aspe.hhs.gov/admnsimp/pl104191.htm

U.S. Department of Health and Human Services Medicaid Commission
[USDHHS MC]. (2005, September 1). *Report to the Honorable Secretary Michael
O. Leavitt.* Retrieved November 2, 2005, from http://www.cms.hhs.gov/faca/
mc/090105rpt.pdf

U.S. Department of Health and Human Services Health Resources and Services
Administration, Maternal and Child Health Bureau [USDHHS HRSA MCHB].
(2004). *The National Survey of Children with Special Health Care Needs Chartbook
2001—Health care needs and access to care.* Retrieved on October 31, 2005,
from http://www.mchb.hrsa.gov/chscn/pages/needs.htm

U.S. Department of Health and Human Services Health Resources and Services
Administration Maternal and Child Health Bureau [USDHHS HRSA MCHB].
(2005a). *MCHB TVIS, Health Systems Capacity Indicator #08.* Retrieved September 11, 2005, from https://performance.hrsa.gov/mchb/mchreports/Search/
HSI/HSIschCore01.aspat

U.S. Department of Health and Human Services Health Resources and Services
Administration Maternal and Child Health Bureau [USDHHS HRSA MCHB].
(2005b). *Search TVIS: National performance measures.* Retrieved October 30,
2005, from https://performance.hrsa.gov/mchb/mchreports/Search/core/
corschSpecial.asp

van Dyck, P.C., Kogan, M.D., McPherson, M.G., Weissman, G.R., & Newacheck,
P.W. (2004). Prevalence and characteristics of children with special health
care needs. *Archives of Pediatrics & Adolescent Medicine, 158*(9), 884–890.

Wehr, E. (2001). Evidence-based health care coverage for children: Proceed
with caution. *Ambulatory Pediatrics, 1*(1), 23–27.

Wehr, E., & Jameson, E.J. (1994). Beyond benefits: The importance of a pediatric standard in private insurance contracts to ensuring health care access for
children. *The Future of Children, 4*(3), 115–133.

Weil, A. (2004). Chipping away at the uninsured. *Health Affairs (Millwood)*,
23(5), 153–154.

White House. (1999). *Interagency Children's Health Outreach Task Force.* Retrieved
October 31, 2005, from http://www.cms.hhs.gov/schip/whitehouse/wh-
chip7.asp

Williams, T.V., Schone, E.M., Archibald, N.D., & Thompson, J.W. (2004). A
national assessment of children with special health care needs: Prevalence
of special needs and use of health care services among children in the military
health system. *Pediatrics, 114*(2), 384–393.

Wright, B.J., Carlson, M.J., Edlund, T., DeVoe, J., Gallia, C., & Smith, J. (2005). The impact of increased cost sharing on Medicaid enrollees. *Health Affairs (Millwood), 24*(4), 1106–1116.

Yu, S.M., Huang, Z.J., Schwalberg, R.H., & Kogan, M.D. (2005). Parental awareness of health and community resources among immigrant families. *Maternal Child Health Journal, 9*(1), 27–34.

Zaslavsky, A.M., Hochheimer, J.N., Schneider, E.C., Cleary, P.D., Seidman, J.J., McGlynn, et al. (2000). Impact of sociodemographic case mix on the HEDIS measures of health plan quality. *Medical Care, 38*(10), 981–992.

Zhan, C., Sangl, J., Meyer, G.S., & Zaslavsky, A.M. (2002). Consumer assessments of care for children and adults in health plans: How do they compare? *Medical Care, 40*(2), 145

INDEX

Page numbers followed by *f* indicate figures; those followed by *t* indicate tables.